Advanced Imaging in Orthopedic Biomechanics

Advanced Imaging in Orthopedic Biomechanics

Editors

Claudio Belvedere
Sorin Siegler

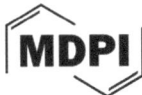

Basel • Beijing • Wuhan • Barcelona • Belgrade • Novi Sad • Cluj • Manchester

Editors

Claudio Belvedere
Movement Analysis Laboratory
IRCCS Istituto Ortopedico Rizzoli
Bologna
Italy

Sorin Siegler
Department of Mechanical Engineering
Drexel University
Philadelphia, PA
USA

Editorial Office
MDPI AG
Grosspeteranlage 5
4052 Basel, Switzerland

This is a reprint of articles from the Special Issue published online in the open access journal *Applied Sciences* (ISSN 2076-3417) (available at: https://www.mdpi.com/journal/applsci/special_issues/Orthopedic_Biomechanics).

For citation purposes, cite each article independently as indicated on the article page online and as indicated below:

Lastname, A.A.; Lastname, B.B. Article Title. *Journal Name* **Year**, *Volume Number*, Page Range.

ISBN 978-3-7258-2497-7 (Hbk)
ISBN 978-3-7258-2498-4 (PDF)
doi.org/10.3390/books978-3-7258-2498-4

© 2024 by the authors. Articles in this book are Open Access and distributed under the Creative Commons Attribution (CC BY) license. The book as a whole is distributed by MDPI under the terms and conditions of the Creative Commons Attribution-NonCommercial-NoDerivs (CC BY-NC-ND) license.

Contents

About the Editors vii

Claudio Belvedere and Sorin Siegler
Special Issue "Advanced Imaging in Orthopedic Biomechanics"
Reprinted from: *Appl. Sci.* 2024, 14, 8193, doi:10.3390/app14188193 1

Elena Campagnoli, Sorin Siegler, Maria Ruiz, Alberto Leardini and Claudio Belvedere
Effect of Ligament Mapping from Different Magnetic Resonance Image Quality on Joint
Stability in a Personalized Dynamic Model of the Human Ankle Complex
Reprinted from: *Appl. Sci.* 2022, 12, 5087, doi:10.3390/app12105087 5

Edoardo Bori and Bernardo Innocenti
Biomechanical Analysis of Femoral Stem Features in Hinged Revision TKA with Valgus or
Varus Deformity: A Comparative Finite Elements Study
Reprinted from: *Appl. Sci.* 2023, 13, 2738, doi:10.3390/app13042738 14

**Gilda Durastanti, Claudio Belvedere, Miriana Ruggeri, Davide Maria Donati,
Benedetta Spazzoli and Alberto Leardini**
A Pelvic Reconstruction Procedure for Custom-Made Prosthesis Design of Bone Tumor Surgical
Treatments
Reprinted from: *Appl. Sci.* 2022, 12, 1654, doi:10.3390/app12031654 27

**Michele Conconi, Filippo De Carli, Matteo Berni, Nicola Sancisi, Vincenzo Parenti-Castelli
and Giuseppe Monetti**
In-Vivo Quantification of Knee Deep-Flexion in Physiological Loading Condition trough
Dynamic MRI
Reprinted from: *Appl. Sci.* 2023, 13, 629, doi:10.3390/app13010629 39

**François Lintz, Cesar de Cesar Netto, Claudio Belvedere, Alberto Leardini,
Alessio Bernasconi and on behalf of the International Weight-bearing CT Society**
Recent Innovations Brought about by Weight-Bearing CT Imaging in the Foot and Ankle:
A Systematic Review of the Literature
Reprinted from: *Appl. Sci.* 2024, 14, 5562, doi:10.3390/app14135562 51

**Thibaut Dhont, Manu Huyghe, Matthias Peiffer, Noortje Hagemeijer, Bedri Karaismailoglu,
Nicola Krahenbuhl, et al.**
Ins and Outs of the Ankle Syndesmosis from a 2D to 3D CT Perspective
Reprinted from: *Appl. Sci.* 2023, 13, 10624, doi:10.3390/app131910624 73

**Eun-Sang Moon, Seora Kim, Nathan Kim, Minjoung Jang, Toru Deguchi, Fengyuan Zheng,
et al.**
Aging Alters Cervical Vertebral Bone Density Distribution: A Cross-Sectional Study
Reprinted from: *Appl. Sci.* 2022, 12, 3143, doi:10.3390/app12063143 90

**Daniel Maya-Anaya, Guillermo Urriolagoitia-Sosa, Beatriz Romero-Ángeles,
Miguel Martinez-Mondragon, Jesús Manuel German-Carcaño, Martin Ivan Correa-Corona,
et al.**
Numerical Analysis Applying the Finite Element Method by Developing a Complex
Three-Dimensional Biomodel of the Biological Tissues of the Elbow Joint Using Computerized
Axial Tomography
Reprinted from: *Appl. Sci.* 2023, 13, 8903, doi:10.3390/app13158903 100

Piotr Nowak, Mikołaj Dąbrowski, Adam Druszcz and Łukasz Kubaszewski
The Spatial Characteristics of Intervertebral Foramina within the L4/L5 and L5/S1 Motor Segments of the Spine
Reprinted from: *Appl. Sci.* **2024**, *14*, 2263, doi:10.3390/app14062263 118

Jesus Alejandro Serrato-Pedrosa, Guillermo Urriolagoitia-Sosa, Beatriz Romero-Ángeles, Guillermo Manuel Urriolagoitia-Calderón, Salvador Cruz-López, Alejandro Urriolagoitia-Luna, et al.
Biomechanical Evaluation of Plantar Pressure Distribution towards a Customized 3D Orthotic Device: A Methodological Case Study through a Finite Element Analysis Approach
Reprinted from: *Appl. Sci.* **2024**, *14*, 1650, doi:10.3390/app14041650 131

Alfonso Trejo-Enriquez, Guillermo Urriolagoitia-Sosa, Beatriz Romero-Ángeles, Miguel Ángel García-Laguna, Martín Guzmán-Baeza, Jacobo Martínez-Reyes, et al.
Numerical Evaluation Using the Finite Element Method on Frontal Craniocervical Impact Directed at Intervertebral Disc Wear
Reprinted from: *Appl. Sci.* **2023**, *13*, 11989, doi:10.3390/app132111989 152

Nurhusna Najeha Amran, Khairul Salleh Basaruddin, Muhammad Farzik Ijaz, Haniza Yazid, Shafriza Nisha Basah, Nor Amalina Muhayudin and Abdul Razak Sulaiman
Spine Deformity Assessment for Scoliosis Diagnostics Utilizing Image Processing Techniques: A Systematic Review
Reprinted from: *Appl. Sci.* **2023**, *13*, 11555, doi:10.3390/app132011555 167

About the Editors

Claudio Belvedere

Claudio Belvedere earned a master's degree in electronic– biomedical engineering from the Faculty of Engineering of the University of Bologna, where he also earned a Ph.D. in bioengineering. He joined the IRCCS Istituto Ortopedico Rizzoli, Bologna, Italy, in 2003, where he is a senior researcher and laboratory manager. His research interests include joint biomechanics and multi-instrumental analysis for pre-/intra-/post-operative functional assessments..

Sorin Siegler

Sorin Siegler earned a bachelor's degree in aeronautical engineering from the Technion, Israel Institute of Technology, a master's degree in biomedical engineering from Texas A&M University, and a Ph.D in biomedical engineering from Drexel University, Philadelphia, Pennsylvania, USA. He joined Drexel University in 1982, where he is now professor emeritus. His research interests include orthopedic biomechanics, human motion analysis, and applied dynamics.

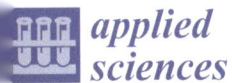

Editorial

Special Issue "Advanced Imaging in Orthopedic Biomechanics"

Claudio Belvedere [1,*] and Sorin Siegler [2]

1. Movement Analysis Laboratory, IRCCS Istituto Ortopedico Rizzoli, 40136 Bologna, Italy
2. Department of Mechanical Engineering, Drexel University, Philadelphia, PA 19104, USA; sieglers@drexel.edu
* Correspondence: belvedere@ior.it

Citation: Belvedere, C.; Siegler, S. Special Issue "Advanced Imaging in Orthopedic Biomechanics". *Appl. Sci.* 2024, 14, 8193. https://doi.org/10.3390/app14188193

Received: 30 August 2024
Accepted: 10 September 2024
Published: 12 September 2024

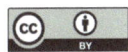

Copyright: © 2024 by the authors. Licensee MDPI, Basel, Switzerland. This article is an open access article distributed under the terms and conditions of the Creative Commons Attribution (CC BY) license (https://creativecommons.org/licenses/by/4.0/).

Continued advances in medical imaging are increasingly resulting in promising developments, for example in producing high-resolution visualization of musculoskeletal systems and thus having a high impact in clinical assessments [1–5]. This is accompanied by a significant reduction in invasiveness, for example in ionizing radiation [6,7], as well as a decrease in cost and improved device ergonomics [8,9]. As such, advanced imaging techniques have become increasingly popular clinical diagnostic tools among orthopedists, physiatrists, and physical therapists [4,5]. They are also becoming an integral part of many biomechanical studies in orthopedics due to their potential positive developments regarding functional assessments, as well as for many new and original highly innovative applications [10–12]. The latter includes the planning and the execution of personalized and minimally invasive surgeries supported by three-dimensional printing of implantable medical devices [13–16]. Advanced imaging also indicates the necessity for representative computational models of highly complex musculoskeletal systems for use in clinical applications or to understand biomechanical behaviors that are still controversial or not entirely clear [17,18]. To this end, the purpose of this Special Issue was to gather studies in which the biomechanics of the human body are highly supported by new, more advanced and accurate medical imaging systems [19,20] and relevant data processing techniques [21–24]. Taking into consideration the entire kinetic chain of the human body, including the totality of interconnected parts (i.e., joints, muscles, and ligaments) and how they work together to execute a specific movement, advanced imaging has been involved in every area and application with interesting and original implications. Starting from the trunk of the human body, including the spine, numerical simulations using finite element analysis based on cranio-cervical computed tomography data have enabled observations of how intervertebral disc wear has affected the biomechanical response of the cervical region, providing useful information on possible force-related injuries to potentially be used to propose better physiotherapy procedures [Contributions 1]. In a very multifactorial way, it is possible to relate the shape of the intervertebral foramina to factors such as age, sex, and motor neuron level to improve conservative and surgical treatment of spinal pathologies using computed tomography [Contributions 2]. Staying in the context of the spine, guidelines can be identified for the development of a more accurate spinal deformity assessment method to improve the diagnosis of scoliosis [Contributions 3]. Cervical vertebral bone mineral density and related age-dependent changes can be detected with alternative tools based on cone-beam computed tomography to diagnose osteoporosis [Contributions 4]. Moving down to the hip, and specifically to related bone oncology, the combined use of computed tomography and magnetic resonance imaging allows for consistent overall surgical procedures, through pre-surgical virtual planning and design of patient-specific surgical instrumentation, for massive hip reconstruction with safer margins for tumor removal [Contributions 5]. Regarding the knee, a joint that should be more appropriately studied under loaded conditions, dynamic MRI represents an emerging technology that should be given much more consideration for safe investigations of the functional interaction between the hard and soft tissues of the joint [Contributions 6]. On the other hand, it has again been confirmed that knee MRI data can be used in finite element analysis to obtain interesting information on the effect of varus/valgus loading configurations in bones after total knee arthroplasty with a hinged implant design [Contributions 7]. By moving even further distally, the overall biomechanics of the ankle–foot complex can be further studied and more thoroughly understood with the help of cutting-edge medical imaging techniques. Indeed, it has been shown that, in the context of dynamic modeling of the human ankle, the mechanical behavior of the joint obtained with the ligament attachment sites of the ankle detected by MRI at 3.0 T is closer to that obtained by direct observation than that obtained by MRI at 1.5 T [Contributions 8]. On the other hand, the importance of cone-beam technology for computed tomography under weight-bearing conditions in the foot and ankle has been extensively reported in two reviews. In detail, a critical discussion of the evidence provided so far in terms of advantages, limitations, and future areas of development is provided [Contributions 9], as well as promising advances in new three-dimensional techniques for automated measurements and bias reduction, particularly for syndesmotic measurements [Contributions 10]. Remaining in the context of the foot, due to the ability of computational models to accurately predict tissue behavior under concrete circumstances, more precise knowledge of foot pressure behavior has been provided through engineering methods that rely on medical imaging data, such as computed tomography, to create customized prosthetic devices and orthoses [Contributions 11]. Similar conclusions can be extended to the upper extremities, particularly the elbow and its biomechanics [Contributions 12].

Through this Special Issue, the guest editors hope to have drawn attention to the relevance of new and more accurate advanced medical imaging techniques, both in orthopedics and related biomechanical evaluations. The authors' contributions covered different anatomical compartments and various data processing methodologies, highlighting the multidisciplinary and translational nature of investigative procedures. This not only confirms that medical imaging is broadly supportive of biomechanical research but that the two are synergistic with each other in identifying better treatments for patients, with psychosocial and economic benefits for the population as a whole.

Author Contributions: C.B.: Conceptualization, Writing—original draft, Writing—review and editing. S.S.: Conceptualization, Writing—original draft, Writing—review and editing. All authors have read and agreed to the published version of the manuscript.

Conflicts of Interest: The authors declare that there are no personal or commercial relationships related to this work that would lead to conflicts of interest.

List of Contributions:

1. Trejo-Enriquez, A.; Urriolagoitia-Sosa, G.; Romero-Ángeles, B.; García-Laguna, M.; Guzmán-Baeza, M.; Martínez-Reyes, J.; Rojas-Castrejon, Y.; Gallegos-Funes, F.; Patiño-Ortiz, J.; Urriolagoitia-Calderón, G. Numerical Evaluation Using the Finite Element Method on Frontal Craniocervical Impact Directed at Intervertebral Disc Wear. *Appl. Sci.* **2023**, *13*, 11989. https://doi.org/10.3390/app132111989.
2. Nowak, P.; Dąbrowski, M.; Druszcz, A.; Kubaszewski, Ł. The Spatial Characteristics of Intervertebral Foramina within the L4/L5 and L5/S1 Motor Segments of the Spine. *Appl. Sci.* **2024**, *14*, 2263. https://doi.org/10.3390/app14062263.
3. Amran, N.; Basaruddin, K.; Ijaz, M.; Yazid, H.; Basah, S.; Muhayudin, N.; Sulaiman, A. Spine Deformity Assessment for Scoliosis Diagnostics Utilizing Image Processing Techniques: A Systematic Review. *Appl. Sci.* **2023**, *13*, 11555. https://doi.org/10.3390/app132011555.
4. Moon, E.; Kim, S.; Kim, N.; Jang, M.; Deguchi, T.; Zheng, F.; Lee, D.; Kim, D. Aging Alters Cervical Vertebral Bone Density Distribution: A Cross-Sectional Study. *Appl. Sci.* **2022**, *12*, 3143. https://doi.org/10.3390/app12063143.
5. Durastanti, G.; Belvedere, C.; Ruggeri, M.; Donati, D.; Spazzoli, B.; Leardini, A. A Pelvic Reconstruction Procedure for Custom-Made Prosthesis Design of Bone Tumor Surgical Treatments. *Appl. Sci.* **2022**, *12*, 1654. https://doi.org/10.3390/app12031654.
6. Conconi, M.; De Carli, F.; Berni, M.; Sancisi, N.; Parenti-Castelli, V.; Monetti, G. In-Vivo Quantification of Knee Deep-Flexion in Physiological Loading Condition trough Dynamic MRI. *Appl. Sci.* **2023**, *13*, 629. https://doi.org/10.3390/app13010629.

7. Bori, E.; Innocenti, B. Biomechanical Analysis of Femoral Stem Features in Hinged Revision TKA with Valgus or Varus Deformity: A Comparative Finite Elements Study. *Appl. Sci.* **2023**, *13*, 2738. https://doi.org/10.3390/app13042738.
8. Campagnoli, E.; Siegler, S.; Ruiz, M.; Leardini, A.; Belvedere, C. Effect of Ligament Mapping from Different Magnetic Resonance Image Quality on Joint Stability in a Personalized Dynamic Model of the Human Ankle Complex. *Appl. Sci.* **2022**, *12*, 5087. https://doi.org/10.3390/app12105087.
9. Dhont, T.; Huyghe, M.; Peiffer, M.; Hagemeijer, N.; Karaismailoglu, B.; Krahenbuhl, N.; Audenaert, E.; Burssens, A. Ins and Outs of the Ankle Syndesmosis from a 2D to 3D CT Perspective. *Appl. Sci.* **2023**, *13*, 10624. https://doi.org/10.3390/app131910624.
10. Lintz, F.; de Cesar Netto, C.; Belvedere, C.; Leardini, A.; Bernasconi, A.; on behalf of the International Weight-Bearing CT Society. Recent Innovations Brought about by Weight-Bearing CT Imaging in the Foot and Ankle: A Systematic Review of the Literature. *Appl. Sci.* **2024**, *14*, 5562. https://doi.org/10.3390/app14135562.
11. Serrato-Pedrosa, J.; Urriolagoitia-Sosa, G.; Romero-Ángeles, B.; Urriolagoitia-Calderón, G.; Cruz-López, S.; Urriolagoitia-Luna, A.; Carbajal-López, D.; Guereca-Ibarra, J.; Murillo-Aleman, G. Biomechanical Evaluation of Plantar Pressure Distribution towards a Customized 3D Orthotic Device: A Methodological Case Study through a Finite Element Analysis Approach. *Appl. Sci.* **2024**, *14*, 1650. https://doi.org/10.3390/app14041650.
12. Maya-Anaya, D.; Urriolagoitia-Sosa, G.; Romero-Ángeles, B.; Martinez-Mondragon, M.; German-Carcaño, J.; Correa-Corona, M.; Trejo-Enríquez, A.; Sánchez-Cervantes, A.; Urriolagoitia-Luna, A.; Urriolagoitia-Calderón, G. Numerical Analysis Applying the Finite Element Method by Developing a Complex Three-Dimensional Biomodel of the Biological Tissues of the Elbow Joint Using Computerized Axial Tomography. *Appl. Sci.* **2023**, *13*, 8903. https://doi.org/10.3390/app13158903.

References

1. Rego, J.; Tan, K. Advances in imaging-the changing environment for the imaging specialist. *Perm. J.* **2006**, *10*, 26–28. [CrossRef]
2. Huang, H.K.; Aberle, D.R.; Lufkin, R.; Grant, E.G.; Hanafee, W.N.; Kangarloo, H. Advances in medical imaging. *Ann. Intern. Med.* **1990**, *112*, 203–220. [CrossRef]
3. Ritt, P. Recent Developments in SPECT/CT. *Semin. Nucl. Med.* **2022**, *52*, 276–285. [CrossRef] [PubMed]
4. Trevino, M.; Birdsong, G.; Carrigan, A.; Choyke, P.; Drew, T.; Eckstein, M.; Fernandez, A.; Gallas, B.D.; Giger, M.; Hewitt, S.M.; et al. Advancing Research on Medical Image Perception by Strengthening Multidisciplinary Collaboration. *JNCI Cancer Spectr.* **2022**, *6*, pkab099. [CrossRef]
5. Fazal, M.I.; Patel, M.E.; Tye, J.; Gupta, Y. The past, present and future role of artificial intelligence in imaging. *Eur. J. Radiol.* **2018**, *105*, 246–250. [CrossRef]
6. Lee, T.Y.; Chhem, R.K. Impact of new technologies on dose reduction in CT. *Eur. J. Radiol.* **2010**, *76*, 28–35. [CrossRef]
7. Raslau, F.D.; Escott, E.J.; Smiley, J.; Adams, C.; Feigal, D.; Ganesh, H.; Wang, C.; Zhang, J. Dose Reduction While Preserving Diagnostic Quality in Head CT: Advancing the Application of Iterative Reconstruction Using a Live Animal Model. *AJNR Am. J. Neuroradiol.* **2019**, *40*, 1864–1870. [CrossRef]
8. Sailer, A.M.; van Zwam, W.H.; Wildberger, J.E.; Grutters, J.P. Cost-effectiveness modelling in diagnostic imaging: A stepwise approach. *Eur. Radiol.* **2015**, *25*, 3629–3637. [CrossRef]
9. Glover, A.M.; Whitman, G.J.; Shin, K. Ergonomics in Radiology: Improving the Work Environment for Radiologists. *Curr. Probl. Diagn. Radiol.* **2022**, *51*, 680–685. [CrossRef]
10. van der Velden, B.H.M.; Kuijf, H.J.; Gilhuijs, K.G.A.; Viergever, M.A. Explainable artificial intelligence (XAI) in deep learning-based medical image analysis. *Med. Image Anal.* **2022**, *79*, 102470. [CrossRef]
11. Bucking, T.M.; Hill, E.R.; Robertson, J.L.; Maneas, E.; Plumb, A.A.; Nikitichev, D.I. From medical imaging data to 3D printed anatomical models. *PLoS ONE* **2017**, *12*, e0178540. [CrossRef] [PubMed]
12. Panayides, A.S.; Amini, A.; Filipovic, N.D.; Sharma, A.; Tsaftaris, S.A.; Young, A.; Foran, D.; Do, N.; Golemati, S.; Kurc, T.; et al. AI in Medical Imaging Informatics: Current Challenges and Future Directions. *IEEE J. Biomed. Health Inform.* **2020**, *24*, 1837–1857. [CrossRef] [PubMed]
13. Gargiulo, P.; Helgason, T.; Ramon, C.; Jonsson, H., Jr.; Carraro, U. CT and MRI Assessment and Characterization Using Segmentation and 3D Modeling Techniques: Applications to Muscle, Bone and Brain. *Eur. J. Transl. Myol.* **2014**, *24*, 3298. [CrossRef]
14. Fokas, G.; Vaughn, V.M.; Scarfe, W.C.; Bornstein, M.M. Accuracy of linear measurements on CBCT images related to presurgical implant treatment planning: A systematic review. *Clin. Oral Implant. Res.* **2018**, *29* (Suppl. S16), 393–415. [CrossRef] [PubMed]
15. Barg, A.; Bailey, T.; Richter, M.; de Cesar Netto, C.; Lintz, F.; Burssens, A.; Phisitkul, P.; Hanrahan, C.J.; Saltzman, C.L. Weightbearing Computed Tomography of the Foot and Ankle: Emerging Technology Topical Review. *Foot Ankle Int.* **2018**, *39*, 376–386. [CrossRef] [PubMed]

16. Scarfe, W.C.; Li, Z.; Aboelmaaty, W.; Scott, S.A.; Farman, A.G. Maxillofacial cone beam computed tomography: Essence, elements and steps to interpretation. *Aust. Dent. J.* **2012**, *57* (Suppl. S1), 46–60. [CrossRef]
17. Fleming, B.C. Imaging and Biomechanics. *Am. J. Sports Med.* **2019**, *47*, 19–21. [CrossRef]
18. Galbusera, F.; Cina, A.; Panico, M.; Albano, D.; Messina, C. Image-based biomechanical models of the musculoskeletal system. *Eur. Radiol. Exp.* **2020**, *4*, 49. [CrossRef]
19. Wang, L.; Chen, K.C.; Gao, Y.; Shi, F.; Liao, S.; Li, G.; Shen, S.G.; Yan, J.; Lee, P.K.; Chow, B.; et al. Automated bone segmentation from dental CBCT images using patch-based sparse representation and convex optimization. *Med. Phys.* **2014**, *41*, 043503. [CrossRef]
20. Hussain, S.; Mubeen, I.; Ullah, N.; Shah, S.; Khan, B.A.; Zahoor, M.; Ullah, R.; Khan, F.A.; Sultan, M.A. Modern Diagnostic Imaging Technique Applications and Risk Factors in the Medical Field: A Review. *BioMed Res. Int.* **2022**, *2022*, 5164970. [CrossRef]
21. Scarfe, W.C.; Farman, A.G.; Sukovic, P. Clinical applications of cone-beam computed tomography in dental practice. *J. Can. Dent. Assoc.* **2006**, *72*, 75–80. [PubMed]
22. Rathnayaka, K.; Momot, K.I.; Noser, H.; Volp, A.; Schuetz, M.A.; Sahama, T.; Schmutz, B. Quantification of the accuracy of MRI generated 3D models of long bones compared to CT generated 3D models. *Med. Eng. Phys.* **2012**, *34*, 357–363. [CrossRef] [PubMed]
23. Biedert, R.; Sigg, A.; Gal, I.; Gerber, H. 3D representation of the surface topography of normal and dysplastic trochlea using MRI. *Knee* **2011**, *18*, 340–346. [CrossRef] [PubMed]
24. Inoue, A.; Ohnishi, T.; Kohno, S.; Nishida, N.; Nakamura, Y.; Ohtsuka, Y.; Matsumoto, S.; Ohue, S. Usefulness of an Image Fusion Model Using Three-Dimensional CT and MRI with Indocyanine Green Fluorescence Endoscopy as a Multimodal Assistant System in Endoscopic Transsphenoidal Surgery. *Int. J. Endocrinol.* **2015**, *2015*, 694273. [CrossRef]

Disclaimer/Publisher's Note: The statements, opinions and data contained in all publications are solely those of the individual author(s) and contributor(s) and not of MDPI and/or the editor(s). MDPI and/or the editor(s) disclaim responsibility for any injury to people or property resulting from any ideas, methods, instructions or products referred to in the content.

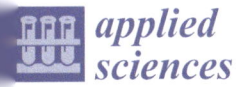

Article

Effect of Ligament Mapping from Different Magnetic Resonance Image Quality on Joint Stability in a Personalized Dynamic Model of the Human Ankle Complex

Elena Campagnoli [1], Sorin Siegler [2], Maria Ruiz [2], Alberto Leardini [1,*] and Claudio Belvedere [1]

1. Movement Analysis Laboratory, IRCCS Istituto Ortopedico Rizzoli, 40136 Bologna, Italy; elena.campagnoli96@gmail.com (E.C.); belvedere@ior.it (C.B.)
2. Department of Mechanical Engineering and Mechanics, Drexel University, Philadelphia, PA 19104, USA; sieglers@drexel.edu (S.S.); mr3393@drexel.edu (M.R.)
* Correspondence: leardini@ior.it; Tel.: +39-051-6366522; Fax: +39-051-6366561

Abstract: Background. Mechanical models of the human ankle complex are used to study the stabilizing role of ligaments. Identification of ligament function may be improved via image-based personalized approach. The aim of this study is to compare the effect of the ligament origin and insertion site definitions obtained with different magnetic resonance imaging (MRI) modalities on the mechanical behaviour of a dynamic model of the ankle complex. Methods. MRI scans, both via 1.5 T and 3.0 T, were performed on a lower-limb specimen, free from anatomical defects, to obtain morphological information on ligament-to-bone attachment sites. This specimen was used previously to develop the dynamic model. A third ligament attachment site mapping scheme was based on anatomical dissection of the scanned specimen. Following morphological comparison of the ligament attachment sites, their effect on the mechanical behaviour of the ankle complex, expressed by three-dimensional load–displacement properties, was assessed through the model. Results. Large differences were observed in the subtalar ligament attachment sites between those obtained through the two MRI scanning modalities. The 3.0 T MRI mapping was more consistent with dissection than the 1.5 T MRI. Load–displacement curves showed similar mechanical behaviours between the three mappings in the frontal plane, but those obtained from the 3.0 T MRI mapping were closer to those obtained from dissection. Conclusions. The state-of-the-art 3.0 T MRI image analysis resulted in more realistic mapping of ligament fibre origin and insertion site definitions; corresponding load–displacement predictions from a subject-specific model of the ankle complex showed a mechanical behaviour more similar to that using direct ligament attachment observations.

Keywords: ankle complex modelling; MRI; ligament origin and insertion; tibio-talar joint; subtalar joint

Citation: Campagnoli, E.; Siegler, S.; Ruiz, M.; Leardini, A.; Belvedere, C. Effect of Ligament Mapping from Different Magnetic Resonance Image Quality on Joint Stability in a Personalized Dynamic Model of the Human Ankle Complex. *Appl. Sci.* 2022, 12, 5087. https://doi.org/10.3390/app12105087

Academic Editor: Vladislav Toronov

Received: 17 February 2022
Accepted: 14 May 2022
Published: 18 May 2022

Publisher's Note: MDPI stays neutral with regard to jurisdictional claims in published maps and institutional affiliations.

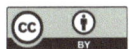

Copyright: © 2022 by the authors. Licensee MDPI, Basel, Switzerland. This article is an open access article distributed under the terms and conditions of the Creative Commons Attribution (CC BY) license (https://creativecommons.org/licenses/by/4.0/).

1. Introduction

Ligaments play a crucial role for the mobility and stability of the human ankle complex, which includes the tibiotalar joint above, between tibia–fibula–talus, and the subtalar joint below, between talus–calcaneus [1,2]. Ankle sprains represent one of the most common musculoskeletal injuries (about 25%) [3,4] and can imply partial or complete tear of the ligaments. Severe ankle sprains frequently result in chronic ankle instability [5,6]. About 10–25% of these patients also present subtalar joint instability [7,8]. When conservative techniques prove to be ineffective, surgery is indicated to restore overall joint functions [5,6,9] by ligament repair and reconstruction procedures.

The knowledge of ankle complex anatomy, and in particular of the geometrical arrangement of the ligament fibres, is fundamental for a correct diagnosis and for successful treatments. In this context, the existing computational models represent useful tools for a better comprehension of the mechanical behaviour of this anatomical complex [10] and can offer a valuable clinical support [11], particularly when tailored to the specific case of interest. From medical images of the patient's ankle complex (via CT and MRI), information about origin and insertion areas (hereinafter all together referred to also as attachments) and dimension of the ligaments can be obtained. Different types of models have been developed: those on passive kinematics [12–14] are meant to replicate joint motion in unloaded conditions; dynamic [11,14–17] and finite element [10,18,19] models may estimate the mechanical behaviour of the joints under external loads, thus approximating realistic conditions. All these models represent the ankle complex with its bones and ligaments, but with a certain level of approximation when compared to the complexity of its real anatomical structures. Unfortunately, with the exception of a few studies [12], the current literature still lacks models that include accurate ligament mapping on a subject-specific basis. A previous attempt from the present authors proposed a 3D dynamic model of the human ankle joint complex with a careful ligament mapping validated against experiment evidence [12] and it was recently extended to a larger cohort of specimens [17]. It consists of the three rigid bone segments, i.e., the tibia–fibula, talus, and calcaneus, segmented from CT images, and nine ligaments approximated from the observation of anatomical atlases and MRIs, by visually selecting the corresponding points on the surface of the bones. The model predictions compared well with related experimental observations [20], but for a thorough customization of the model, more accurate ligament characterisation is necessary [17]. Tibio–talar, tibio–calcaneal, and fibula–calcaneal ligaments geometry and configuration have been studied extensively in the past [1,21,22]. However, the subtalar ligaments were much less investigated, likely because of their difficult accessibility [23,24], particularly for those in the sinus tarsi. The most suitable medical imaging technology for the identification of soft tissues, i.e., the ligaments, is definitely MRI [25–27]. Some authors have compared 1.5 T versus 3.0 T MRI for the visualisation of cartilage, tendons, and ligaments of different anatomical joints, but the results were controversial. Among these studies, some [28–31] did not find considerable improvements from 1.5 T to 3.0 T. On the other hand, other investigations [32–34] demonstrated higher image quality and better diagnostic performance of the 3.0 T MRI. From a technical point of view, the 3.0 T MRI has higher signal strength, but introduces artefacts due to field inhomogeneities [35]. In addition, the 3D Cube sequences offered by both MRI systems provide the opportunity to observe less accessible anatomical structures, such as subtalar ligaments, from any direction. However, the resulting visualization depends on the overall image quality, which is generally better from the 3.0 T MRI systems [36,37]. This feature has rarely been used in the past for this purpose.

The aim of this study is to compare the effect of ligament attachment sites obtained with different MRI modalities (i.e., 1.5 T and 3.0 T MRI) on the mechanical behaviour of a previously validated dynamic model of the human ankle complex [12,17], for which subject-specific mapping of the origin and insertion of the ligaments is essential. In addition, direct observations of ligament attachment sites from careful anatomical dissection were performed. Model predictions derived from the two MRI modalities were compared to those obtained from dissection, here used as a reference. The comparison was based on the load–displacement (i.e., joint torque–joint rotation) properties predicted by the model. We hypothesized that the mechanical behaviour of the model obtained with the ligament attachment sites detected through the 3.0 T MRI is closer to that obtained from direct observation than that from the 1.5 T MRI.

2. Material and Methods

2.1. The Model

The original model consisted of the ankle complex bones (i.e., the tibia–fibula as a single rigid body, the talus, and the calcaneus) and relevant ligaments [12] with their mechanical properties [38,39]. The ligaments were modelled as pre-strained, non-linear, viscoelastic springs, and the number of fibres was chosen depending on their thickness [12]. The model included nine ligaments [17]: Anterior Talo-Fibular (ATFL), Posterior Talo-Fibular (PTFL),

Calcaneo-Fibular (CFL), Anterior Tibio-Talar (ATTL), Posterior Tibio-Talar (PTTL), Tibio-Calcaneal (TCL), Tibio Spring (TSL), Interosseus Talo-Calcaneal (ITCL), and Cervical Ligament (CL). The morphology of the bones was obtained from CT (DE Rev HD 1700 GSI, GE; 0.6 mm slicing space) after segmentation (Analyze Direct^{TM}, Overland Park, KS, USA), smoothing, and 3D rendering (Geomagic^{TM}, 3D Systems, Morrisville, NC, USA). The contact between the bones was modelled according to classical contact mechanics, with maximum local penetration, speed of penetration, stiffness, and damping ratio properties taken from the human articular cartilage [12].

2.2. Identification of 1.5 T MRI-Based Ligament Attachments

2D and 3D sequences were acquired with 1.5 T MRI (SIGNA EXCITE HDxt, GE Healthcare, Chicago, IL, USA). In detail, 3D Cube acquisition was executed using a Quad Knee coil with 0.5 mm slice thickness and $0.6 \times 0.6 \times 0.5$ mm voxel size; 2D Fat-Sat axial, coronal and sagittal were also acquired with 3.3 mm slice thickness and $0.3 \times 0.3 \times 3.3$ mm voxel size.

The ligament attachment areas were segmented starting from the 3D sequence. However, due to the low overall image quality resulting from this scan, morphological reconstruction was obtained by combining relevant information with that derived from the 2D sequences. The obtained ligament attachment areas were then compared to those present in the original model [12]. When differences in attachment sites were observed, they were transferred to the dynamic model to replace the original ones.

2.3. Identification of 3.0 T MRI-Based Ligament Attachments

2D and 3D sequences were acquired with 3.0 T MRI (MR750W GEM ENAB, GE Healthcare, Chicago, IL, USA). In detail, 3D Cube acquisition was executed using a 16-ch gem flex medium coil, with 0.4 mm slice thickness and $0.4 \times 0.4 \times 0.4$ mm voxel size; 2D Fat-Sat axial, coronal, and sagittal were acquired with 3.0 mm slice thickness and $0.5 \times 0.5 \times 3.0$ mm voxel size.

The ligament attachment areas were segmented from the 3D Cube sequence which, in this case, provided high quality images, although 2D sequences were always analysed for completeness. Thanks to the overall better resolution of the 3D Cube of 3.0 T MRI scan when compared to the corresponding from 1.5 T MRI scan, several reslicing were here performed to best identify the regions of origin and insertion of the different ligaments. The reslicing process maintained full resolution since no deterioration resulted from the adopted process. The obtained ligament attachment areas were then compared to those present in the original model [12]. When differences in attachment sites were observed, they were transferred to the dynamic model to replace the original ones.

3. Dissection

The same specimen, a below knee amputation from a fresh frozen cadaver, was dissected to provide direct access and visualization of the morphology of the ligament attachment sites, and these were used as a reference for the image-based assessments. All soft tissues were removed, and the ligaments of interest were exposed. Each ligament was photographed and marked with a surgical marking pen. The ligament attachment sites of data were compared to those present in the original model [12]. When differences in attachment sites were observed, they were transferred to the dynamic model to replace the original ones.

Model Simulations with Updated Mapping

Three different models were derived from the original model [12] for this specific specimen used in this study. Two models were based on MRI (1.5 T and 3.0 T) and one on the dissection-based observations. The only difference between each of these models and the original one was in the attachment sites of some of the ligaments, but they used loading and boundary conditions identical to those described earlier [20]. Simulations were performed (MSC ADAMS™, Newport Beach, CA, USA) by imposing 100 N axial compression and applying loading/unloading cycles in the frontal plane and axial plane. Load–displacement properties were obtained in inversion–eversion and internal–external rotation for the tibiotalar joint (TTJ), the subtalar joint (STJ), and the ankle joint complex (AJC) for each of the three models.

4. Results

The ligaments attachment sites obtained from the 3.0 T MRI were better visualized than those from 1.5 T MRI and their locations were more consistent with those obtained from direct observations. All these three definition schemes provided similar data on the origin and insertion sites for the ankle complex ligaments, except for those of the subtalar joint, particularly for the ITCL. In the 1.5 T MRI, the ITCL consisted of two branches with a common insertion on the calcaneus (Figure 1A), which split in two distinguished origins on the lower surface of the talus (Figure 1B), one more lateral and the other more medial. In the 3.0 T MRI, the common origin was on the talus (Figure 1D) and then the two branches divided into a more anterior insertion area and a more posterior one on the lateral part of the lower surface of the calcaneus (Figure 1C). Overall, ligament attachment sites from the 3.0 T MRI were consistent with the direct observations from dissection (compare Figures 1E,F and 2 left and right).

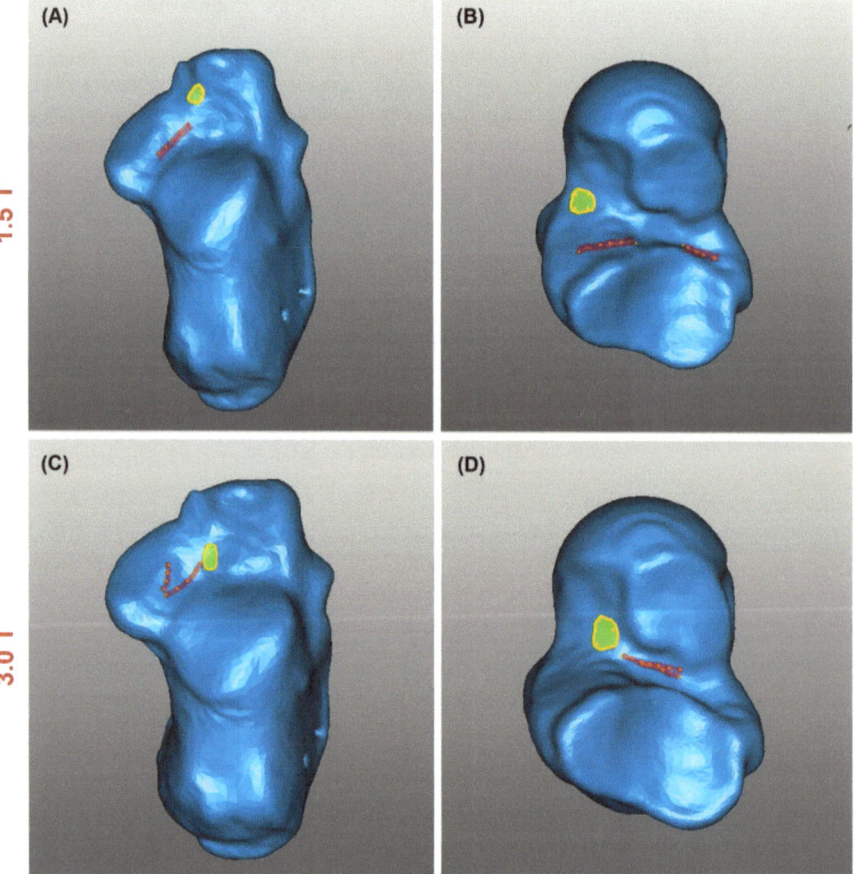

Figure 1. *Cont.*

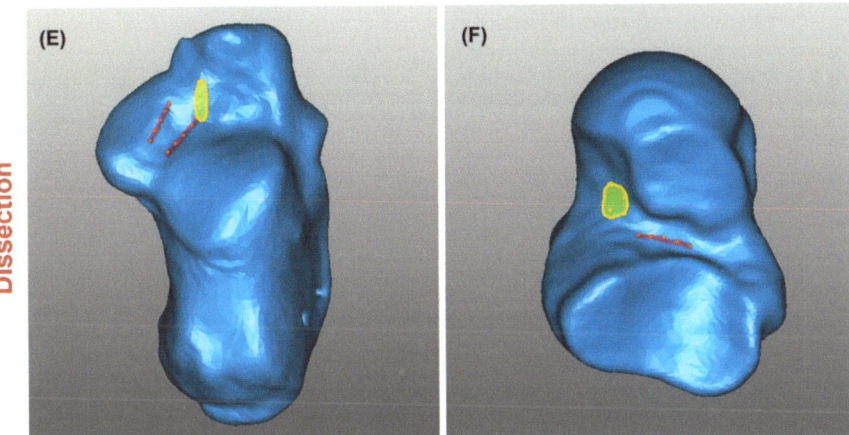

Figure 1. Maps of the subtalar ligaments from 1.5 T MRI (**A,B**), 3.0 T MRI (**C,D**), and from dissection (**E,F**): CL (yellow), ITCL (red). Origin areas on the bottom of the talus bone (**B,D,F**) and insertion areas on the top of the calcaneus bone (**A,C,E**).

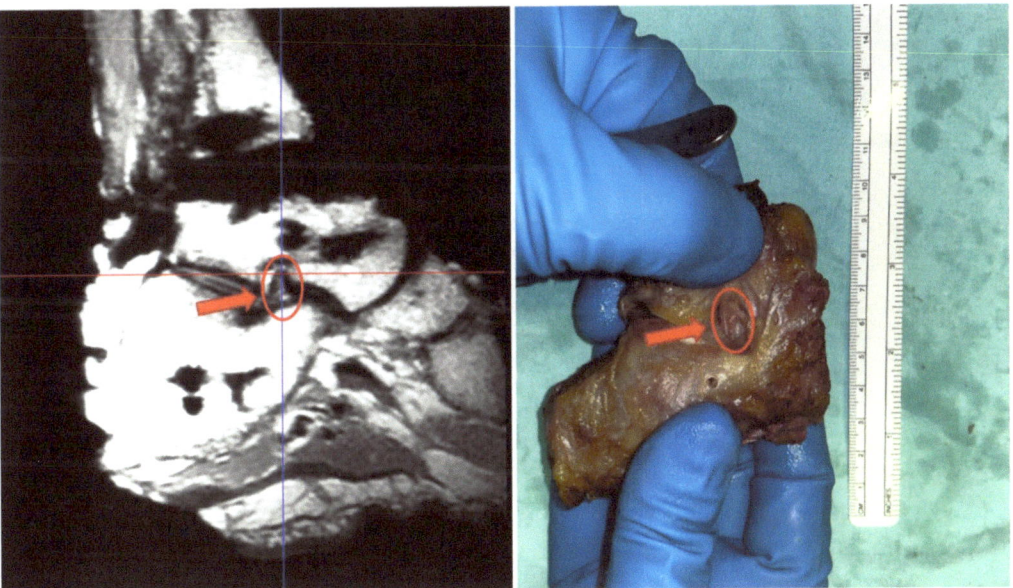

Figure 2. ITCL from 3.0 T MRI (**left**) and from direct observation (**right**).

In Figure 3, the load–displacement curves for the TTJ, STJ, and AJC in internal–external rotation and inversion–eversion were obtained from the three different schemes. For the AJC, similar load–displacement patterns were observed in the frontal plane (Figure 3B). In the transverse plane (Figure 3A), 1.5 T MRI model produced a different pattern when compared to the other two, reaching about 40° of internal rotation as compared to only 25°.

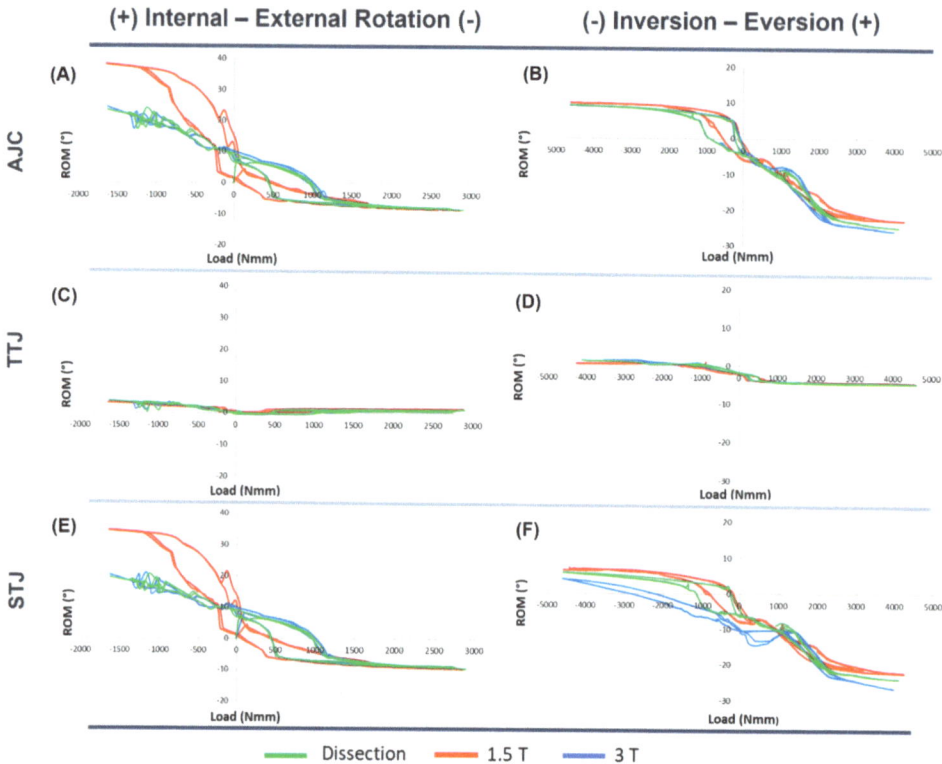

Figure 3. Superimposition of the load–displacement curves resulting from the three mappings of the ligament attachment sites obtained via 1.5 T (red curves), 3.0 T (blue curves), and direct observation from the dissection of the specimen (green curves). Curves associated to Internal–External Rotation (**A,C,E**) and Inversion–Eversion (**B,D,F**) are reported for the AJC (**A,B**), TTJ (**C,D**), and STJ (**E,F**).

For TTJ (Figure 3C,D) the three schemes resulted in similar load–displacement patterns in both the frontal and axial plane.

The differences in the load–displacement properties between the three different schemes for the STJ (Figure 3E,F) are similar to those for the AJC, i.e., with 3.0 T MRI generally replicating results from the dissection map.

5. Discussion

The attachment areas of ankle and subtalar ligaments were identified using 1.5 T and 3.0 T MRI systems via both 2D and 3D sequences, and also via direct observations used as a reference. After relevant redistribution of the ligament fibres, a dynamic analysis of an ankle complex model showed load–displacement curves based on the 3.0 T MRI observations more consistent with those curves based on direct observations of the specimen.

A number of papers in radiologic anatomy have addressed MRI imaging for ankle complex ligaments [40–43]. However, these have not dealt with careful definition of origin and insertion areas of the ligaments, and this is particularly true for the subtalar ligaments. Additionally, not a single paper has compared geometrical and morphological features of these ligaments with corresponding direct observations. Also very limited is the analysis of the effects of resulting ligament mapping on dynamic computer models of the ankle joint complex. A recent paper from these authors has addressed medical imaging of the ankle complex by different modalities [44], but with a focus on the articular cartilage.

The comparison of the ligament attachment sites obtained using the two MRI modalities with the direct observations demonstrated the superiority of the 3.0 T MRI over the 1.5 T MRI in imaging ligaments and identifying their regions of origin and insertion on bones. The main reason for these differences was that the 3D Cube sequence in 3.0 T MRI allows for a clearer visualization and revisualization of the ligaments and their attachment areas without losing resolution. In addition, 3.0 T MRI provides twice the signal-to-noise ratio compared to 1.5 T MRI, resulting in better image quality and higher spatial resolution [35].

Visualization through imaging of the subtalar ligament morphology is very difficult [23,40]. This study demonstrated that this difficulty may be overcome by more advanced imaging modalities and may offer a solution for accurate diagnosis of subtalar ligament injuries [8,24]. Furthermore, this study demonstrated that visualizing the subtalar ligaments from different orientations without loss of resolution provides an important imaging advantage over non-cubic sequences where high resolution is only available in one direction.

The 3.0 T MRI-based dynamic model produced load–displacement behaviour similar to that resulting from the model based on direct observations of the ligaments attachment sites. The 1.5 T MRI-based model, on the other hand, produced different results. This demonstrates the importance of using higher resolution 3D Cube sequence, as by 3.0 T MRI, in developing accurate models of the ankle complex and its ligamentous support.

This study is not without limitations. The study relied on one single specimen so that inter-subject variability was not considered. In addition, direct observation, even from very careful anatomical dissections by experienced anatomists and surgeons, is difficult and subject to controversies due to the complex structure of these ligaments and their hard-to-access location. This also applies to identification by radiologists in image-based observations. In addition, no inter-observer assessment was included. The present relevant findings can be certainly strengthened in the future with other specimens, other MRI devices, and other ligament mapping definitions.

6. Conclusions

The present study offers an enhancement for subject-specification of a previously validated 3D dynamic model of the ankle complex [12,17] through MRI-based mappings of the ligaments from a single representative specimen. The results obtained from the two MRI systems and the anatomical dissection of the same specimen demonstrated how essential the identification of ligaments origin and insertion sites is for subject-specific modelling of the ankle complex. In particular, the better quality of the state-of-the-art 3.0 T MRI images, with respect to traditional 1.5 T MRI, resulted in definitions of these attachment sites closer to the direct observations, and in more similar load–displacement curves from the computer model.

Author Contributions: Conceptualization: S.S., C.B. and A.L.; methodology: E.C., M.R. and C.B.; software: E.C., S.S. and M.R.; validation: E.C., S.S. and C.B.; formal analysis: E.C.; investigation: E.C., C.B. and A.L.; resources: S.S. and A.L.; writing—original draft preparation: E.C., C.B. and A.L.; writing—review and editing: E.C., S.S., C.B., M.R. and A.L.; visualization: E.C.; supervision: C.B. and A.L.; project administration: S.S. and A.L.; funding acquisition: A.L. All authors have read and agreed to the published version of the manuscript.

Funding: This study was funded by the Italian Ministry of Economy and Finance, program "5 per mille".

Institutional Review Board Statement: Local IRB approval is not required for this type of study.

Informed Consent Statement: Patient consent was waived due to the cadaver specimen from Tissue Bank, according to National regulation.

Data Availability Statement: The datasets generated during the current study are not publicly available but are available from the corresponding author on reasonable request.

Conflicts of Interest: All authors declare that there are no personal or commercial relationships related to this work that would lead to a conflict of interest.

References

1. Leardini, A.; O'Connor, J.J.; Catani, F.; Giannini, S. The role of the passive structures in the mobility and stability of the human ankle joint: A literature review. *Foot Ankle Int.* **2000**, *21*, 602–615. [CrossRef] [PubMed]
2. Stagni, R.; Leardini, A.; O'Connor, J.J.; Giannini, S. Role of passive structures in the mobility and stability of the human subtalar joint: A literature review. *Foot Ankle Int.* **2003**, *24*, 402–409. [CrossRef] [PubMed]
3. Petersen, W.; Rembitzki, I.V.; Koppenburg, A.G.; Ellermann, A.; Liebau, C.; Bruggemann, G.P.; Best, R. Treatment of acute ankle ligament injuries: A systematic review. *Arch. Orthop. Trauma. Surg.* **2013**, *133*, 1129–1141. [CrossRef] [PubMed]
4. Van den Bekerom, M.P.; Kerkhoffs, G.M.; McCollum, G.A.; Calder, J.D.; van Dijk, C.N. Management of acute lateral ankle ligament injury in the athlete. *Knee Surg. Sports Traumatol. Arthrosc. Off. J. ESSKA* **2013**, *21*, 1390–1395. [CrossRef]
5. Guillo, S.; Bauer, T.; Lee, J.W.; Takao, M.; Kong, S.W.; Stone, J.W.; Mangone, P.G.; Molloy, A.; Perera, A.; Pearce, C.J.; et al. Consensus in chronic ankle instability: Aetiology, assessment, surgical indications and place for arthroscopy. *Orthop. Traumatol. Surg. Res.* **2013**, *99*, S411–S419. [CrossRef]
6. Michels, F.; Pereira, H.; Calder, J.; Matricali, G.; Glazebrook, M.; Guillo, S.; Karlsson, J.; Group, E.-A.A.I.; Acevedo, J.; Batista, J.; et al. Searching for consensus in the approach to patients with chronic lateral ankle instability: Ask the expert. *Knee Surg. Sports Traumatol. Arthrosc. Off. J. ESSKA* **2018**, *26*, 2095–2102. [CrossRef]
7. Yamaguchi, R.; Nimura, A.; Amaha, K.; Yamaguchi, K.; Segawa, Y.; Okawa, A.; Akita, K. Anatomy of the Tarsal Canal and Sinus in Relation to the Subtalar Joint Capsule. *Foot Ankle Int.* **2018**, *39*, 1360–1369. [CrossRef]
8. Kim, T.H.; Moon, S.G.; Jung, H.G.; Kim, N.R. Subtalar instability: Imaging features of subtalar ligaments on 3D isotropic ankle MRI. *BMC Musculoskelet. Disord.* **2017**, *18*, 475. [CrossRef]
9. Leardini, A.; O'Connor, J.J.; Giannini, S. Biomechanics of the natural, arthritic, and replaced human ankle joint. *J. Foot Ankle Res.* **2014**, *7*, 8. [CrossRef]
10. Nie, B.; Panzer, M.B.; Mane, A.; Mait, A.R.; Donlon, J.P.; Forman, J.L.; Kent, R.W. Determination of the in situ mechanical behavior of ankle ligaments. *J. Mech. Behav. Biomed. Mater.* **2017**, *65*, 502–512. [CrossRef]
11. Iaquinto, J.M.; Wayne, J.S. Computational model of the lower leg and foot/ankle complex: Application to arch stability. *J. Biomech. Eng.* **2010**, *132*, 021009. [CrossRef] [PubMed]
12. Imhauser, C.W.; Siegler, S.; Udupa, J.K.; Toy, J.R. Subject-specific models of the hindfoot reveal a relationship between morphology and passive mechanical properties. *J. Biomech.* **2008**, *41*, 1341–1349. [CrossRef] [PubMed]
13. Leardini, A.; O'Connor, J.J.; Catani, F.; Giannini, S. A geometric model of the human ankle joint. *J. Biomech.* **1999**, *32*, 585–591. [CrossRef]
14. Forlani, M.; Sancisi, N.; Parenti-Castelli, V. A three-dimensional ankle kinetostatic model to simulate loaded and unloaded joint motion. *J. Biomech. Eng.* **2015**, *137*, 061005. [CrossRef] [PubMed]
15. Liacouras, P.C.; Wayne, J.S. Computational modeling to predict mechanical function of joints: Application to the lower leg with simulation of two cadaver studies. *J. Biomech. Eng.* **2007**, *129*, 811–817. [CrossRef]
16. Purevsuren, T.; Kim, K.; Batbaatar, M.; Lee, S.; Kim, Y.H. Influence of ankle joint plantarflexion and dorsiflexion on lateral ankle sprain: A computational study. *Proc. Inst. Mech. Eng. Part H* **2018**, *232*, 458–467. [CrossRef]
17. Palazzi, E.; Siegler, S.; Balakrishnan, V.; Leardini, A.; Caravaggi, P.; Belvedere, C. Estimating the stabilizing function of ankle and subtalar ligaments via a morphology-specific three-dimensional dynamic model. *J. Biomech.* **2020**, *98*, 109421. [CrossRef]
18. Li, J.; Wei, Y.; Wei, M. Finite Element Analysis of the Effect of Talar Osteochondral Defects of Different Depths on Ankle Joint Stability. *Med. Sci. Monit.* **2020**, *26*, e921823. [CrossRef]
19. Haraguchi, N.; Armiger, R.S.; Myerson, M.S.; Campbell, J.T.; Chao, E.Y. Prediction of three-dimensional contact stress and ligament tension in the ankle during stance determined from computational modeling. *Foot Ankle Int.* **2009**, *30*, 177–185. [CrossRef]
20. Belvedere, C.; Siegler, S.; Ensini, A.; Toy, J.; Caravaggi, P.; Namani, R.; Giannini, G.; Durante, S.; Leardini, A. Experimental evaluation of a new morphological approximation of the articular surfaces of the ankle joint. *J. Biomech.* **2017**, *53*, 97–104. [CrossRef]
21. Golano, P.; Vega, J.; de Leeuw, P.A.; Malagelada, F.; Manzanares, M.C.; Gotzens, V.; van Dijk, C.N. Anatomy of the ankle ligaments: A pictorial essay. *Knee Surg. Sports Traumatol. Arthrosc. Off. J. ESSKA* **2010**, *18*, 557–569. [CrossRef] [PubMed]
22. Anand Prakash, A. Anatomy of Ankle Syndesmotic Ligaments: A Systematic Review of Cadaveric Studies. *Foot Ankle Spec.* **2020**, *13*, 341–350. [CrossRef] [PubMed]
23. Michels, F.; Matricali, G.; Vereecke, E.; Dewilde, M.; Vanrietvelde, F.; Stockmans, F. The intrinsic subtalar ligaments have a consistent presence, location and morphology. *Foot Ankle Surg.* **2021**, *27*, 101–109. [CrossRef] [PubMed]
24. Poonja, A.J.; Hirano, M.; Khakimov, D.; Ojumah, N.; Tubbs, R.S.; Loukas, M.; Kozlowski, P.B.; Khan, K.H.; DiLandro, A.C.; D'Antoni, A.V. Anatomical Study of the Cervical and Interosseous Talocalcaneal Ligaments of the Foot with Surgical Relevance. *Cureus* **2017**, *9*, e1382. [CrossRef]
25. Sconfienza, L.M.; Orlandi, D.; Lacelli, F.; Serafini, G.; Silvestri, E. Dynamic high-resolution US of ankle and midfoot ligaments: Normal anatomic structure and imaging technique. *Radiographics* **2015**, *35*, 164–178. [CrossRef]

26. Ngai, S.S.; Tafur, M.; Chang, E.Y.; Chung, C.B. Magnetic Resonance Imaging of Ankle Ligaments. *Can. Assoc. Radiol. J.* **2016**, *67*, 60–68. [CrossRef]
27. Chen, E.T.; Borg-Stein, J.; McInnis, K.C. Ankle Sprains: Evaluation, Rehabilitation, and Prevention. *Curr. Sports Med. Rep.* **2019**, *18*, 217–223. [CrossRef]
28. Van Dyck, P.; Kenis, C.; Vanhoenacker, F.M.; Lambrecht, V.; Wouters, K.; Gielen, J.L.; Dossche, L.; Parizel, P.M. Comparison of 1.5-and 3-T MR imaging for evaluating the articular cartilage of the knee. *Knee Surg. Sports Traumatol. Arthrosc. Off. J. ESSKA* **2014**, *22*, 1376–1384. [CrossRef]
29. Van Dyck, P.; Vanhoenacker, F.M.; Lambrecht, V.; Wouters, K.; Gielen, J.L.; Dossche, L.; Parizel, P.M. Prospective comparison of 1.5 and 3.0-T MRI for evaluating the knee menisci and ACL. *J. Bone Jt. Surg.* **2013**, *95*, 916–924. [CrossRef]
30. Nouri, N.; Bouaziz, M.C.; Riahi, H.; Mechri, M.; Kherfani, A.; Ouertatani, M.; Ladeb, M.F. Traumatic Meniscus and Cruciate Ligament Tears in Young Patients: A Comparison of 3T Versus 1.5T MRI. *J. Belg. Soc. Radiol.* **2017**, *101*, 14. [CrossRef]
31. Grossman, J.W.; De Smet, A.A.; Shinki, K. Comparison of the accuracy rates of 3-T and 1.5-T MRI of the knee in the diagnosis of meniscal tear. *AJR Am. J. Roentgenol.* **2009**, *193*, 509–514. [CrossRef] [PubMed]
32. Barr, C.; Bauer, J.S.; Malfair, D.; Ma, B.; Henning, T.D.; Steinbach, L.; Link, T.M. MR imaging of the ankle at 3 Tesla and 1.5 Tesla: Protocol optimization and application to cartilage, ligament and tendon pathology in cadaver specimens. *Eur. Radiol.* **2007**, *17*, 1518–1528. [CrossRef] [PubMed]
33. Oehler, N.; Ruby, J.K.; Strahl, A.; Maas, R.; Ruether, W.; Niemeier, A. Hip abductor tendon pathology visualized by 1.5 versus 3.0 Tesla MRIs. *Arch. Orthop. Trauma. Surg.* **2020**, *140*, 145–153. [CrossRef] [PubMed]
34. Bauer, J.S.; Barr, C.; Henning, T.D.; Malfair, D.; Ma, C.B.; Steinbach, L.; Link, T.M. Magnetic resonance imaging of the ankle at 3.0 Tesla and 1.5 Tesla in human cadaver specimens with artificially created lesions of cartilage and ligaments. *Investig. Radiol.* **2008**, *43*, 604–611. [CrossRef]
35. Bauer, J.S.; Monetti, R.; Krug, R.; Matsuura, M.; Mueller, D.; Eckstein, F.; Rummeny, E.J.; Lochmueller, E.M.; Raeth, C.W.; Link, T.M. Advances of 3T MR imaging in visualizing trabecular bone structure of the calcaneus are partially SNR-independent: Analysis using simulated noise in relation to micro-CT, 1.5T MRI, and biomechanical strength. *J. Magn. Reson. Imaging* **2009**, *29*, 132–140. [CrossRef]
36. Neri, E.; Caramella, D.; Bartolozzi, C. *Image Processing in Radiology: Current Applications*; Springer: Berlin, Germany; New York, NY, USA, 2008; p. x, 434p.
37. Stevens, K.J.; Busse, R.F.; Han, E.; Brau, A.C.; Beatty, P.J.; Beaulieu, C.F.; Gold, G.E. Ankle: Isotropic MR imaging with 3D-FSE-cube–initial experience in healthy volunteers. *Radiology* **2008**, *249*, 1026–1033. [CrossRef]
38. Siegler, S.; Block, J.; Schneck, C.D. The mechanical characteristics of the collateral ligaments of the human ankle joint. *Foot Ankle* **1988**, *8*, 234–242. [CrossRef]
39. Funk, J.R.; Hall, G.W.; Crandall, J.R.; Pilkey, W.D. Linear and quasi-linear viscoelastic characterization of ankle ligaments. *J. Biomech. Eng.* **2000**, *122*, 15–22. [CrossRef]
40. Lopez-Ben, R. Imaging of the subtalar joint. *Foot Ankle Clin.* **2015**, *20*, 223–241. [CrossRef]
41. Sormaala, M.J.; Ruohola, J.P.; Mattila, V.M.; Koskinen, S.K.; Pihlajamaki, H.K. Comparison of 1.5T and 3T MRI scanners in evaluation of acute bone stress in the foot. *BMC Musculoskelet. Disord.* **2011**, *12*, 128. [CrossRef]
42. Cledera, T.H.C.; Flores, D.V. Magnetic Resonance Imaging of Ankle Ligaments. *Contemp. Diagn. Radiol.* **2021**, *44*, 1–7. [CrossRef]
43. Fritz, B.; Fritz, J.; Sutter, R. 3D MRI of the Ankle: A Concise State-of-the-Art Review. *Semin. Musculoskelet. Radiol.* **2021**, *25*, 514–526. [CrossRef] [PubMed]
44. Durastanti, G.; Leardini, A.; Siegler, S.; Durante, S.; Bazzocchi, A.; Belvedere, C. Comparison of cartilage and bone morphological models of the ankle joint derived from different medical imaging technologies. *Quant. Imaging Med. Surg.* **2019**, *9*, 1368–1382. [CrossRef] [PubMed]

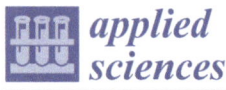 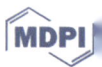

Article

Biomechanical Analysis of Femoral Stem Features in Hinged Revision TKA with Valgus or Varus Deformity: A Comparative Finite Elements Study

Edoardo Bori and Bernardo Innocenti *

BEAMS Department (Bio Electro and Mechanical Systems), Université Libre de Bruxelles, 1050 Brussels, Belgium
* Correspondence: bernardo.innocenti@ulb.be; Tel.: +32-(0)-2650-3531

Featured Application: The present study intends to help and support clinicians and specialists in the decision process concerning the length and type of stems to use in case varus–valgus deformity is present in a patient.

Abstract: Hinged total knee arthroplasty (TKA) is a valid option to treat patients during revision of an implant; however, in case of varus/valgus deformity, the force transmission from the femur to the tibia could be altered and therefore the performance of the implant could be detrimental. To be able to evaluate this, the goal of this study was to investigate, using a validated finite element analysis, the effect of varus/valgus load configurations in the bones when a hinged TKA is used. In detail, short and long stem lengths (50 mm, and 120 mm), were analyzed both under cemented or press-fit fixation under the following varus and valgus deformity: 5°, 10°, 20°, and 30°. The main outputs of the study were average bone stress in different regions of interest, together with tibio-femoral contact pressure and force. Results demonstrated that changes in the varus or valgus deformity degrees induce a change in the medio-lateral stress and force distribution, together with a change in the contact area. The effect of stem length and cement do not alter the tibio-femoral contact biomechanics but its effect is mainly localized in the distal femoral region, and it is negligible in the proximal regions.

Keywords: hinged TKA; varus deformity; valgus deformity; finite element; stem length; cemented; press fit; biomechanics

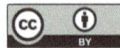

1. Introduction

Achieving the correct alignment in total knee arthroplasty (TKA) is an important factor to restore biomechanical functions of the knee (such as soft tissue balancing and joint line) and prevent early implant failure, thus guaranteeing long-term survival of the implant [1–3]. In detail, the alignment of the prosthesis components on the frontal plane strongly influences the distribution of tibio-femoral contact forces between the two tibial plateau compartments: biomechanical studies report that varus misalignment causes overload on the medial side while valgus misalignment leads to increased tibio-femoral force in the lateral side [4]. As a result of these deviations, the non-physiological loading of the knee enhances degeneration of the joint and causes overloads on the bone-implant interface and in the bone itself.

Alterations of the natural alignment, therefore, may lead to early aseptic loosening, polyethylene wear, erroneous patellofemoral tracking, instability and infection [2,5]; all of these factors are usually associated with TKA failure, which consequently leads to the need of a revision total knee replacement.

Together with alignment, the choice of an adequate level of constraint is essential to ensure successful clinical outcomes and long-term TKA survival [6]; this is even more important when dealing with revision surgeries.

The rotating hinge (RH) prosthesis represents a common solution among the different models available for revision procedures, as thanks to this degree of freedom around the tibial axis, this model is able to achieve reduced shear stress at the bone-cement interface, compared to other devices [7–11]. It is important to mention that this kind of implant can also be used as an alternative to primary TKA, in case of complex situations, such as extreme joint deformities [7,12].

The main issues addressed with the use of a RH TKA are therefore large ligamentous instability, severe bone loss, distal femoral or proximal tibial defects (resulting from injury or tumor) and severe varus or valgus deformities [13–15].

The design of a rotating hinge prosthesis usually consists of a femoral component and a tibial one (constrained among each other with a rotating hinge mechanism) and of a polyethylene insert placed between these two elements, in order to prevent luxation without reducing the range of motion [16].

The current designs are available in multiple sizes and present modularity, with sets of different features/stem lengths to allow for the different possible fixation techniques; this variety of possibilities represents thus a worthwhile opportunity, especially in revision patients where deficiencies of the bone cannot be totally predicted [17].

Stem length, among the other parameters, covers a crucial role in the overall success of the reconstruction. Usually, the choice of which length to use is largely determined by the stem fixation technique selected: in modern revision TKA, the options are usually fully cemented and press-fit fixation [18–21].

Despite its advantages, this kind of implant also implies the relative risks of mechanical failure and infection [9,22–24], which can furthermore increase in case of eventual patient joint deformities. The level of constraint provided by the rotating hinge, paired with the use of different stems and/or fixation approached, may therefore lead to eventual over-constraining issues affecting the tibio-femoral and/or the bone-implant interactions; a more comprehensive guideline on the suggested use and optimal configuration of these implants (when mainly aimed to address high deformities) is however still missing.

The present study intends to help and support clinicians and specialists, assisting the decision process concerning the length and type of stems to use in case varus–valgus deformity is present in a patient. A numerical biomechanical study was therefore performed in order to evaluate the effects and performances of different configurations of RH TKA prosthesis in patients with severe valgus and varus deformities, in terms of distribution of forces and relative contact areas on the polyethylene insert when different lengths of femoral stems are used, considering both fixation types (cemented and press-fit) and in terms of average bone stress in different regions of interests.

2. Materials and Methods

The model was developed based on an already validated and published knee finite element model [25–27].

Finite elements analysis approach was selected since it guarantees a great comparative potential, allowing to change any single parameter of the model in order to precisely analyze its influence on the outcomes while leaving the other boundary conditions unchanged [28–30].

The following features were implemented in the models.

2.1. Geometry & Configurations

The three-dimensional model of a femur, divided in cortical and cancellous bone, was obtained from CT scans of a right-side Sawbone synthetic bone (Sawbones Europe AB, Limhamn, Sweden), following an approach widely used for numerical and experimental tests [2,31–36].

A right side, medium size endo-model rotating hinge knee prosthesis (Waldemar Link GMBH & Co., Hamburg, Germany) was considered for the study and the relative geometries were obtained from a previous study [21].

Different angles of valgus and varus deformities of the femur were considered (5°, 10°, 20°, and 30°, considering a 0° configuration as the physiological control) and the relative models were implemented. For each configuration, two femoral stem lengths (50, 120 mm) and two types of fixations (cemented or press-fit) were tested; tibial tray component and polyethylene insert sizes were kept the same in each configuration, together with the tibial stem of 50 mm length. For each of the configurations analyzed, the prosthesis was virtually implanted into the femoral bone following the manufacturer's surgical technique (therefore considered to be the ideal positioning of the implant, according to the patient configuration [21]). In the cemented configuration, the stem was positioned in the center of the intramedullary canal and surrounded by a homogeneous cement mantle, obtained by filling a previously reamed hole and subtracting the stem volume, simulating thus the ideal cementing technique [32].

2.2. Material Properties

According to the literature [2,32,37–39], the materials used in this study were assumed to be linear elastic; this was chosen to obtain a better approximation of all materials, in order to achieve a qualitative comparison among different configurations [2]. In particular, the material for the femoral component and the tibial tray was considered as cobalt-chromium (CoCr), whereas the material of the tibial insert was ultra-high-molecular-weight-polyethylene (UHMWPE). These materials were assumed to be homogeneous and isotropic [2,32,40]. The material used for the bone cement (Polymethyl-methacrylate, PMMA) in the relative configurations was considered homogeneous and isotropic [2,11]. The material properties in terms of Young's modulus (E) and Poisson's ratio (ν) are available in Table 1 [2,32,37].

Table 1. Material properties of the implant components: CoCr = cobalt-chromium alloy, UHMWE = ultra-high-molecular-weight-polyethylene, PMMA = polymethyl-methacrylate.

Material	Material Model	Elastic Modulus (MPa)	Poisson Ratio
CoCr	Isotropic	240,000	0.30
UHMW	Isotropic	685	0.40
PMMA	Isotropic	3000	0.30

The cortical bone, according to previous studies, was considered transversely isotropic [2,8,41,42]; the cancellous bone was instead considered linear isotropic [2,32,43]. The material properties used are reported in Table 2.

Table 2. Material properties of the femoral bone used for all models; the third axis was taken parallel with the anatomical axis of the femur.

Material	Material Model	Elastic Modulus (MPa)			Poisson Ratio		
		E_1	E_2	E_3	ν_{12}	ν_{23}	ν_{31}
Cortical Bone	Transversely Isotropic	11,500	11,500	17,000	0.51	0.31	031
Cancellous Bone	Isotropic	2130			0.30		

2.3. Finite Element Analysis and Boundary Conditions

Abaqus/Standard version 6.19 (Dassault Systèmes, Vélizy-Villacoublay, France) was used to assemble all parts of the prosthesis with femur bone, in order to perform all the finite element simulations.

Each model was meshed using tetrahedral elements with a size between 1 mm and 3 mm. A refinement of mesh was performed in the contact area of the internal components of the implant, and in the tibio-femoral and bone-implant interface sections to make sure that the selected mesh was the proper one to achieve the sought after results: to check the quality of the mesh and the proper size, a convergence test was thus performed [2,20] and is available in the Supplementary Materials.

According to the previously published study [21], surface-to-surface contacts were implemented for the definition of all contacts, i.e., among the components involved in the hinge mechanism, between the insert and the femoral component of the prosthesis and between the implant and the bone.

Each configuration analyzed was tested under the same total load conditions, i.e., the proximal part of the femur constrained and a total vertical compressive force of 1000 N applied to the inferior face of the tibial tray. The subdivision of this total force on the two sides of the tibial tray was then used as a parameter in order to model the different levels of varus/valgus deformities: a simplified model in the literature [11] allowed indeed to obtain the percentage of force distribution in the medial and lateral regions of the tibial component for each angle of deformity (based on the equilibrium of forces and moments in the frontal plane), and was therefore taken as reference. The percentages of force distribution in the medial and lateral compartments obtained from this mathematical model are reported in Table 3.

Table 3. Percentages of the total force applied in the different configurations analyzed in the study [11].

Configuration	Medial Force	Lateral Force
30° Varus	91%	9%
20° Varus	82%	18%
10° Varus	64%	36%
5° Varus	60%	40%
Well Aligned	55%	45%
5° Valgus	43%	57%
10° Valgus	38%	62%
20° Valgus	8%	92%
30° Valgus	1%	99%

These percentages were therefore used in the present study to determine the subdivision of the total force on the medial and lateral sides, and the resulting forces were applied on the respective side of the tibial tray plateau (see Figure 1), as input loads for the FE simulations.

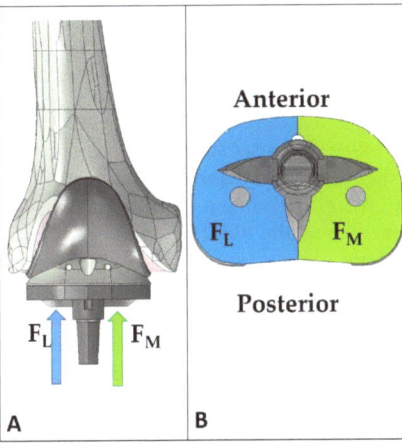

Figure 1. Load conditions applied to the model, (**A**) frontal view, reporting the direction of the forces applied; (**B**) distal view, reporting the area used for the applied force. FL = lateral force (in blue), FM = medial force (in green).

Each varus/valgus aligned configuration was statically analyzed in full extension, analyzing two femoral stem lengths (50, and 120 mm) and considering both types of fixations examined (cemented or press-fit).

For all of the configurations tested, the output for the finite element analysis was the medial and lateral tibio-femoral contact force and the relative contact area in the polyethylene insert, together with the average von Mises stress [44–48] in different regions of interest of the bone; in detail, in agreement with previous studies [20,21], the femoral shaft was subdivided in eight regions of interest, each with a height of 30 mm (Figure 2).

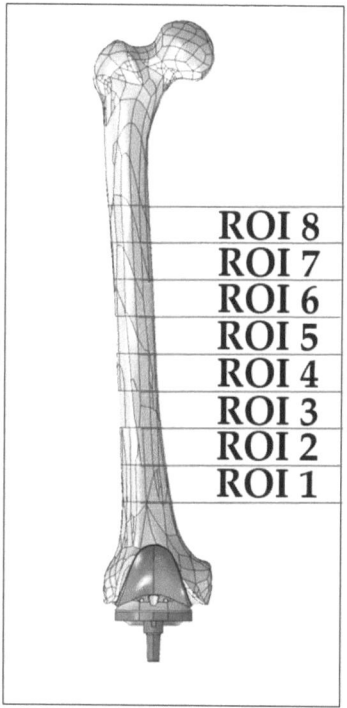

Figure 2. Regions of interest defined for the present study. All of the regions have a height of 30 mm measured along the femoral anatomical axis.

3. Results

Figure 3 concerns the cemented stem of 50 mm length, and reports the graphical overview of the average von Mises stress and contact pressure and area on the polyethylene insert for the different angles of deformity addressed.

From the figure, it is possible to note a change in the distribution of the stress and of the contact pressure on the tibial insert, that translates from lateral to medial when switching from valgus to varus configurations. Addressing the position of the contact point, the results show that the lateral contact is mainly located in the posterior section of the compartment while the medial contact point is mainly in the anterior one.

From a quantitative point of view, Tables 4 and 5 report, respectively, the values of medial and lateral contact forces and the values of the medial and lateral contact areas for the different configurations and for different stem lengths and cementing techniques.

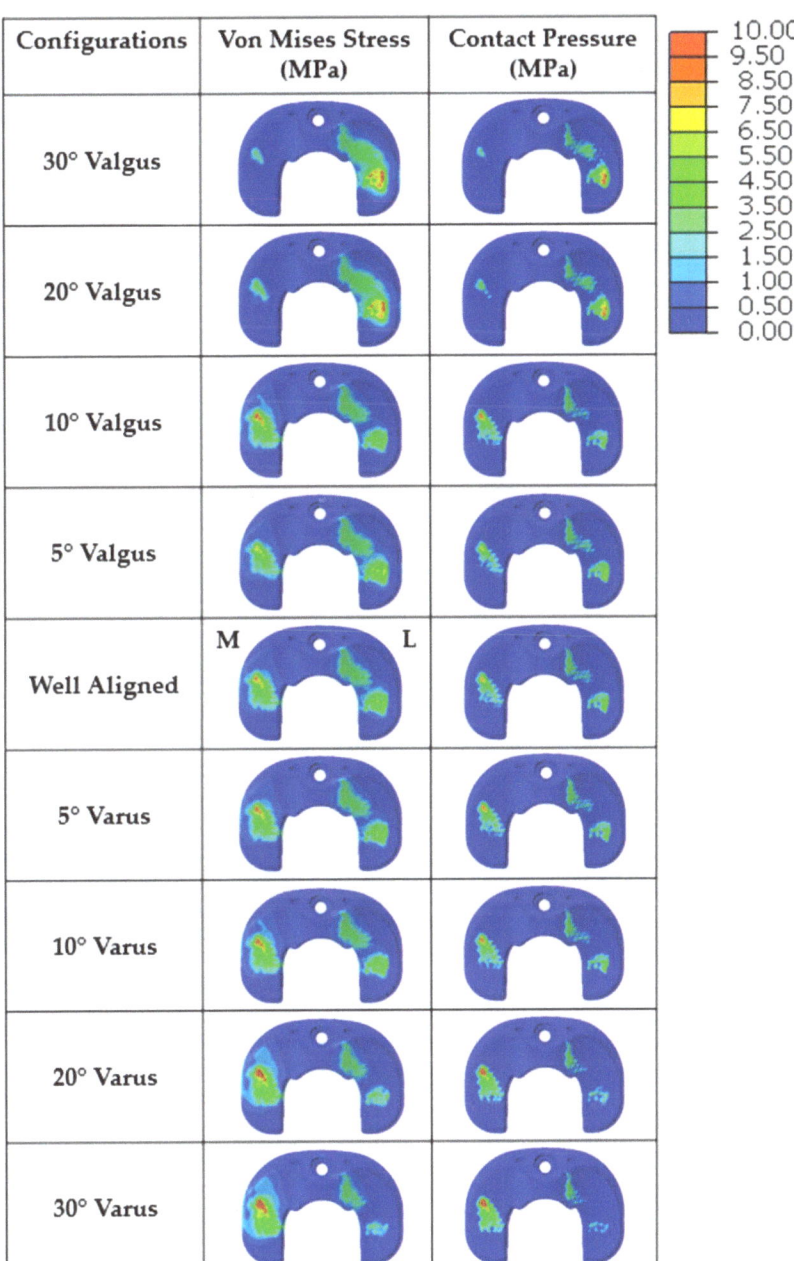

Figure 3. Qualitative overview of the von Mises stress distribution (in MPa) on the polyethylene insert and of the contact pressure (in MPa) and area on the polyethylene insert for the different varus/valgus configurations analyzed in the study, for a stem length of 50 mm cemented. M = medial, L = lateral.

Table 4. Medial and lateral contact forces for the different configurations and for different stem lengths and cementing techniques.

Configuration	Press Fit 50		Cemented 50		Press Fit 120		Cemented 120	
	Medial Force(N)	Lateral Force (N)	Medial Force(N)	Lateral Force(N)	Medial Force (N)	Lateral Force(N)	Medial Force (N)	Lateral Force (N)
30° Valgus	43	906	41	911	43	905	40	911
20° Valgus	89	860	86	867	87	858	86	864
10° Valgus	307	651	307	659	310	655	308	657
5° Valgus	350	619	347	618	348	620	345	620
Well Alligned	442	532	447	532	443	528	445	532
5° Varus	484	497	486	495	484	488	484	495
10° Varus	517	469	516	462	515	456	517	464
20° Varus	657	314	660	315	660	316	663	316
30° Varus	726	243	726	244	728	243	731	246

Table 5. Medial and lateral contact areas for the different configurations and for the different stem lengths and cementing techniques.

Configuration	Press Fit 50		Cemented 50		Press Fit 120		Cemented 120	
	Medial Area (mm^2)	Lateral Area (mm^2)	Medial Area (mm^2)	Lateral Area (mm^2)	Medial Area (mm^2)	Lateral Area (mm^2)	Medial Area (mm^2)	Lateral Area (mm^2)
30° Valgus	15	157	15	158	15	159	15	158
20° Valgus	28	156	28	156	28	155	28	156
10° Valgus	62	132	63	132	62	132	63	132
5° Valgus	71	130	71	130	71	130	70	130
Well Alligned	79	115	79	115	79	115	79	115
5° Varus	81	110	81	110	81	109	81	109
10° Varus	83	107	83	106	83	106	83	106
20° Varus	95	91	96	91	95	91	96	91
30° Varus	103	74	105	74	105	74	105	74

From these two tables, it is possible to note that the differences in terms of tibio-femoral contact relative to a change of stem lengths or fixation approach are negligible if compared to the changes induced by a different varus/valgus angle.

Figure 4 then reports, for the cemented 50 mm stem, different results relative to the medial side expressed as a percentage of their total on both sides; in detail, the different tibio-femoral contact forces and areas are represented in relation to the varus/valgus angles, together with the values of the input forces applied on the distal surface of the tibial insert (as a control for a comparative point of view).

It is possible to notice that each parameter presents a different trend, with the contact area being less sensible to changes of the varus/valgus angle (with a range of 9–58%) while the contact force is more sensible (with a range of 5–75%).

While the tibio-femoral contact forces and areas returned to be mostly insensible to variations of the stem length and fixation approach, the femoral bone showed to be influenced by these variations in terms of bone stress distributions in the different regions of interest addressed. Figure 5 reports the variations in terms of the average von Mises stress for ROI 1, 3, 5, and 7, according to the different configurations of stem length, fixation, and varus–valgus angle.

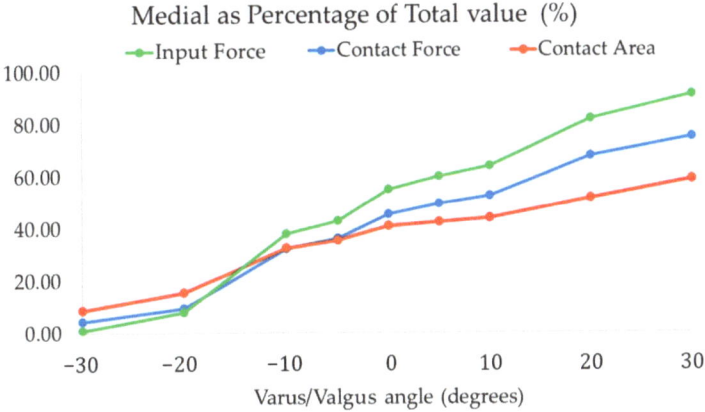

Figure 4. Input force, contact force and contact area relative to different varus/valgus angles for the cemented 50 mm stem.

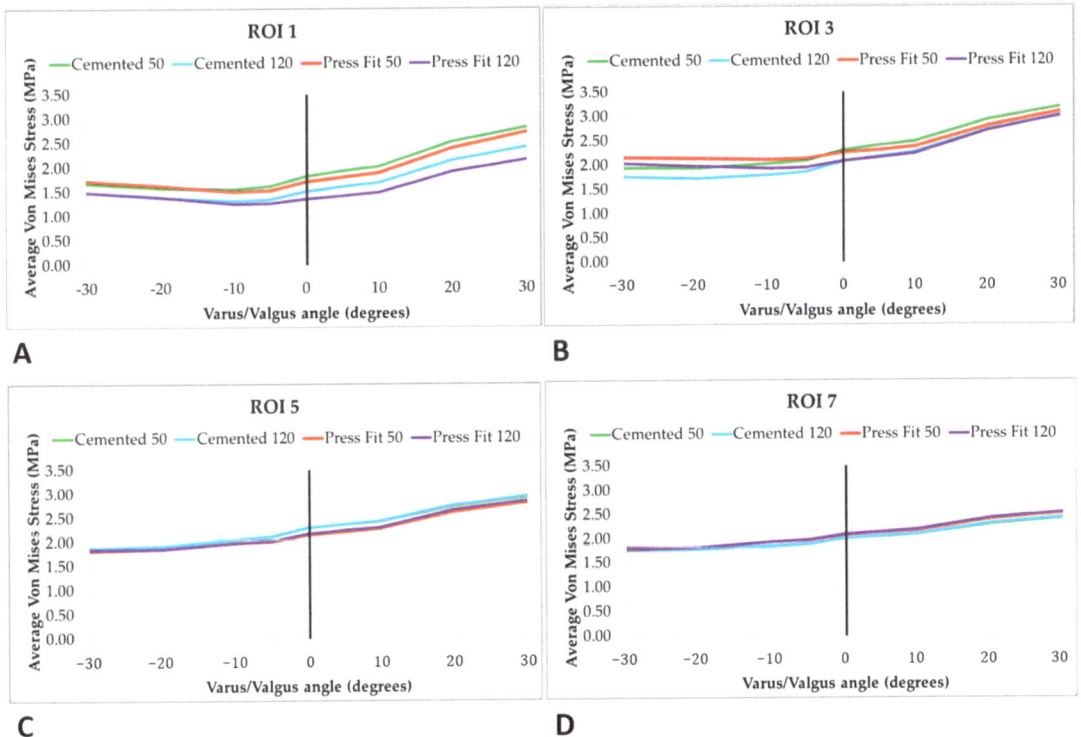

Figure 5. Average von Mises stresses in four regions of interest ((**A**): ROI 1, (**B**): ROI 3, (**C**): ROI 5, (**D**): ROI 7) for the different prosthesis features, according to the varus/valgus angles addressed.

The detailed values for the four different models are reported in Tables 6–9.

Table 6. Average von Mises stresses (in MPa) in the different ROIs for the 50 mm press-fit stem.

Configuration	Press-Fit 50—Average von Mises Stress (MPa)							
	ROI 1	ROI 2	ROI 3	ROI 4	ROI 5	ROI 6	ROI 7	ROI 8
30° Valgus	1.73	1.88	2.15	1.82	1.83	1.72	1.79	1.83
20° Valgus	1.62	1.80	2.14	1.81	1.86	1.73	1.81	1.84
10° Valgus	1.50	1.73	2.10	1.81	1.97	1.75	1.93	1.87
5° Valgus	1.52	1.77	2.12	1.85	2.01	1.78	1.96	1.87
Well Aligned	1.70	1.99	2.24	2.01	2.15	1.89	2.06	1.92
5° Varus	1.79	2.09	2.29	2.10	2.21	1.95	2.11	1.94
10° Varus	1.88	2.18	2.36	2.18	2.27	2.00	2.16	1.96
20° Varus	2.39	2.69	2.79	2.63	2.61	2.28	2.39	2.08
30° Varus	2.71	3.01	3.08	2.90	2.80	2.44	2.51	2.14

Table 7. Average von Mises stresses in the different ROIs for the 120 mm press-fit stem.

Configuration	Press-Fit 120—Average von Mises Stress (MPa)							
	ROI 1	ROI 2	ROI 3	ROI 4	ROI 5	ROI 6	ROI 7	ROI 8
30° Valgus	1.49	1.65	2.03	1.84	1.85	1.74	1.81	1.81
20° Valgus	1.39	1.57	1.97	1.82	1.86	1.72	1.81	1.81
10° Valgus	1.25	1.46	1.92	1.82	1.98	1.75	1.93	1.83
5° Valgus	1.26	1.50	1.94	1.86	2.02	1.78	1.96	1.85
Well Aligned	1.35	1.67	2.07	2.03	2.16	1.90	2.07	1.89
5° Varus	1.41	1.77	2.14	2.12	2.23	1.96	2.13	1.92
10° Varus	1.48	1.85	2.22	2.21	2.30	2.02	2.18	1.94
20° Varus	1.90	2.32	2.70	2.68	2.65	2.31	2.40	2.06
30° Varus	2.15	2.60	3.00	2.95	2.84	2.47	2.53	2.13

Table 8. Average von Mises stresses in the different ROIs for the 50 mm cemented stem.

Configuration	Cemented 50—Average von Mises Stress (MPa)							
	ROI 1	ROI 2	ROI 3	ROI 4	ROI 5	ROI 6	ROI 7	ROI 8
30° Valgus	1.67	1.73	1.94	1.65	1.87	1.76	1.75	1.67
20° Valgus	1.57	1.70	1.93	1.69	1.90	1.77	1.77	1.67
10° Valgus	1.56	1.83	2.02	1.89	2.05	1.86	1.83	1.65
5° Valgus	1.61	1.90	2.08	1.97	2.11	1.91	1.87	1.67
Well Aligned	1.81	2.14	2.29	2.21	2.29	2.06	1.99	1.72
5° Varus	1.92	2.26	2.40	2.32	2.36	2.12	2.04	1.74
10° Varus	2.02	2.36	2.48	2.40	2.42	2.17	2.08	1.76
20° Varus	2.52	2.84	2.91	2.82	2.73	2.43	2.28	1.88
30° Varus	2.81	3.13	3.18	3.06	2.92	2.58	2.40	1.95

Table 9. Average von Mises stresses in the different ROIs for the 120 mm cemented stem.

Configuration	Cemented 120—Average von Mises Stress (MPa)							
	ROI 1	ROI 2	ROI 3	ROI 4	ROI 5	ROI 6	ROI 7	ROI 8
30° Valgus	1.49	1.53	1.75	1.66	1.88	1.76	1.76	1.67
20° Valgus	1.38	1.48	1.72	1.69	1.91	1.78	1.77	1.67
10° Valgus	1.30	1.56	1.79	1.89	2.05	1.87	1.84	1.65
5° Valgus	1.34	1.62	1.85	1.97	2.11	1.91	1.88	1.67
Well Aligned	1.50	1.84	2.06	2.21	2.29	2.05	1.99	1.72
5° Varus	1.60	1.95	2.16	2.32	2.36	2.12	2.04	1.74
10° Varus	1.68	2.04	2.25	2.41	2.43	2.18	2.09	1.77
20° Varus	2.14	2.50	2.70	2.83	2.75	2.44	2.30	1.89
30° Varus	2.40	2.78	2.99	3.08	2.94	2.60	2.42	1.96

From Figure 5, it is thus possible to see that each model induces a different stress distribution, especially in the distal femoral region (ROI 1), and that the differences are instead lower in the proximal regions (ROI 7). Moreover, it is also possible to see that, for each configuration analyzed, the change in average von Mises stress is mostly insensible to changes of the valgus angle (with a variation curve almost horizontal) while it is moderately sensible to changes in terms of the varus angle.

Analyzing the proximal regions in detail, it is possible to see that in ROI 1 the short stem is characterized by a higher average stress (almost the same for cemented and press-fit fixation) while the press-fit long stem is characterized by lower stresses, especially in the varus conditions: this outcome is reasonably due to the stress shielding effect related to the longer stems, which consequently leads to slightly higher stresses in the regions close to the stem tip.

4. Discussion

In this study, a series of finite element simulations was performed in order to evaluate the effects on the insert and bones of different configurations of RH TKA prosthesis, in terms of valgus and varus deformities, lengths of femoral stems, and fixation approaches.

The results found returned that, overall, the tibio-femoral contact forces and areas are not considerably influenced by variations of stem length and fixation approach while varus/valgus variations lead to relative changes (varying according to the parameter analyzed and to the gravity of the deformity). Moreover, the femoral bone stress distribution was determined to be influenced by the variations in the prosthesis design and fixation, with further differences found in relation to the region of interest considered.

Addressing more in depth, the outcomes of the tibio-femoral interface, the reason behind the lower sensibility of the contact area to varus/valgus angles and the overall insensibility to the variations in stem length and fixation approach is indeed to be found in the design of the RH TKA itself. In detail the central constraint, which allows internal-external rotations and superior-inferior translations, does not enable any other degree of freedom and thus contributes to maintain the tibio-femoral interactions to be more constant. For this reason, indeed, changes in the contact area are remarkably low in varus deformities ranging from 0° to 30° (less than 20% variation in terms of contact area, while slightly higher values are found in terms of force), even if the difference in the input forces is greater than 35%. These outcomes are then in agreement with several clinical studies focused on endo-model hinged TKAs, which reported its stability and absence of cases of wear due to overloading of the polyethylene [13,15,49]. Moreover, a recently published study [50] on the use of the rotating hinge and followed over 10-years concluded that using a specific RH TKA design with less rotational constraint has better clinical and survival outcomes than implants with greater rotational constraint (such as one specific CCK addressed in the study) in case of varus and valgus deformities.

Addressing then the outcomes in terms of femoral bone stress, the results highlighted how these values are influenced more by the stem length and fixation rather than the values of varus and valgus deformities; these results are indeed in agreement with that found in the literature concerning the effects of stem design [20,21] and moreover demonstrate the ability of this prosthesis to maintain similar outcomes in terms of bone-prosthesis interactions, despite the different levels of deformity of the patient joint.

It is however to be mentioned that this study presents a series of limitations. Firstly, only one implant model was considered, with a single size and typology being analyzed; a single angle of flection was then simulated for all of the configurations. These two restrictions may indeed represent a limitation for the generalization of the results, but it is to be highlighted that these choices allowed to perform a comparative study focused on the specific parameters taken into consideration, thus obtaining meaningful information that can therefore represent an interesting insight for the surgeons during the decision-making process. Addressing the finite element models, it is to be mentioned that the material models used to simulate the bones in this study implied a series of assumptions: indeed, no bone activity was considered in the simulations and therefore the variations in femoral mechanic characteristic, usually occurring in response to the different loading conditions the joint undergoes [51–54], are not taken into account. Despite these latter limitations, however, these models were developed based on previously published and validated ones [21] and therefore the results they provided can be considered reliable, as they are furthermore in agreement with the literature [2,20,21].

Concerning the validation of the model, it is to be mentioned that no direct validation was performed for this study; however, it is to be considered that the model used was implemented starting from validated models that can be found in previously published studies [21,25–27], and therefore can be considered as reliable in its results.

5. Conclusions

This study provided interesting information on the influence of varus/valgus deformities of different levels of severity on the performances of different configurations of rotating hinged TKA, showing how the prosthesis design features mainly alter the bone stress distribution while varus/valgus deformities are the main responsible factors for variations in tibio-femoral contact forces and areas.

This result represents an interesting information for the surgeons: for implants characterized by high level of constraint, indeed, alterations in the bending and torsional stiffness and moments might occur if the stem length and fixation are modified, and they would therefore be transferred to the tibio-femoral interface of the implant; this eventuality may thus condition the surgeon's choice, which may aim for a compromise in order to avoid any tibio-femoral issues deriving from these alterations. The results of this study showed instead that, in the case of the rotating hinge analyzed, no remarkable mechanical consequences on the tibio-femoral interface are found despite variations in stem and fixation configuration; the surgeon can therefore focus their decisions on optimizing the bone-implant interface, without the need for finding a compromise in the fear of altering excessively the tibio-femoral biomechanics.

Supplementary Materials: The following supporting information can be downloaded at: https://www.mdpi.com/article/10.3390/app13042738/s1, Convergence Test.

Author Contributions: Conceptualization, E.B. and B.I.; methodology, B.I.; software, B.I.; formal analysis, E.B. and B.I.; investigation, E.B. and B.I.; data curation, B.I.; writing—original draft preparation, E.B. and B.I.; writing—review and editing, E.B.; visualization, B.I.; supervision, B.I.; project administration, B.I. All authors have read and agreed to the published version of the manuscript.

Funding: This research received no external funding.

Institutional Review Board Statement: Not applicable.

Informed Consent Statement: Not applicable.

Data Availability Statement: Not applicable.

Conflicts of Interest: The authors declare no conflict of interest.

References

1. Ritter, M.A.; Davis, K.E.; Meding, J.B.; Pierson, J.L.; Berend, M.E.; Malinzak, R.A. The Effect of Alignment and BMI on Failure of Total Knee Replacement. *J. Bone Jt. Surg.* **2011**, *93*, 1588–1596. [CrossRef] [PubMed]
2. Innocenti, B.; Bellemans, J.; Catani, F. Deviations from Optimal Alignment in TKA: Is There a Biomechanical Difference Between Femoral or Tibial Component Alignment? *J. Arthroplast.* **2016**, *31*, 295–301. [CrossRef] [PubMed]
3. Innocenti, B. Knee Prosthesis: Biomechanics and Design. In *Human Orthopaedic Biomechanics*; Elsevier: Amsterdam, The Netherlands, 2022; pp. 377–407.
4. Sharma, L.; Song, J.; Dunlop, D.; Felson, D.; Lewis, C.E.; Segal, N.; Torner, J.; Cooke, T.D.V.; Hietpas, J.; Lynch, J.; et al. Varus and Valgus Alignment and Incident and Progressive Knee Osteoarthritis. *Ann. Rheum. Dis.* **2010**, *69*, 1940–1945. [CrossRef] [PubMed]
5. Becker, R.; Tandogan, R.; Violante, B. Alignment in Total Knee Arthroplasty. *Knee Surg. Sport. Traumatol. Arthrosc.* **2016**, *24*, 2393–2394. [CrossRef]
6. Castellarin, G.; Bori, E.; Rapallo, L.; Pianigiani, S.; Innocenti, B. Biomechanical Analysis of Different Levels of Constraint in TKA during Daily Activities. *Arthroplasty* **2023**, *5*, 3. [CrossRef]

7. Guenoun, B.; Latargez, L.; Freslon, M.; Defossez, G.; Salas, N.; Gayet, L.-E. Complications Following Rotating Hinge Endo-Modell (Link®) Knee Arthroplasty. *Orthop. Traumatol. Surg. Res.* **2009**, *95*, 529–536. [CrossRef]
8. Andreani, L.; Pianigiani, S.; Bori, E.; Lisanti, M.; Innocenti, B. Analysis of Biomechanical Differences Between Condylar Constrained Knee and Rotating Hinged Implants: A Numerical Study. *J. Arthroplast.* **2020**, *35*, 278–284. [CrossRef]
9. Sanguineti, F.; Mangano, T.; Formica, M.; Franchin, F. Total Knee Arthroplasty with Rotating-Hinge Endo-Model Prosthesis: Clinical Results in Complex Primary and Revision Surgery. *Arch. Orthop. Trauma Surg.* **2014**, *134*, 1601–1607. [CrossRef]
10. Zhao, D.; Banks, S.A.; D'Lima, D.D.; Colwell, C.W.; Fregly, B.J. In Vivo Medial and Lateral Tibial Loads during Dynamic and High Flexion Activities. *J. Orthop. Res.* **2007**, *25*, 593–602. [CrossRef]
11. Halder, A.; Kutzner, I.; Graichen, F.; Heinlein, B.; Beier, A.; Bergmann, G. Influence of Limb Alignment on Mediolateral Loading in Total Knee Replacement. *J. Bone Jt. Surg.* **2012**, *94*, 1023–1029. [CrossRef]
12. Dauwe, J.; Vandenneucker, H. Indications for Primary Rotating-Hinge Total Knee Arthroplasty. Is There Consensus? *Acta Orthop. Belg.* **2018**, *84*, 245–250.
13. Gehrke, T.; Mommsen, P. 55 Hinged Implants for Revision Total Knee Replacement. In *The Unhappy Total Knee Replacement*; Springer International Publishing: Cham, Switzerland, 2015; pp. 663–669.
14. Hernández-Vaquero, D.; Sandoval-García, M.A. Hinged Total Knee Arthroplasty in the Presence of Ligamentous Deficiency. *Clin. Orthop. Relat. Res.* **2010**, *468*, 1248–1253. [CrossRef] [PubMed]
15. Mavrodontidis, A.N.; Andrikoula, S.I.; Kontogeorgakos, V.A.; Babis, G.C.; Xenakis, T.A.; Beris, A.E.; Soucacos, P.N. Application of the Endomodel Rotating Hinge Knee Prosthesis for Knee Osteoarthritis. *J. Surg. Orthop. Adv.* **2008**, *17*, 179–184. [PubMed]
16. Rong, Q.; Bai, J.; Huang, Y.; Lin, J. Biomechanical Assessment of a Patient-Specific Knee Implant Design Using Finite Element Method. *Biomed Res. Int.* **2014**, *2014*, 353690. [CrossRef]
17. Manning, D.W.; Chiang, P.P.; Freiberg, A.A. Hinge Implants. In *Revision Total Knee Arthroplasty*; Springer-Verlag: New York, NY, USA; pp. 219–236.
18. Patel, A.R.; Barlow, B.; Ranawat, A.S. Stem Length in Revision Total Knee Arthroplasty. *Curr. Rev. Musculoskelet. Med.* **2015**, *8*, 407–412. [CrossRef]
19. Conlisk, N.; Gray, H.; Pankaj, P.; Howie, C.R. The Influence of Stem Length and Fixation on Initial Femoral Component Stability in Revision Total Knee Replacement. *Bone Jt. Res.* **2012**, *1*, 281–288. [CrossRef]
20. Innocenti, B.; Bori, E.; Pianigiani, S. Biomechanical Analysis of the Use of Stems in Revision Total Knee Arthroplasty. *Bioengineering* **2022**, *9*, 259. [CrossRef]
21. Bori, E.; Armaroli, F.; Innocenti, B. Biomechanical Analysis of Femoral Stems in Hinged Total Knee Arthroplasty in Physiological and Osteoporotic Bone. *Comput. Methods Programs Biomed.* **2022**, *213*, 106499. [CrossRef]
22. Bourbotte-Salmon, F.; Ferry, T.; Cardinale, M.; Servien, E.; Rongieras, F.; Fessy, M.-H.; Bertani, A.; Laurent, F.; Buffe-Lidove, M.; Batailler, C.; et al. Rotating Hinge Knee Arthroplasty for Revision Prosthetic-Knee Infection: Good Functional Outcomes but a Crucial Need for Superinfection Prevention. *Front. Surg.* **2021**, *8*, 388. [CrossRef]
23. Utting, M.R.; Newman, J.H. Customised Hinged Knee Replacements as a Salvage Procedure for Failed Total Knee Arthroplasty. *Knee* **2004**, *11*, 475–479. [CrossRef] [PubMed]
24. Rodríguez-Merchán, E.C. Total Knee Arthroplasty Using Hinge Joints: Indications and Results. *EFORT Open Rev.* **2019**, *4*, 121–132. [CrossRef] [PubMed]
25. Innocenti, B.; Bilgen, Ö.F.; Labey, L.; van Lenthe, G.H.; Vander Sloten, J.; Catani, F. Load Sharing and Ligament Strains in Balanced, Overstuffed and Understuffed UKA. A Validated Finite Element Analysis. *J. Arthroplast.* **2014**, *29*, 1491–1498. [CrossRef]
26. van Jonbergen, H.-P.W.; Innocenti, B.; Gervasi, G.; Labey, L.; Verdonschot, N. Differences in the Stress Distribution in the Distal Femur between Patellofemoral Joint Replacement and Total Knee Replacement: A Finite Element Study. *J. Orthop. Surg. Res.* **2012**, *7*, 28. [CrossRef]
27. Catani, F.; Innocenti, B.; Belvedere, C.; Labey, L.; Ensini, A.; Leardini, A. The Mark Coventry Award Articular: Contact Estimation in TKA Using In Vivo Kinematics and Finite Element Analysis. *Clin. Orthop. Relat. Res.* **2010**, *468*, 19–28. [CrossRef] [PubMed]
28. Heller, M.O. Finite Element Analysis in Orthopedic Biomechanics. In *Human Orthopaedic Biomechanics*; Elsevier: Amsterdam, The Netherlands, 2022; pp. 637–658.
29. Innocenti, B.; Bori, E.; Armaroli, F.; Schlager, B.; Jonas, R.; Wilke, H.-J.; Galbusera, F. The Use of Computational Models in Orthopedic Biomechanical Research. In *Human Orthopaedic Biomechanics*; Elsevier: Amsterdam, The Netherlands, 2022; pp. 681–712.
30. Pianigiani, S.; Innocenti, B. *The Use of Finite Element Modeling to Improve Biomechanical Research on Knee Prosthesis*; Nova Science Publishers: Hauppauge, NY, USA, 2015.
31. Brihault, J.; Navacchia, A.; Pianigiani, S.; Labey, L.; De Corte, R.; Pascale, V.; Innocenti, B. All-Polyethylene Tibial Components Generate Higher Stress and Micromotions than Metal-Backed Tibial Components in Total Knee Arthroplasty. *Knee Surg. Sport. Traumatol. Arthrosc.* **2016**, *24*, 2550–2559. [CrossRef] [PubMed]
32. El-Zayat, B.F.; Heyse, T.J.; Fanciullacci, N.; Labey, L.; Fuchs-Winkelmann, S.; Innocenti, B. Fixation Techniques and Stem Dimensions in Hinged Total Knee Arthroplasty: A Finite Element Study. *Arch. Orthop. Trauma Surg.* **2016**, *136*, 1741–1752. [CrossRef] [PubMed]
33. Soenen, M.; Baracchi, M.; De Corte, R.; Labey, L.; Innocenti, B. Stemmed TKA in a Femur With a Total Hip Arthroplasty. *J. Arthroplast.* **2013**, *28*, 1437–1445. [CrossRef]

34. Viceconti, M.; Casali, M.; Massari, B.; Cristofolini, L.; Bassini, S.; Toni, A. The "Standardized Femur Program" Proposal for a Reference Geometry to Be Used for the Creation of Finite Element Models of the Femur. *J. Biomech.* **1996**, *29*, 1241. [CrossRef]
35. van Eijnatten, M.; van Dijk, R.; Dobbe, J.; Streekstra, G.; Koivisto, J.; Wolff, J. CT Image Segmentation Methods for Bone Used in Medical Additive Manufacturing. *Med. Eng. Phys.* **2018**, *51*, 6–16. [CrossRef]
36. McNamara, B.P.; Cristofolini, L.; Toni, A.; Taylor, D. Relationship between Bone-Prosthesis Bonding and Load Transfer in Total Hip Reconstruction. *J. Biomech.* **1997**, *30*, 621–630. [CrossRef]
37. Innocenti, B.; Pianigiani, S.; Ramundo, G.; Thienpont, E. Biomechanical Effects of Different Varus and Valgus Alignments in Medial Unicompartmental Knee Arthroplasty. *J. Arthroplast.* **2016**, *31*, 2685–2691. [CrossRef] [PubMed]
38. Kayabasi, O.; Ekici, B. The Effects of Static, Dynamic and Fatigue Behavior on Three-Dimensional Shape Optimization of Hip Prosthesis by Finite Element Method. *Mater. Des.* **2007**, *28*, 2269–2277. [CrossRef]
39. Sarathi Kopparti, P.; Lewis, G. Influence of Three Variables on the Stresses in a Three-Dimensional Model of a Proximal Tibia-Total Knee Implant Construct. *Biomed. Mater. Eng.* **2007**, *17*, 19–28. [PubMed]
40. Ingrassia, T.; Nalbone, L.; Nigrelli, V.; Tumino, D.; Ricotta, V. Finite Element Analysis of Two Total Knee Joint Prostheses. *Int. J. Interact. Des. Manuf.* **2013**, *7*, 91–101. [CrossRef]
41. Heiner, A.D. Structural Properties of Fourth-Generation Composite Femurs and Tibias. *J. Biomech.* **2008**, *41*, 3282–3284. [CrossRef] [PubMed]
42. Rho, J.-Y.; Kuhn-Spearing, L.; Zioupos, P. Mechanical Properties and the Hierarchical Structure of Bone. *Med. Eng. Phys.* **1998**, *20*, 92–102. [CrossRef]
43. Castellarin, G.; Pianigiani, S.; Innocenti, B. Asymmetric Polyethylene Inserts Promote Favorable Kinematics and Better Clinical Outcome Compared to Symmetric Inserts in a Mobile Bearing Total Knee Arthroplasty. *Knee Surg. Sport. Traumatol. Arthrosc.* **2019**, *27*, 1096–1105. [CrossRef]
44. Quilez, M.P.; Seral, B.; Pérez, M.A. Biomechanical Evaluation of Tibial Bone Adaptation after Revision Total Knee Arthroplasty: A Comparison of Different Implant Systems. *PLoS ONE* **2017**, *12*, e0184361. [CrossRef]
45. Jang, Y.W.; Kwon, S.-Y.; Kim, J.S.; Yoo, O.S.; Lee, M.C.; Lim, D. Alterations in Stress Distribution and Micromotion Characteristics Due to an Artificial Defect within a Composite Tibia Used for Mechanical/Biomechanical Evaluation of Total Knee Arthroplasty. *Int. J. Precis. Eng. Manuf.* **2015**, *16*, 2213–2218. [CrossRef]
46. Apostolopoulos, V.; Tomáš, T.; Boháč, P.; Marcián, P.; Mahdal, M.; Valoušek, T.; Janíček, P.; Nachtnebl, L. Biomechanical Analysis of All-Polyethylene Total Knee Arthroplasty on Periprosthetic Tibia Using the Finite Element Method. *Comput. Methods Programs Biomed.* **2022**, *220*, 106834. [CrossRef]
47. Kang, K.; Jang, Y.W.; Yoo, O.S.; Jung, D.; Lee, S.-J.; Lee, M.C.; Lim, D. Biomechanical Characteristics of Three Baseplate Rotational Arrangement Techniques in Total Knee Arthroplasty. *Biomed Res. Int.* **2018**, *2018*, 9641417. [CrossRef]
48. Du, M.; Sun, J.; Liu, Y.; Wang, Y.; Yan, S.; Zeng, J.; Zhang, K. Tibio-Femoral Contact Force Distribution of Knee Before and After Total Knee Arthroplasty: Combined Finite Element and Gait Analysis. *Orthop. Surg.* **2022**, *14*, 1836–1845. [CrossRef] [PubMed]
49. Pradhan, N.R.; Bale, L.; Kay, P.; Porter, M.L. Salvage Revision Total Knee Replacement Using the Endo-Model® Rotating Hinge Prosthesis. *Knee* **2004**, *11*, 469–473. [CrossRef] [PubMed]
50. Sanz-Ruiz, P.; León-Román, V.E.; Matas-Diez, J.A.; Villanueva-Martínez, M.; Vaquero, J. Long-Term Outcomes of One Single-Design Varus Valgus Constrained versus One Single-Design Rotating Hinge in Revision Knee Arthroplasty after over 10-Year Follow-Up. *J. Orthop. Surg. Res.* **2022**, *17*, 135. [CrossRef] [PubMed]
51. Zhang, L.; Liu, H.; Chen, T.; Yuan, F. Initial Damage Analysis in Bone Cement-Stem Debonding Procession of Cemented Hip Arthropsty. *Mater. Des.* **2023**, *225*, 111486. [CrossRef]
52. Buccino, F.; Colombo, C.; Vergani, L.M. A Review on Multiscale Bone Damage: From the Clinical to the Research Perspective. *Materials* **2021**, *14*, 1240. [CrossRef]
53. Doblaré, M.; Garcıa, J.M. Application of an Anisotropic Bone-Remodelling Model Based on a Damage-Repair Theory to the Analysis of the Proximal Femur before and after Total Hip Replacement. *J. Biomech.* **2001**, *34*, 1157–1170. [CrossRef]
54. Buccino, F.; Zagra, L.; Savadori, P.; Colombo, C.; Grossi, G.; Banfi, G.; Vergani, L. Mapping Local Mechanical Properties of Human Healthy and Osteoporotic Femoral Heads. *SSRN Electron. J.* **2021**, *20*, 101229. [CrossRef]

Disclaimer/Publisher's Note: The statements, opinions and data contained in all publications are solely those of the individual author(s) and contributor(s) and not of MDPI and/or the editor(s). MDPI and/or the editor(s) disclaim responsibility for any injury to people or property resulting from any ideas, methods, instructions or products referred to in the content.

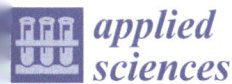

Article

A Pelvic Reconstruction Procedure for Custom-Made Prosthesis Design of Bone Tumor Surgical Treatments

Gilda Durastanti [1], Claudio Belvedere [1], Miriana Ruggeri [1,*], Davide Maria Donati [2], Benedetta Spazzoli [2] and Alberto Leardini [1]

[1] Movement Analysis Laboratory, IRCCS Istituto Ortopedico Rizzoli, 40136 Bologna, Italy; gilda.durastanti@gmail.com (G.D.); belvedere@ior.it (C.B.); leardini@ior.it (A.L.)
[2] III Clinical Department, IRCCS Istituto Ortopedico Rizzoli, 40136 Bologna, Italy; davidemaria.donati@ior.it (D.M.D.); benedetta.spazzoli@ior.it (B.S.)
* Correspondence: miriana.ruggeri@ior.it; Tel.: +39-051-636-6570; Fax: +39-051-636-6561

Abstract: In orthopaedic oncology, limb salvage procedures are becoming more frequent thanks to recent major improvements in medical imaging, biomechanical modelling and additive manufacturing. For the pelvis, surgical reconstruction with metal implants after tumor resection remains challenging, because of the complex anatomical structures involved. The aim of the present work is to define a consistent overall procedure to guide surgeons and bioengineers for proper implant design. All relevant steps from medical imaging to an accurate 3D anatomical-based model are here reported. In detail, the anatomical 3D models include bone shapes from CT on the entire pelvic bone, i.e., including both affected and unaffected sides, and position and extension of the tumor and soft tissues from MRI on the affected side. These models are then registered in space, and an initial shape of the personalized implant for the affected side can be properly designed and dimensioned based on the information from the unaffected side. This reported procedure can be fundamental also for virtual pre-surgical planning, and the design of patient-specific cutting guides, which would result is a safe margin for tumor cut. The entire procedure is here shown by describing the results in a single real case.

Keywords: multimodal medical imaging; DICOM segmentation; anatomical modelling; model registration; distance mapping; pelvic reconstruction; personalised implant design; surgical planning; orthopaedic oncology

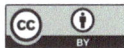

1. Introduction

In orthopaedic oncology, limb salvage procedures for the pelvis requires tumor resection by an appropriate excision followed by careful corresponding reconstruction of the affected bone and soft tissues [1]. Pelvic resections and reconstructions are classified by tumor extension and the section of bone to be resected, i.e., iliac or periacetabular or pubic location [2]. In particular, according to the Enneking and Dunham classification [2], type I involves the iliac region, type II the periacetabular region, type III the pubis or ischium, and type IV the lateral part of the sacrum. Most of these reconstructions involve the acetabulum, which implies the replacement of the hip joint [3,4]. For all pelvic resection and reconstruction procedures, the primary goals are the restoration of the physiologic joint motion and the maintenance of good quality of life [4]. To date, surgical reconstruction after tumor resection in the pelvis remains a challenge, because of the critical and complex anatomical structures involved. A major critical aspect is the bone cut, which must be performed to achieve an adequate margin around the tumor, but also to preserve as much skeletal structure and joint function as possible, including adequate bone stock and soft tissues such as ligaments and tendons [1,5–7].

Important advancements in pelvic reconstruction using biological reconstruction such as structural pelvic allografts or autografts, arthrodesis and endoprostheses have been shown [8], though a high rate of complications, including infection, dislocation and mechanical failure, have been reported [5,9–12]. More recently, there has been a strong interest in custom-made prostheses, particularly after the great developments of additive manufacturing, also known as 3D-printing. A custom-made prosthesis is a fully personalized implant, which is aimed at achieving a more anatomical reconstruction, i.e., more respectful of the original anatomy, and a better match with patient's residual bone, and thus a smaller risk of loosening, infection, fractures, and any possible mechanical failure. It also allows a precise pre-operative planning of the surgical procedure, this including the positioning of the prosthesis, and the setting of corresponding bone cuts. The potential better long-term clinical and functional results are supported by the good short-term results [3,5,7,13–24]. 3D printed implants have attracted much attention nowadays also because of faster production and lower costs, together with the accurate optimization and control of the overall geometry, both in terms of the external roughness and internal topology [25].

Surgical reconstructions at the pelvis using custom-made implants are showing encouraging results, both at the acetabulum, ileum, and sacrum sections, with low complication rates, although wound healing problems have been reported [17,26]. On the other hand, any custom-made implant requires careful medical imaging and time-consuming modelling and design [6]. Nevertheless, this digital process allows a precise identification of the tumor and, thus, a careful computer-based pre-surgical planning of the bone resection [5,24,27], though this virtual surgery depends on the quality of medical imaging and the software tools utilized and the experience and ability of the surgical team. As mentioned, computer-based design and 3D printing of these implants have the potential to result in advanced porous metal implants, with different geometries of the internal and external structures, and with no limits to their complexity. It is also possible to use a number of different materials, with mechanical properties similar to those of the natural anatomical structures [25,28,29]. This further technical advancement has been assessed already also in custom-made implants for complex pelvic reconstructions [13,17,30,31]. The final surgical result of these reconstructions, also in term of an accurate prosthesis-to-bone contact, largely relies also on how bone resections are performed, and thus on the design and manufacturing of the so-called patient-specific cutting guides [1,15,30,32–35].

The anatomical design of these implants based on digital bone models should imply the knowledge of the shape of both the affected and unaffected hemipelvis; the former must provide an accurate location and extension of the tumor, the latter should be considered a best possible target for the final reconstruction [15,27,36,37]. The exact definition of the tumor, together with the skeletal and soft tissue structures, requires complete computer-based anatomical models, to be obtained via multimodal medical image scans using computed tomography (CT) and magnetic resonance imaging (MRI), and accurate 3D reconstructions. These final 3D models, observed separately and also registered superimposed on one another in 3D space, allow visualization, identification and localization of all important anatomical structures, necessary for a careful pre-surgical planning and implant design [3,38,39]. For these procedures, and for the following virtual surgery planning, a close collaboration between surgeons, radiologists, bioengineers, and technicians is necessary. Despite these techniques must have been exploited massively for modern custom-made implants, only a few papers have reported in detail the procedures implied in this modelling part of the personalisation [15,27,30].

The aim of the present work is to report on an original procedure in orthopaedic oncology for the 3D design of custom-made implants for the pelvis. In particular, the procedure is here shown for a single clinical case and follows the full process from medical imaging to final 3D computer-based models of the tumor resection and bone reconstruction. All these steps are based on personalised models of the pelvis of the patient, including the bones and the tumor, as derived from of CT and MRI images using state-of-the-art semi-automatic segmentation tools. The steps of this procedure are also defined under careful indication of the surgical team, including of course the critical decision on the osteotomies for tumor resection. This technical procedure includes for the first-time spatial registrations and also mirroring of the unaffected hemipelvis to the affected one, as a reliable subject-specific homologous reference for a possible most accurate definition of these cutting planes. In every step, the main accuracy parameters are tracked.

2. Methods

The technical steps here reported refer to a female patient, a 54 year-old woman (height: 168 cm; weight: 70 Kg; body mass index: 24.8 kg/m^2) affected by a malignant bone tumor in the left pelvic bone, in particular a condrosarcome grade II. According to the Enneking and Dunham classification [2], this patient had a type I + II + III partial lesion, due to the extension of the tumor on the iliac region, in the acetabulum and, partially, also in the pubic and ischiatic area. The patient had not received chemotherapy at the time of medical imaging data collection.

2.1. Image Processing: Image Segmentation and Geometrical Modelling

The patient underwent pre-operative computed tomography (CT) of the pelvis, sacrum and proximal femur, and magnetic resonance imaging (MRI) of the pelvis regions involved in the tumor lesion. The acquired images were exported in Digital Imaging and Communications in Medicine (DICOM) files and imported into an image visualization and processing software, Amira (Zuse Institute Berlin ZIB, Dahlem, Berlin, Germany—Thermo Fisher Scientific, Waltham, MA, USA). A semi-automatic segmentation was performed (Figure 1A) [40], for anatomical structure reconstructions. For every slice of the scan, the external surface of the bones and the tumor were identified and depicted, to obtain their 3D models (Figure 1B) by merging these 2D segmented silhouettes.

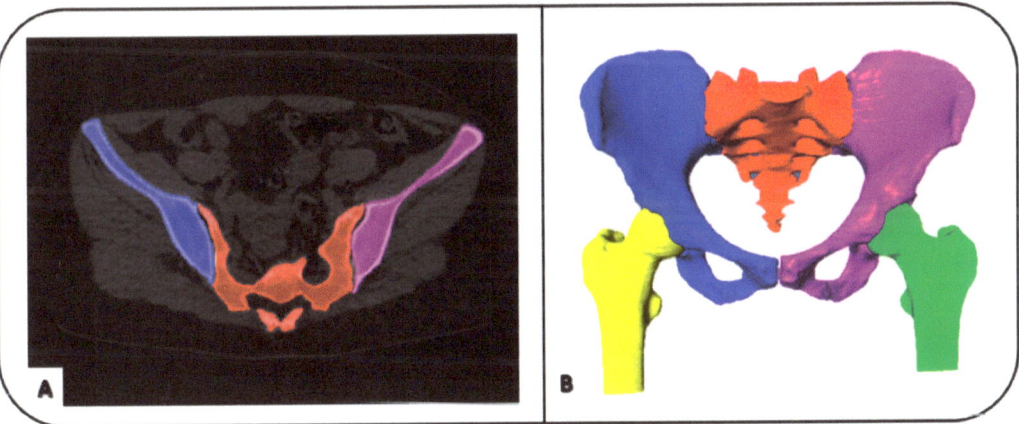

Figure 1. The process of geometrical modeling of the bone shape: image segmentation in the 2D images (**A**) and the final 3D model (**B**) via Amira software.

Several tools of the Amira software package were used to obtain accurate patient-specific models of the above reported anatomical structures. In more details, among these tools, thresholding was preferred, according to the Hounsfield Unit (HU) values for the bones and the tumor, which was set slice by slice, also depending on the quality of the corresponding CT or MRI medical image. The 3D model of the bones was generated from segmentation of the former (Figure 2A), the 3D model of the bones and tumor was generated from segmentation of the latter (Figure 2B). The full segmentation and modelling process was performed by a single expert operator. These two 3D models were exported in binary stereolithography format (STL), and then imported into a reverse engineering software, Geomagic Control (2014.3.0.1781, 3D Systems, Rock Hill, SC, USA).

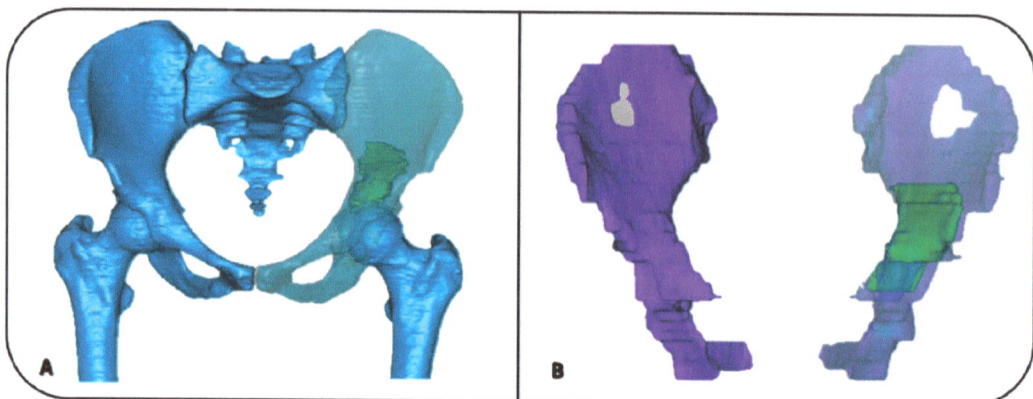

Figure 2. (**A**) 3D bone models (blue) obtained by segmentation from CT images, including pelvis, sacrum and femur bones. (**B**) 3D model of the pelvis (purple) obtained by segmentation from MRI images. In both the 3D models of the tumor on the left hemipelvis is depicted in green.

2.2. Registrations of 3D Models

To obtain a complete model of the pelvis suitable for the planning of the bone cuts and the design of the implant device, which must include shapes of both bones and tumor, registrations between CT-based and MRI-based models were performed in Geomagic as well as the following steps. These registrations in general were executed via best-fit spatial alignments based on 3D models of rigid objects achieved by the established iterative closest point (ICP) algorithm [41]. This best-fit registration of two objects, i.e., the so-called "reference" and the "test", consists of an optimal spatial matching to minimize an overall distance error between their surfaces. This results in a transformation matrix, together with the estimation of the mean and root mean square (RMS) errors of the transformation.

Two major such registration procedures were performed, both bone-to-bone. A first registration was between the CT-based and the MRI-based models, as the goal is to take the 3D shape of the tumor on the bone model of the affected hemipelvis (Figure 3). Because the bone is poorly represented in MRI-based models, the final result is to superimpose exactly the tumor, which better identified in MRI, with the best representation of the bone, which is best obtained from CT. In other words, the portion of bone from MRI is registered to the corresponding from CT; the same transformation is then applied to the tumor to get the final bone plus tumor model.

A second registration then is between the affected and the unaffected hemipelvis. To get a first anatomical shape to the metal implant meant to replace the resected bone stock, the unaffected hemipelvis is mirrored and registered to the affected hemipelvis. A mirroring plane is defined at the pubic symphysis (Figure 4A), and the unaffected is mirrored by spatial registration. This can be performed by considering the whole hemipelvis, as well as any part of it; several such trials can be performed, and the transformation with the lowest registration error can be selected (Figure 4A). Eventually a model with the two hemipelvis superimposed and the tumor in the correct position is obtained (Figure 4B). In this model, the same 3D planes representing bone cuts at the affected hemipelvis are used also to cut the unaffected hemipelvis, and thus to separate a most accurate possible shape of the implant for the replacement.

2.3. Design of Bone Resection Planes

The cutting planes were defined on this 3D anatomical model under strict indications by the surgical team members. They very carefully identify the tumor also by looking at relevant original MRI images, and then plan its excision by setting the relevant bone resection cuts. Locations and orientations of these resection planes in the computer model were decided by identifying the exact position and extension of the tumor and by considering a sufficient safety margin, here taken initially at about 20 mm, which takes into account also the resolution of MRI and CT scans. Additional more surgical and clinical criteria are also considered for a final compromise for this value, such as the smallest possible bone stock to be removed, a best preservation of the critical soft tissues, and a best large contact between the host bone and the implant, for its optimal final integration. In case of resection of the iliac bone (type I + II), it is preferred to define a so-called "roof" cut, with an angle of about $100° \approx 110°$ with respect to the anatomical frontal plane of the pelvis, for a best fit of the prosthesis on the host bone, as well as for a secure support to the vertical forces exchanged over the hip.

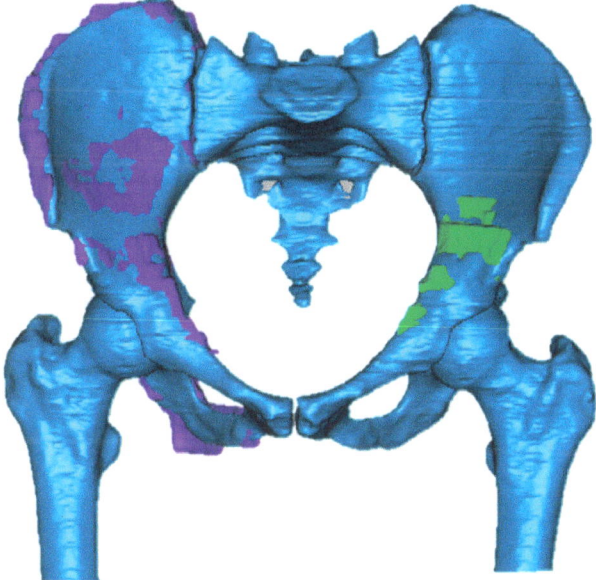

Figure 3. The 3D result after a best-fit registration of the MRI-based models to CT-based models; again, the model of the tumor from MRI is depicted in green.

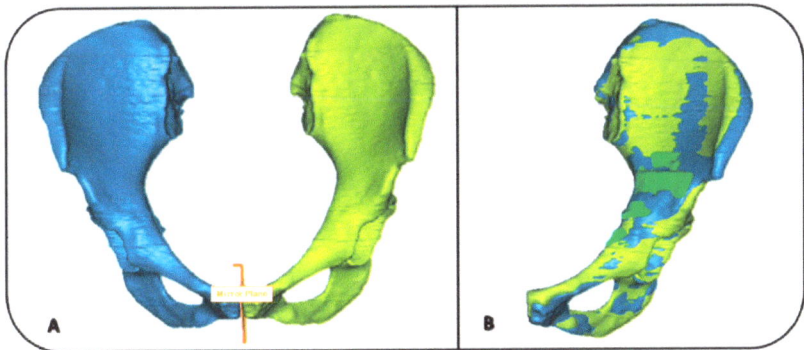

Figure 4. Bone models to depict the procedure for mirroring (**A**) and spatial matching of the two hemipelvis (**B**). In (**A**), the unaffected hemipelvis (in blue, on the left) is to be mirrored to the affected one (in yellow, on the right). This latter model, the affected one, is then matched (**B**) to the unaffected one (blue); the tumor in the affected hemipelvis (from the registration as in Figure 3) is depicted in green.

The defined resection planes are introduced into the model, and, according to these, cuts of the bone models are performed, both on the affected hemipelvis, i.e., left, and on the mirrored and registered unaffected hemipelvis. In the present case, this virtual surgical planning involves the iliac region, the acetabulum and partially the pubic and ischiatic regions, for a total of four cutting planes (Figure 5).

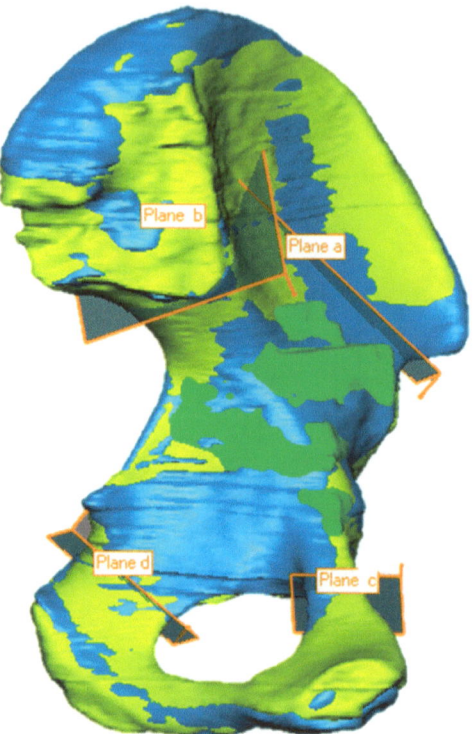

Figure 5. The four cutting planes (a-b-c-d) defined for the four osteotomies necessary to remove the bone stock with the tumor (in green). These virtual osteotomies are performed on both the affected (in yellow) and unaffected (in blue) hemipelvis, after registration as in Figure 4B.

2.4. Creation of the Models for the Final Surgery

Additional bone models are thus defined from virtually performing these bone cuts. The resection of the affected left hemipelvis results in the model of the region of the bone containing the tumor, to be removed during surgery (Figure 6A), and the model of the part of the pelvis meant to host the implant, i.e., the pelvis bone on which the implant will be fixed (Figure 6B).

A third new model is obtained by the virtual bone cuts performed on the mirrored and registered right hemipelvis; the part in correspondence of the tumor is meant to represent a best possible shape of the implant, to be implanted in the host bone as defined in Figure 6C.

2.5. Virtual Planning Analysis and Post-Operative Evaluations

From these models, a great deal of relevant information can be taken, such as tumor volume and areas of the hosting bone sections (Figure 7), in case to amend position and orientation of the planes and to start with a new overall surgical plan. A suitable surgical approach and optimal location and orientation of the fixation elements, such as screws and plates, can also be adjusted. This overall procedure ensures that the design of the initial shape of the implant is based on the exact patient-specific bone and tumor morphology, to obtain a full custom-made limb salvage plan.

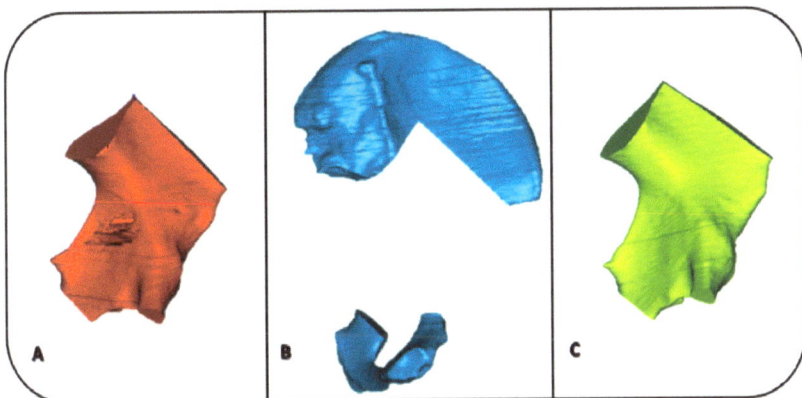

Figure 6. The three relevant models defined at the end of the procedure, after the registration as in Figure 4B and the bone cuts as in Figure 5: (**A**) the model of the hemipelvis section containing the tumor; (**B**) the model of the affected hemipelvis without A, thus intended as the bone to host the prosthesis; (**C**) the model representing a first shape of the implant, because derived from registered unaffected hemipelvis after applying the same cuts. Because of the overall procedure, the section areas in (**B**,**C**) have exactly the same position and orientation.

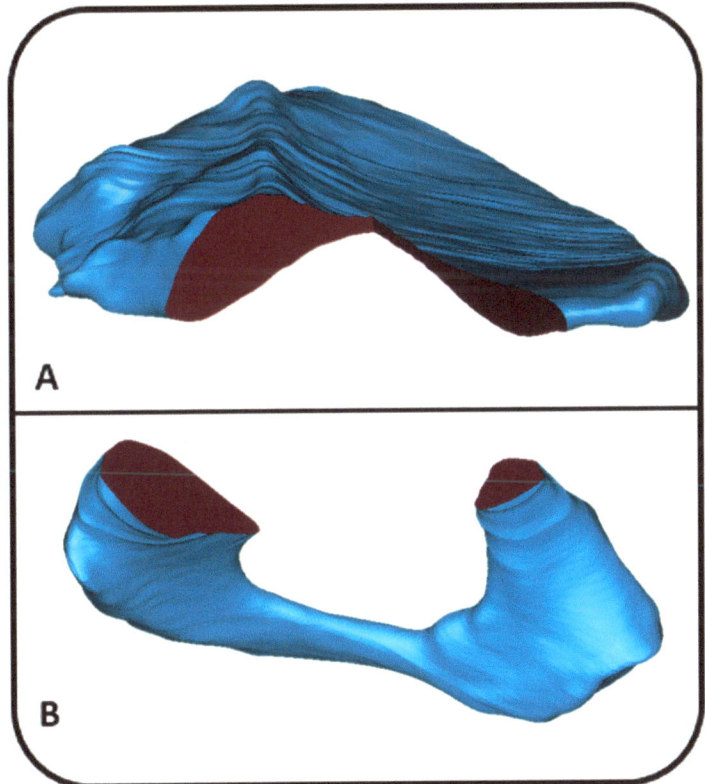

Figure 7. Depiction of the sections (in red) at the affected hemipelvis, supposed to host the implant, the upper part in the ilium (**A**), and the lower part in the ischium and pubis (**B**).

3. Results

The best-fit registration gives as results a transformation matrix, besides the mean error and the root mean square (RMS) of the registration.

3.1. Registration of 3D Models

The mean error and RMS value of the first best-fit registration, i.e., from MRI-based to CT-based models, are 0.98 and 1.44 mm, respectively.

3.2. Creation of Final Models for Implant Design

The corresponding results for the second best-fit registration, i.e., between the affected hemipelvis and the unaffected hemipelvis after mirroring and matching procedures, are 0.87 and 1.16 mm, respectively.

3.3. Virtual Planning Analysis and Post-Operative Evaluations

The results of the virtual planning analysis are shown in Table 1. In particular, the area of cutting sections in the second model defined in the current procedure (the affected hemipelvis meant to host the implant) and its volume, the volume of the first model (the hemipelvis section containing the tumor) and the volume of the third model (the model representing a first possible shape of the implant).

Table 1. Area of the cutting sections and volume of the final models obtained.

	FIRST MODEL - Affected Hemipelvis Meant to Host the Implant	SECOND MODEL - Hemipelvis Section Containing the Tumor	THIRD MODEL - Model of the First Shape of the Implant
SECTION AREA (mm^2)	2454.8	2454.8	2489.6
VOLUME (mm^3)	178,601.5	103,961.6	135,535.6

4. Discussion

Limb salvage for pelvic tumor is a complex surgical treatment and represents a challenge for orthopaedic oncology surgeons. The primary goal in the removal of the tumor and replacement with an implant is to achieve an adequate margin and to preserve the relationship between the remaining tissues [5,8]. The recent advent of 3D printing technology, together with the use of CT and MRI, provides an important solution for these problems [7,14,15,38,42]. In the present study, an original procedure is defined, with all steps from these medical imaging to an accurate 3D anatomical—based model with the shape of the implant; this would be fundamental also for virtual pre-surgical planning, and the design of patient-specific cutting guides. The entire procedure is here shown by depicting the results in a single real case.

These guides are fundamental, for the surgeons to achieve the result designed in the pre-operative planning, in particular the perfect intra-operative positioning and fixation of the prosthesis, which would result also in a safe margin for full tumor removal [3]. Knowing from the virtual models the exact shape of the bones, and the exact position and orientation of the cuts, together with the experience of the surgical access and overall room, the design of these cutting guides and their additive manufacturing with suitable material is straightforward. In the operating theatre, their correct position is usually checked with the help of drawings from pre-operative planning and also with sterile bone models from the case. Once the cutting guides are placed in the correct position, bone is cut with oscillating saw, and then bone and guides are removed.

The anatomical 3D computer models include bone shapes from CT, and position and extension of the tumor and soft tissues from MRI. These models, in their digital format, are registered in space (Figure 3), i.e., positioned in corresponding locations; from this, a process starts for an initial shape of the personalized implant to be obtained (Figures 4–7, Table 1). The major originality of the present procedure is the definition of a best possible initial virtual model for the final personalized implant (Figure 6C). This is designed to restore skeletal anatomy as best as possible, by mirroring the corresponding contralateral part (Figure 4) and thus it matches well with the remaining bone to host the implant (Figure 6B) by definition. These two models do come from different hemipelvis, but the cuts are performed once, when these hemipelvis are mirrored and registered one over the other (Figures 4B and 5). In other words, the same virtual bone cuts (planes a-b-c-d in Figure 5) identify the bone-stock with the tumor (to be removed, in the affected hemipelvis) and the corresponding contralateral part (for the replacement, in the unaffected hemipelvis), respectively parts A and C in Figure 6. This guarantees a perfect match between these models, for a final successful replacement in the operating theatre, apart of course the anatomical asymmetry also caused by the tumor and the spatial registration error, which are expected however to be small. These are the only sources of the present very small difference (about 35 mm^2—Table 1) of the matching faces in the corresponding resection areas, which is clinically acceptable. In any case, the very final design of the implant can cope and adjust this mismatch easily.

These operations were all performed at the computer, using suitable software tools, but can also be replicated by using physical models, thanks to current accessible 3D printers, able to manufacture corresponding objects by the additive technology, now in a fast and cheap way [14]. These physical models are very important both for surgeons and bioengineers, to handle and check the virtual planning by using an exact replica of the case; final recommendations can be made, and refinements can still be performed to the design of the implant and of the treatment. In particular, the fixation elements of the implant and the bone cutting guides are to be checked carefully. This phase is also suitable for the preparation and training of the team, and in case for the explanation of the anatomical conditions and of the relevant surgery to the patient and relatives. The industry is also involved in this process, to assess the final production of the implant (for instance materials, surfaces, porosity, lattice, etc.).

In this report, the ICP registration between the bone models was performed. These spatial registrations can be performed also via the so-called single value decomposition method [38], but in this case a repeatable procedure to identify corresponding anatomical landmarks must be developed and tested, besides the fact that generally the present ICP registration method resulted in a lower error value [38]. The overall computer models after spatial registration between CT- and MRI- based reconstruction of anatomical structures may also involve the soft tissue. Together with the pelvic bones and the tumor, also the muscle-tendon units and even blood vessels can be included, as their location can possibly have a very critical impact with the implant and the surgical instruments such as guides, drills, and saws.

The overall quality of the planning can be checked preoperatively at the computer but also with the physical models. During surgery, additional checks shall be performed. Postoperatively, additional measurements can be taken to validate quantitatively the overall process of segmentation, modelling, registration between models, designing and implanting. A CT scan of the resected bone affected by the tumor can be performed, and its 3D computer model can be compared to the corresponding model defined in the virtual preoperative planning; after a spatial merging of the two models, a root mean square error would well represent the overall quality of the digital and surgical actions [30]. On the other hand, a larger CT scan of the entire operated pelvis can in theory reveal the quality of the entire plan and surgery, but the presence of large metal implants results in severe image artefacts, these being difficult to be removed.

This study has limitations. First of all, the use of a single patient to better explain the procedure; other cases may correspond to more or less complex situations. This was also run by only one trained operator: the result of the present procedure was certainly influenced by this single implementation, in particular the overall process of segmentation and the identification of the tumor. This is by necessity a generalised procedure, because of the uniqueness of each single clinical case in this area; in other words, established standard procedures cannot be defined, as bone tumor location and extension cannot be known and catalogued precisely [2]. In this respect, the role and involvement of the surgeons are fundamental for tumor identification, location, and treatment, together for the definition of the cutting planes and the overall preoperative surgical planning. These resection planes could be better positioned by taking advantage of more cautious considerations and knowledge of the magnitude and direction of the hip joint contact forces; these can be taken generically from the literature, or even by patient-specific measurements, by using state-of-the-art gait analysis and musculo-skeletal models of the lower limbs.

5. Conclusions

A thorough procedure supporting the custom-made design and manufacturing of implants for the surgical treatment of bone tumors at the pelvis is proposed. A few steps are based on established practice in biomechanical modelling, others on original concepts. All these however have been shared with surgeons and industry, as well as discussed within international teams of experts. The present use of both CT and MRI imaging does allow a careful reproduction of the main anatomical structures, including the tumor, resulting in a more accurate planning and implant designing. The procedure could be easily rearranged also for other anatomical complexes, especially where symmetry restoration represents an important scope.

Author Contributions: Conceptualization: G.D., C.B. and A.L.; methodology: G.D. and C.B.; software: G.D. and M.R.; validation: G.D., C.B. and B.S.; formal analysis: G.D.; investigation: G.D. and B.S; resources: D.M.D. and A.L.; writing–original draft preparation: G.D., C.B. and A.L.; writing–review and editing: G.D., C.B., M.R., D.M.D., B.S. and A.L.; visualization: G.D. and M.R.; supervision: C.B. and A.L.; project administration: D.M.D. and A.L.; funding acquisition: A.L. All authors have read and agreed to the published version of the manuscript.

Funding: This study was funded by the Italian Ministry of Economy and Finance, program "5 per mille".

Institutional Review Board Statement: The study was conducted according to the guidelines of the Declaration of Helsinki, and approved by the Institutional Review Board CE AVEC (number: EM468/2021_47/2014/Oss/IOR_EM1; final amendment approval Prot. Gen 0008191, 27 May 2021).

Informed Consent Statement: Informed consent was obtained from the subject involved in the study.

Data Availability Statement: The datasets generated during the current study are not publicly available but are available from the corresponding author on reasonable request.

Conflicts of Interest: All authors declare that there are no personal or commercial relationships.

References

1. Park, J.W.; Kang, H.G.; Lim, K.M.; Park, D.W.; Kim, J.H.; Kim, H.S. Bone tumor resection guide using three-dimensional printing for limb salvage surgery. *J. Surg. Oncol.* **2018**, *118*, 898–905. [CrossRef]
2. Enneking, W.F.; Dunham, W.K. Resection and reconstruction for primary neoplasms involving the innominate bone. *J. Bone Jt. Surg. Am.* **1978**, *60*, 731–746. [CrossRef]
3. Zhu, D.; Fu, J.; Wang, L.; Guo, Z.; Wang, Z.; Fan, H. Reconstruction with customized, 3D-printed prosthesis after resection of periacetabular Ewing's sarcoma in children using "triradiate cartilage-based" surgical strategy:a technical note. *J. Orthop. Translat.* **2021**, *28*, 108–117. [CrossRef]
4. Angelini, A.; Calabro, T.; Pala, E.; Trovarelli, G.; Maraldi, M.; Ruggieri, P. Resection and reconstruction of pelvic bone tumors. *Orthopedics* **2015**, *38*, 87–93. [CrossRef] [PubMed]
5. Hennessy, D.W.; Santiago, M.E.A.; Lozano-Calderón, A. Complex Pelvic Reconstruction using Patient-Specific Instrumentation and a 3D-Printed Custom Implant following Tumor Resection. *J. Hip Surg.* **2017**, *2*, 061–067. [CrossRef]
6. Matar, H.E.; Selvaratnam, V.; Shah, N.; Wynn Jones, H. Custom triflange revision acetabular components for significant bone defects and pelvic discontinuity: Early UK experience. *J. Orthop.* **2020**, *21*, 25–30. [CrossRef] [PubMed]

7. Dong, E.; Wang, L.; Iqbal, T.; Li, D.; Liu, Y.; He, J.; Zhao, B.; Li, Y. Finite Element Analysis of the Pelvis after Customized Prosthesis Reconstruction. *J. Bionic Eng.* **2018**, *15*, 443–451. [CrossRef]
8. Fujiwara, T.; Medellin Rincon, M.R.; Sambri, A.; Tsuda, Y.; Clark, R.; Stevenson, J.; Parry, M.C.; Grimer, R.J.; Jeys, L. Limb-salvage reconstruction following resection of pelvic bone sarcomas involving the acetabulum. *Bone Jt. J.* **2021**, *103-B*, 795–803. [CrossRef]
9. Ozaki, T.; Hillmann, A.; Bettin, D.; Wuisman, P.; Winkelmann, W. High complication rates with pelvic allografts. Experience of 22 sarcoma resections. *Acta Orthop. Scand.* **1996**, *67*, 333–338. [CrossRef]
10. Abudu, A.; Grimer, R.J.; Cannon, S.R.; Carter, S.R.; Sneath, R.S. Reconstruction of the hemipelvis after the excision of malignant tumours. Complications and functional outcome of prostheses. *J. Bone Jt. Surg. Br.* **1997**, *79*, 773–779. [CrossRef]
11. Gebert, C.; Wessling, M.; Hoffmann, C.; Roedl, R.; Winkelmann, W.; Gosheger, G.; Hardes, J. Hip transposition as a limb salvage procedure following the resection of periacetabular tumors. *J. Surg. Oncol.* **2011**, *103*, 269–275. [CrossRef] [PubMed]
12. Jansen, J.A.; van de Sande, M.A.; Dijkstra, P.D. Poor long-term clinical results of saddle prosthesis after resection of periacetabular tumors. *Clin. Orthop. Relat. Res.* **2013**, *471*, 324–331. [CrossRef] [PubMed]
13. Angelini, A.; Trovarelli, G.; Berizzi, A.; Pala, E.; Breda, A.; Ruggieri, P. Three-dimension-printed custom-made prosthetic reconstructions: From revision surgery to oncologic reconstructions. *Int. Orthop.* **2019**, *43*, 123–132. [CrossRef] [PubMed]
14. Belvedere, C.; Siegler, S.; Fortunato, A.; Caravaggi, P.; Liverani, E.; Durante, S.; Ensini, A.; Konow, T.; Leardini, A. New comprehensive procedure for custom-made total ankle replacements: Medical imaging, joint modeling, prosthesis design, and 3D printing. *J. Orthop. Res.* **2019**, *37*, 760–768. [CrossRef] [PubMed]
15. Park, J.W.; Kang, H.G.; Kim, J.H.; Kim, H.S. The application of 3D-printing technology in pelvic bone tumor surgery. *J. Orthop. Sci.* **2021**, *26*, 276–283. [CrossRef]
16. Sun, W.; Li, J.; Li, Q.; Li, G.; Cai, Z. Clinical effectiveness of hemipelvic reconstruction using computer-aided custom-made prostheses after resection of malignant pelvic tumors. *J. Arthroplast.* **2011**, *26*, 1508–1513. [CrossRef]
17. Liang, H.; Ji, T.; Zhang, Y.; Wang, Y.; Guo, W. Reconstruction with 3D-printed pelvic endoprostheses after resection of a pelvic tumour. *Bone Jt. J.* **2017**, *99-B*, 267–275. [CrossRef]
18. Iqbal, T.; Shi, L.; Wang, L.; Liu, Y.; Li, D.; Qin, M.; Jin, Z. Development of finite element model for customized prostheses design for patient with pelvic bone tumor. *Proc. Inst. Mech. Eng. H* **2017**, *231*, 525–533. [CrossRef]
19. Colen, S.; Dalemans, A.; Schouwenaars, A.; Mulier, M. Outcome of custom-made IMP femoral components of total hip arthroplasty: A follow-up of 15 to 22 years. *J. Arthroplast.* **2014**, *29*, 397–400. [CrossRef]
20. Fan, H.; Fu, J.; Li, X.; Pei, Y.; Li, X.; Pei, G.; Guo, Z. Implantation of customized 3-D printed titanium prosthesis in limb salvage surgery: A case series and review of the literature. *World J. Surg. Oncol.* **2015**, *13*, 308. [CrossRef]
21. Xiu, P.; Jia, Z.; Lv, J.; Yin, C.; Cheng, Y.; Zhang, K.; Song, C.; Leng, H.; Zheng, Y.; Cai, H.; et al. Tailored Surface Treatment of 3D Printed Porous Ti6Al4V by Microarc Oxidation for Enhanced Osseointegration via Optimized Bone In-Growth Patterns and Interlocked Bone/Implant Interface. *ACS Appl. Mater. Interfaces* **2016**, *8*, 17964–17975. [CrossRef] [PubMed]
22. Sing, S.L.; An, J.; Yeong, W.Y.; Wiria, F.E. Laser and electron-beam powder-bed additive manufacturing of metallic implants: A review on processes, materials and designs. *J. Orthop. Res.* **2016**, *34*, 369–385. [CrossRef] [PubMed]
23. Shah, F.A.; Snis, A.; Matic, A.; Thomsen, P.; Palmquist, A. 3D printed Ti6Al4V implant surface promotes bone maturation and retains a higher density of less aged osteocytes at the bone-implant interface. *Acta Biomater.* **2016**, *30*, 357–367. [CrossRef] [PubMed]
24. Angelini, A.; Kotrych, D.; Trovarelli, G.; Szafranski, A.; Bohatyrewicz, A.; Ruggieri, P. Analysis of principles inspiring design of three-dimensional-printed custom-made prostheses in two referral centres. *Int. Orthop.* **2020**, *44*, 829–837. [CrossRef]
25. Attarilar, S.; Ebrahimi, M.; Djavanroodi, F.; Fu, Y.; Wang, L.; Yang, J. 3D Printing Technologies in Metallic Implants: A Thematic Review on the Techniques and Procedures. *Int. J. Bioprint* **2021**, *7*, 306. [CrossRef]
26. Wang, B.; Hao, Y.; Pu, F.; Jiang, W.; Shao, Z. Computer-aided designed, three dimensional-printed hemipelvic prosthesis for peri-acetabular malignant bone tumour. *Int. Orthop.* **2018**, *42*, 687–694. [CrossRef]
27. Fang, C.; Cai, H.; Kuong, E.; Chui, E.; Siu, Y.C.; Ji, T.; Drstvensek, I. Surgical applications of three-dimensional printing in the pelvis and acetabulum: From models and tools to implants. *Unfallchirurg* **2019**, *122*, 278–285. [CrossRef]
28. Sohling, N.; Neijhoft, J.; Nienhaus, V.; Acker, V.; Harbig, J.; Menz, F.; Ochs, J.; Verboket, R.D.; Ritz, U.; Blaeser, A.; et al. 3D-Printing of Hierarchically Designed and Osteoconductive Bone Tissue Engineering Scaffolds. *Materials* **2020**, *13*, 1836. [CrossRef]
29. Pei, X.; Ma, L.; Zhang, B.; Sun, J.; Sun, Y.; Fan, Y.; Gou, Z.; Zhou, C.; Zhang, X. Creating hierarchical porosity hydroxyapatite scaffolds with osteoinduction by three-dimensional printing and microwave sintering. *Biofabrication* **2017**, *9*, 045008. [CrossRef]
30. Wong, K.C.; Kumta, S.M.; Geel, N.V.; Demol, J. One-step reconstruction with a 3D-printed, biomechanically evaluated custom implant after complex pelvic tumor resection. *Comput. Aided Surg.* **2015**, *20*, 14–23. [CrossRef]
31. Chen, X.; Xu, L.; Wang, Y.; Hao, Y.; Wang, L. Image-guided installation of 3D-printed patient-specific implant and its application in pelvic tumor resection and reconstruction surgery. *Comput. Methods Programs Biomed.* **2016**, *125*, 66–78. [CrossRef] [PubMed]
32. Gouin, F.; Paul, L.; Odri, G.A.; Cartiaux, O. Computer-Assisted Planning and Patient-Specific Instruments for Bone Tumor Resection within the Pelvis: A Series of 11 Patients. *Sarcoma 2014* **2014**, 842709. [CrossRef]
33. Cartiaux, O.; Paul, L.; Francq, B.G.; Banse, X.; Docquier, P.L. Improved accuracy with 3D planning and patient-specific instruments during simulated pelvic bone tumor surgery. *Ann. Biomed. Eng.* **2014**, *42*, 205–213. [CrossRef] [PubMed]

34. Wong, K.C.; Sze, K.Y.; Wong, I.O.; Wong, C.M.; Kumta, S.M. Patient-specific instrument can achieve same accuracy with less resection time than navigation assistance in periacetabular pelvic tumor surgery: A cadaveric study. *Int. J. Comput. Assist. Radiol. Surg.* **2016**, *11*, 307–316. [CrossRef] [PubMed]
35. Wong, K.C.; Kumta, S.M.; Sze, K.Y.; Wong, C.M. Use of a patient-specific CAD/CAM surgical jig in extremity bone tumor resection and custom prosthetic reconstruction. *Comput. Aided Surg.* **2012**, *17*, 284–293. [CrossRef] [PubMed]
36. Iqbal, T.; Wang, L.; Li, D.; Dong, E.; Fan, H.; Fu, J.; Hu, C. A general multi-objective topology optimization methodology developed for customized design of pelvic prostheses. *Med. Eng. Phys.* **2019**, *69*, 8–16. [CrossRef] [PubMed]
37. Park, D.W.L.A.; Park, J.W.; Lim, K.M.; Kang, H.G. Biomechanical Evaluation of a New Fixation Type in 3D-Printed Periacetabular Implants using a Finite Element Simulation. *Appl. Sci.* **2019**, *9*, 820. [CrossRef]
38. Durastanti, G.; Leardini, A.; Siegler, S.; Durante, S.; Bazzocchi, A.; Belvedere, C. Comparison of cartilage and bone morphological models of the ankle joint derived from different medical imaging technologies. *Quant. Imaging Med. Surg.* **2019**, *9*, 1368–1382. [CrossRef]
39. De Paolis, M.; Sambri, A.; Zucchini, R.; Frisoni, T.; Spazzoli, B.; Taddei, F.; Donati, D.M. Custom made 3D-printed prosthesis in periacetabular resections through a novel ileoadductor approach. *Orthopedics* **2021**. [CrossRef]
40. Van Eijnatten, M.; van Dijk, R.; Dobbe, J.; Streekstra, G.; Koivisto, J.; Wolff, J. CT image segmentation methods for bone used in medical additive manufacturing. *Med. Eng. Phys.* **2018**, *51*, 6–16. [CrossRef]
41. Besl, P.J.; McKay, N.D. A method for registration of 3-D shapes. *IEEE Trans. Pattern Anal. Mach. Intell.* **1992**, *14*, 239–256. [CrossRef]
42. Bohme, J.; Shim, V.; Hoch, A.; Mutze, M.; Muller, C.; Josten, C. Clinical implementation of finite element models in pelvic ring surgery for prediction of implant behavior: A case report. *Clin. Biomech.* **2012**, *27*, 872–878. [CrossRef] [PubMed]

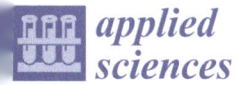

Article

In-Vivo Quantification of Knee Deep-Flexion in Physiological Loading Condition trough Dynamic MRI

Michele Conconi [1,*], Filippo De Carli [2], Matteo Berni [3], Nicola Sancisi [1], Vincenzo Parenti-Castelli [1] and Giuseppe Monetti [2]

1. Department of Industrial Engineering—DIN, University of Bologna, 40139 Bologna, Italy
2. Primus Forlì Medical Center, 47121 Forlì, Italy
3. Medical Technology Laboratory, IRCCS Istituto Ortopedico Rizzoli, 40139 Bologna, Italy
* Correspondence: michele.conconi@unibo.it

Abstract: The in-vivo quantification of knee motion in physiological loading conditions is paramount for the understanding of the joint's natural behavior and the comprehension of articular disorders. Dynamic MRI (DMRI) represents an emerging technology that makes it possible to investigate the functional interaction among all the joint tissues without risks for the patient. However, traditional MRI scanners normally offer a reduced space of motion, and complex apparatus are needed to load the articulation, due to the horizontal orientation of the scanning bed. In this study, we present an experimental and computational procedure that combines an open, weight-bearing MRI scanner with an original registration algorithm to reconstruct the three-dimensional kinematics of the knee from DMRI, thus allowing the investigation of knee deep-flexion under physiological loads in space. To improve the accuracy of the procedure, an MR-compatible rig has been developed to guide the knee flexion of the patient. We tested the procedure on three volunteers. The overall rotational and positional accuracy achieved are 1.8° ± 1.4 and 1.2 mm ± 0.8, respectively, and they are sufficient for the characterization of the joint behavior under load.

Keywords: Dynamic MRI; weight-bearing MRI; knee deep-flexion

Citation: Conconi, M.; De Carli, F.; Berni, M.; Sancisi, N.; Parenti-Castelli, V.; Monetti, G. In-Vivo Quantification of Knee Deep-Flexion in Physiological Loading Condition trough Dynamic MRI. *Appl. Sci.* **2023**, *13*, 629. https://doi.org/10.3390/app13010629

Academic Editor: Arkady Voloshin

Received: 28 November 2022
Revised: 20 December 2022
Accepted: 29 December 2022
Published: 3 January 2023

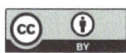

Copyright: © 2023 by the authors. Licensee MDPI, Basel, Switzerland. This article is an open access article distributed under the terms and conditions of the Creative Commons Attribution (CC BY) license (https://creativecommons.org/licenses/by/4.0/).

1. Introduction

Musculoskeletal disorders are the second most common cause of disability worldwide, exceeded only by traffic-related injuries, and they are responsible for the 21.3% of the total years lived with disability [1,2]. Among human articulations, the knee is one of the most susceptible to ligament injuries and to the risk of osteoarthritis development [3]. Understanding and identifying a patient's normal and pathological joint function is, therefore, a high clinical priority.

Static morphological imaging helps the diagnosis and the etiology identification of these disorders [4]. However, the functional characterization of musculoskeletal system in physiological conditions still relies on clinician experience [5]. Indeed, the relation between anatomical structures that can be observed during static imaging may significantly differ from what is measured during dynamic musculoskeletal tasks [6–8]. Several studies showed that evaluating a patient by means of static, non-weight-bearing scans alone may result in misdiagnoses [6–10]. In-vivo imaging of joint motion may fill the gap, providing a tool to better understand the normal joint physiology, investigating the etiology of musculoskeletal diseases, and designing more effective treatments.

Currently, in-vivo analysis of articular motion can be performed by several techniques [11]: ultrasonography [12], fluoroscopy [13], computed tomography (CT) [14], and Magnetic Resonance Imaging (MRI) [6]. Ultrasonography, however, is limited to the evaluation of soft tissues around the joint. Fluoroscopy and CT expose the patient to ionizing radiation and do not allow the direct observation of soft tissues. On the other hand, MRI returns information of both bones and soft tissues without known risk for the patient. This, together with the recent advances in dynamic sequences, boosted the application of Dynamic MRI (DMRI) to the investigation of joint behavior [15].

The goal of this work is to present an experimental-computational procedure for the investigation of the knee deep-flexion under physiological loads. The procedure reconstructs the spatial kinematics of the knee from dynamic planar MR images. To this aim, we employed a weight-bearing MR scanner, in combination with a custom MR compatible rig, to guide the knee flexion during the dynamic scan. Finally, we developed a new registration algorithm to reconstruct the three-dimensional tibio-femoral kinematics from DMRI.

2. Materials and Methods

2.1. Experimental Setup

MR scans were performed with a 0.25 T G-Scan, Esaote SpA. Despite the low magnetic field, this scanner has the advantages of a rotatable bore (Figure 1), allowing for the weight-bearing imaging of the patient. Additionally, the scanner is open, thus making a wider mobility of the patient possible. Loaded knee flexion was performed with the scanner in vertical position and with the aid of an MR-compatible rig specifically designed to guide the knee flexion. The rig is in plastic and consists of a hydraulic step that can be lowered at controlled velocity by regulating the liquid flow from the piston sustaining the step to the accumulation tank (Figure 2). Connectors in the hydraulic circuit were made out of brass to minimize the magnetic field distortion, while the steel-controlling valves were positioned outside the scanner room and controlled by an operator.

During the scans, the volunteers stood with the right leg in the scanner, while the contralateral leg was supported by the step (Figure 2). Lowering the step, the right leg flexed under the weight of the volunteer, resulting in a physiological load comparable with what is experienced during stair climbing.

2.2. Preliminary Static Acquisitions

We analyzed three volunteers (age: 29 ± 7.9 years; height: 174.3 ± 7.6 cm; weight: 71.7 ± 7.6 kg). For each volunteer, an initial MRI of the knee (3D hybrid contrast enhancement, FOV 512×512, pixel spacing 0.5/0.5, slice thickness 0.5 mm, TR = 10 ms, TE = 5 ms, flip angle 60°, hereinafter 3D HYCE) was taken in a supine, non-weight-bearing configuration to provide a reference image for the segmentation of all the main knee structures. In particular, bone models of the femur, tibia, and fibula were segmented through the open software MITK. Anatomical reference systems for the femur and tibia were defined based on the convention proposed by Tashman and co-workers [16], for which x, y, and z are axes respectively pointing anteriorly, proximally and to the right. For the aims of the present study, fibula and tibia were considered as a rigid complex.

2.3. Registration Algorithm

With the employed scanner, DMRI results in a series of subsequent planar acquisitions taken while the subject is moving. More than one plane can be scanned for the same joint pose: for instance, as clarified below, we chose to use two synchronized planes in this case, although the number could be higher. Joint kinematics can, thus, be reconstructed by registering a 3D model of the moving objects on the DMRI planes for each measured joint pose.

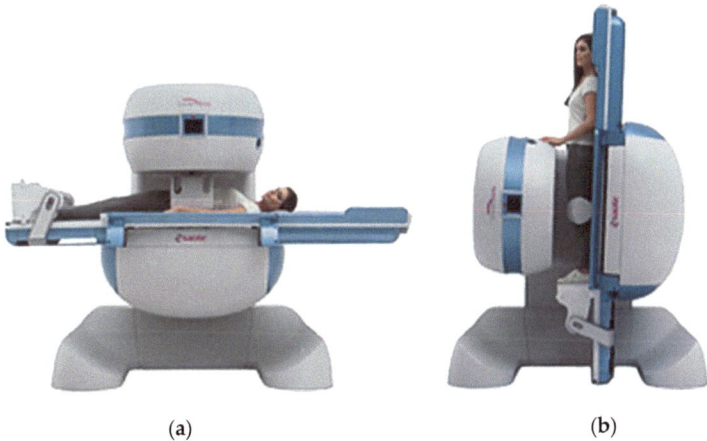

Figure 1. The employed MR scanner in traditional (**a**) and weight-bearing (**b**) configuration.

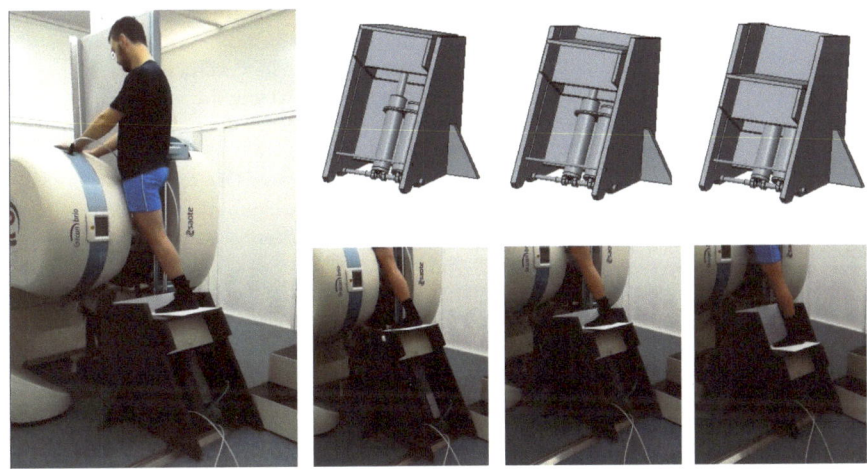

Figure 2. The MR-compatible rig used to guide the knee flexion.

The 2D/3D registration algorithm developed for this study is based on voxel intensity, exploiting the low signal associated with the bone tissue within the MR scans to register 3D bone models on the DMRI images through rigid rototranslations. To this aim, a model of the inner bone, namely the internal surface of the cortical and subchondral bone, was also segmented from the non-weight-bearing MRI with an offset of 0.5 mm. Thanks to this offset, when the model is correctly registered on MRI data, for each image, the intersection between the inner bone model and each DMRI plane will take place inside the cortical bone region, which should correspond to the minimum signal intensity on the DMRI images.

Optimal registration is performed within a proprietary C++ code. Bones are moved within the MR reference system, and the intersection between the DMRI planes and stl model is computed for each pose. Since DMRI has a non-zero thickness, all the stl points whose distance to the scanning plane is less than half the slice thickness are considered as belonging to the intersection and projected on the scanning plane. For each intersection point, the corresponding intensity is computed by bilinear interpolation of the DMRI voxel values. For each frame, optimal bone position is obtained by minimizing the mean of this intensity value extended on the overall intersection between DMRI planes and bone stl model.

The registration process just presented is fully automatic; however, it is affected by the initial registration, i.e., the first guess of the first joint pose. To minimize the impact of the operator, initialization of the registration is partially automatized in a separate step. The first DMRI frame of each plane is processed by means of a Channy edge detection algorithm to identify the bone contours, resulting in a cloud of points. The operator is then requested to refine the detected edges, manually eliminating points that do not correspond to the cortical bone. The operator manually registers the bone stl models to this cloud of points. This initial registration is then refined by means of an ICP algorithm and passed, as a starting point, to the 2D/3D intensity-based registration algorithm. A schematic representation of the overall code workflow is given in Figure 3.

2.4. Identification of the Optimal Scanning Planes and Registration Accuracy

In order to provide a reference motion to test the registration algorithm performance, five additional static scans (3D HYCE) were also taken in weight-bearing configuration, setting the flexion angle, by means of the rig, approximately at $0°$, $15°$, $45°$, $75°$, and $90°$ (Figure 4). Bones were segmented from all the scans, and the femur, tibia, and fibula from non-weight-bearing MRI were registered to the corresponding bones on each scan through an Iterative Closest Point (ICP) algorithm developed in Matlab (Figure 4). Since the anatomical reference frames were defined on the non-weight-bearing MRI, as noted above, in this way, it was possible to define the rototranslational matrixes describing the relative pose of the anatomical reference systems of the femur and tibia at the five static scans. The femoro-tibial motion was derived by parametrizing the rototranslational matrixes, using the center of the femoral reference system to track the translations and the ZXY cardanic angle sequence to represent the rotations [17].

To reduce the scanning time, the number of DMRI planes acquired for each exam was limited to two. To determine which plane combinations would allow for the optimal motion reconstruction, DMRI was simulated from the five static weight-bearing scans of one volunteer by resampling the original MRI in different planes (Figure 5). The set of tested plane pairs is reported in Table 1. For each combination of planes and each static scan, the registration algorithm was run, and the positional and orientational accuracies were evaluated as the mean absolute error (MAE) between the reconstructed and measured tibio-femoral motion. Once the combination resulting in the smallest rotational and translational MAE was identified, plane orientation was further adjusted to minimize the chance of out-of-plane motion during knee flexion. Accuracy was also tested for these optimal planes to ensure no quality loss in bone registration.

Once the optimal scanning planes were determined, DMRI results were simulated from the static scans for all the three volunteers, as described above, and the registration algorithm was run. With respect to the real dynamic imaging described below, the bone spatial pose is known in this case, thus facilitating an accurate validation of the registration algorithm. The overall rotational and translational algorithm accuracies were then defined as the MAE between reconstructed and measured motion, as well as averaged on the three volunteers.

2.5. Dynamic Imaging

For each volunteer, three exams were performed for recording DMRI (2D hybrid contrast enhancement, FOV 200 × 200, pixel spacing 0.68/0.68, slice thickness 5 mm, TR = 20 ms, TE = 10 ms, flip angle $80°$, 2.9 s per frame) of the right leg on the two optimal planes. Each exam required two flexions since the G-Scan Brio allows the acquisition on a single plane at a time. To minimize the variations between subsequent acquisitions, DMRI were taken one after the other using the same step velocity. An additional support was introduced to keep the shank fixed in the scanner during the tests while, at the same time, allowing an unconstrained motion at the knee.

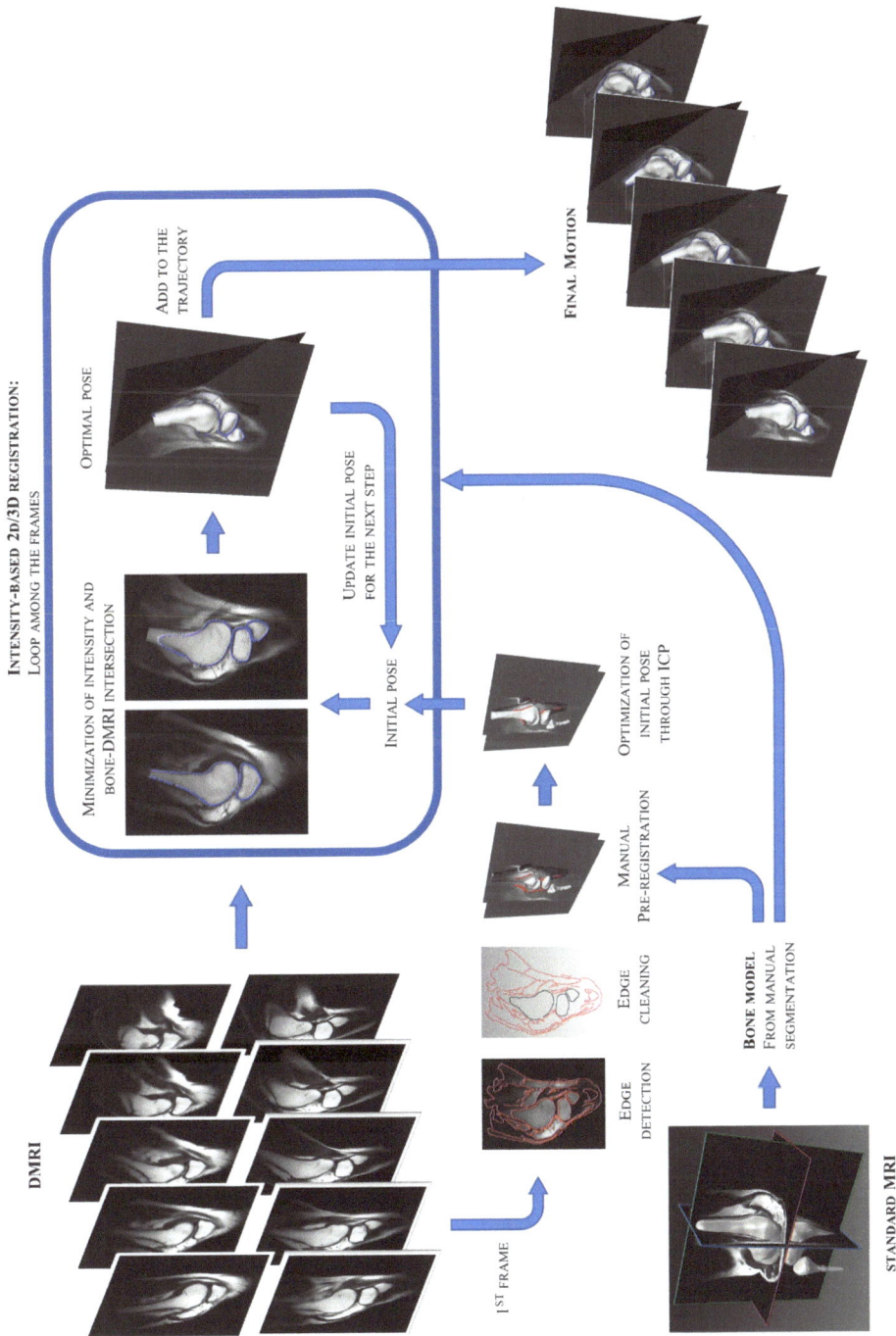

Figure 3. Schematic representation of the registration process to the reconstruction of the knee kinematics from DMRI.

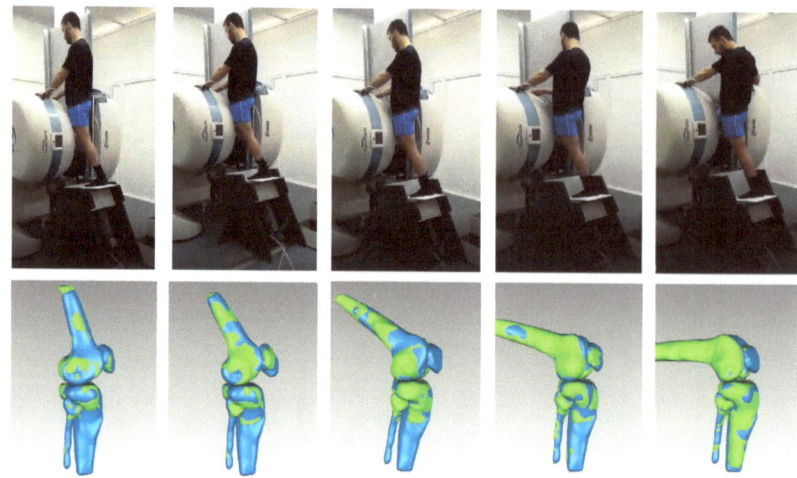

Figure 4. Reconstruction of knee kinematics from five static scans at different knee flexion angles: patient position for each scan (**top row**) and corresponding segmentation of knee bones (**bottom row**). The bones from non-weight-bearing scan are represented in green, registered on the corresponding bones, as segmented from each weight-bearing MRI, in blue.

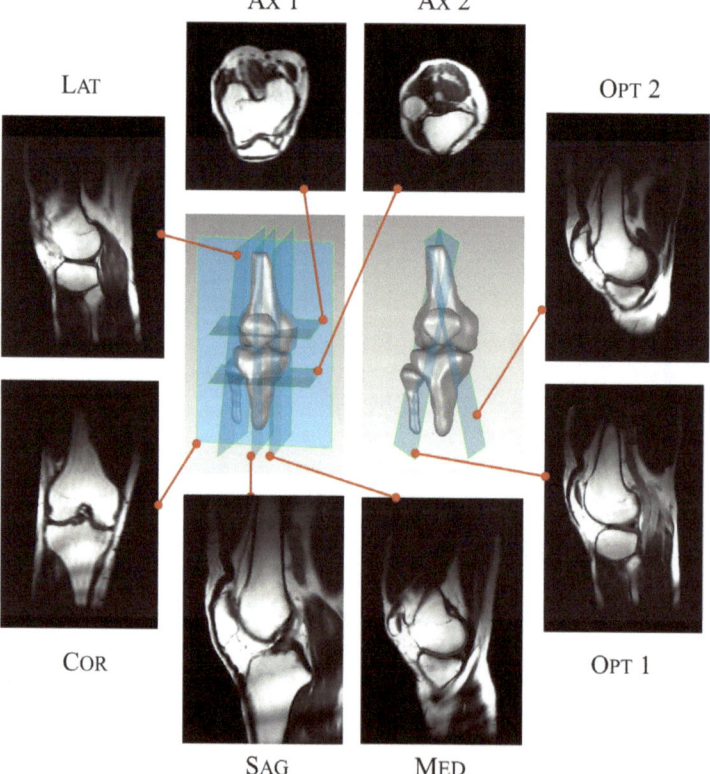

Figure 5. Location of the tested DMRI plane for the optimization of the kinematics reconstruction.

The first two exams were identical, while during the third, a wooden block was positioned below the left foot to increase the starting flexion angle to the volunteer's maximum. For each repetition, 71 frames were recorded.

2.6. Joint Kinematics Reconstruction: Repeatability of the Exam and Sensitivity to the Initial Registration

The registration algorithm was applied to the three repetitions of DMRI performed by each volunteer. To minimize the effect of the initial registration, simulations were run from full extension to flexion, and then, the frame order was inverted to simulate extension. Only the extension cycle was considered.

To test the repeatability of the experimental procedure, the standard deviation among the three repetitions was computed over the common flexion range for each motion component. Rotational and translational repeatability were defined as the mean standard deviation values over all volunteers.

To test the impact of the initial registration on the final reconstructed motion, the algorithm was run by perturbing the pose of the tibia, fibula, and femur (the three considered as a single rigid complex) first by ± 5 and then by ± 10 (mm and °), on each component, for a total of 1456 combinations around the initial registration proposed by the operator. In this case, simulation from full extension to flexion and then back to extension was also run, and only the extension cycle was considered and compared with the motion obtained without perturbation of the initial pose. Trajectories with rotational MAE below 0.5° and translational MAE below 0.5 mm were considered not affected by the considered perturbation.

3. Results

The rotational and translational MAE for the different pairs of tested planes are reported in Table 1, considering this measure as an indicator of the system accuracy. The optimal planes show the lowest errors.

The registration accuracy estimated on the simulated DMRI for the three subjects was 1.8° $\pm$ 1.4 and 1.2 mm $\pm$ 0.8, for rotations and translations, respectively. In Figure 6, the bone registration on the two DMRI planes is depicted.

Figure 7 shows the comparison among knee motion as reconstructed from a real DMRI exam and as estimated through static scans for the three volunteers, while Figure 8a shows the three repetitions for one volunteer. The overall repeatability for the three volunteers was 3.2° and 1.3 mm. Over the 1456 perturbations of the initial registration, 97.6% (1421) resulted in differences below 0.5° and 0.5 mm with respect to the unperturbed motion (Figure 8b). In the remaining 2.4% of cases (35), the reconstruction error was significantly detectable, resulting in average rotational and translational differences of 17.3° $\pm$ 7.7 and 9.7 mm $\pm$ 4.5, respectively.

4. Discussion

We presented an experimental-computational procedure for the in-vivo quantification of the knee kinematics under physiological loads by means of non-invasive DMRI. The procedure combines a weight-bearing, open MR scanner, a MR compatible rig to guide the knee flexion, and a registration algorithm to reconstruct the motion from DMRI. The procedure is non-invasive and, except for some initialization parameters, completely automatic.

Table 1. Rotational and translational MAE for each of the tested combinations of DMRI planes.

Plane Combination	Rotational MAE [°]	Translational MAE [mm]
Sag-Cor	1.8 ± 1.5	1.8 ± 1.7
Sag-Ax1	2.8 ± 2.4	1.8 ± 1.4
Sag-Ax2	1.0 ± 0.7	1.4 ± 0.9
Sag-Med	2.4 ± 1.4	1.6 ± 1.4
Sag-Lat	1.8 ± 1.1	1.3 ± 1.5
Cor-Ax1	3.2 ± 4.6	4.2 ± 4.8
Cor-Ax2	3.0 ± 3.0	2.4 ± 1.9
Cor-Med	2.8 ± 2.5	1.7 ± 1.6
Cor-Lat	2.5 ± 2.1	1.9 ± 1.7
Ax1-Ax2	3.1 ± 2.3	1.4 ± 0.8
Ax1-Med	2.2 ± 1.9	1.4 ± 1.4
Ax1-Lat	3.5 ± 1.9	5.5 ± 5.8
Ax2-Med	5.0 ± 3.2	2.7 ± 2.7
Ax2-Lat	2.3 ± 1.5	2.8 ± 2.5
Med-Lat	1.8 ± 1.1	**1.2 ± 0.6**
Opt1-Opt2	**1.0 ± 0.5**	0.7 ± 0.4

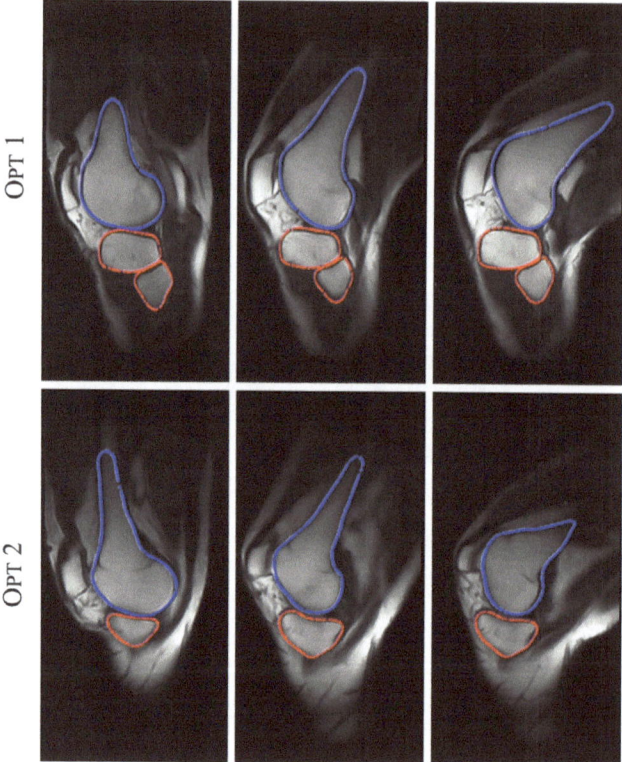

Figure 6. Representation of the bone registration, on the two optimal DMRI planes, at different flexion angles. The registered femur intersection with the planes is depicted in blue, while the tibia–fibula complex intersection is depicted in red.

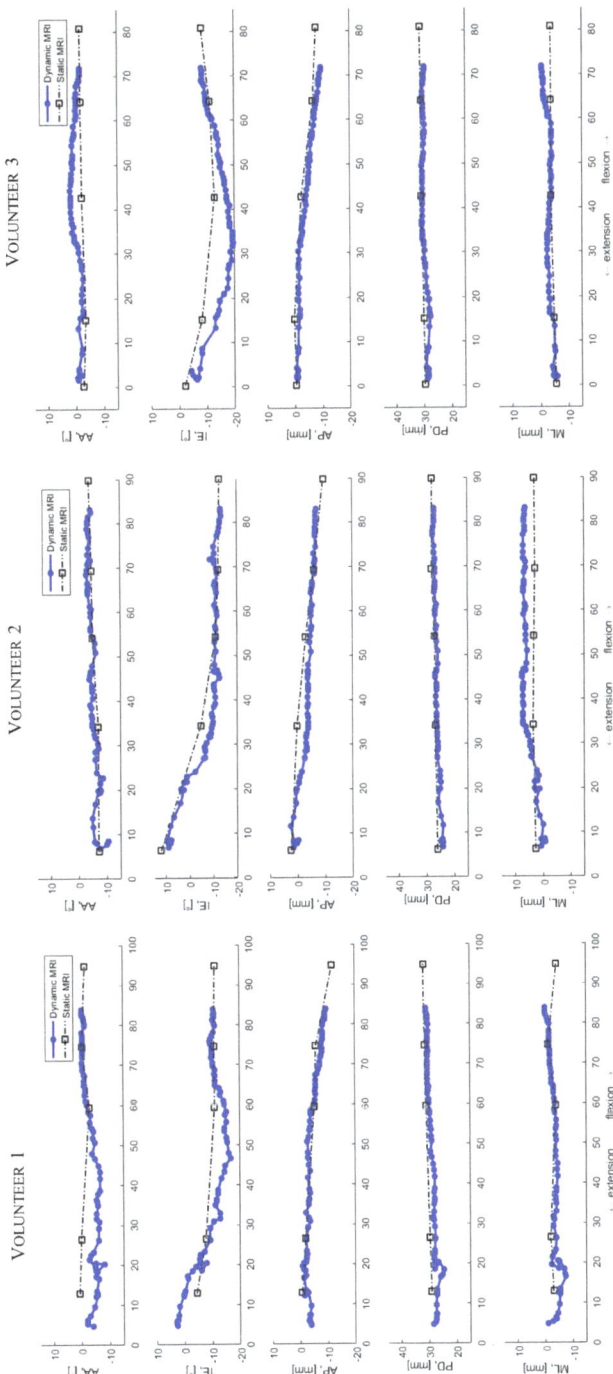

Figure 7. Comparison between knee kinematics reconstructed from dynamic (blue) and static (black) MRI. The Abduction/adduction (AA), internal/external rotation (IE), anterior/posterior (AP), proximal/distal (PD), and medial/lateral (ML) translations are plotted vs. the knee flexion angle.

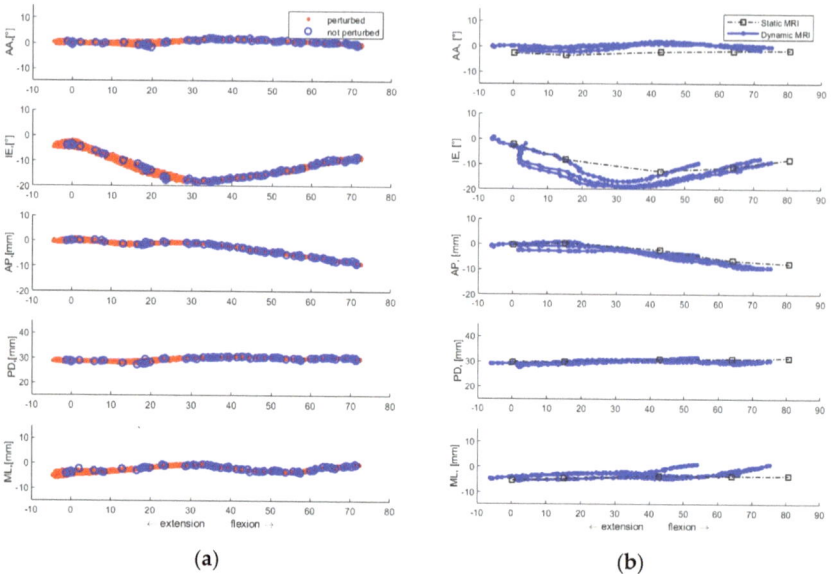

Figure 8. (a) Comparison between knee kinematics reconstructed from three repetition of dynamic (blue) and static (black) MRI for one volunteer. The Abduction/adduction (AA), internal/external rotation (IE), anterior/posterior (AP), proximal/distal (PD), and medial/lateral (ML) translations are plotted. (b) Comparison among the kinematics reconstructed from DMRI without (blue) and with (red) perturbations. In red, the 1421 cases (97.6%) not affected by perturbation of the initial pose are plotted.

The specific scanner employed in this study offers several advantages. Being open, it allows a considerable range of motion. Moreover, the possibility to scan the person in vertical position allows for the analysis of the articulation under the action of the weight and the muscles, thus resulting in a more physiological loading condition.

The 2D/3D registration algorithm shows a rotational and positional accuracy below 2° and 1.5 mm, where the latter is in the order of magnitude of twice the in-plane dimension of the DMRI voxel for this study. The registration accuracy is reasonably limited by the low intensity of the magnetic field of the employed scanner. It has, indeed, been shown that motion tracking through DMRI is proportional both to the strength of the magnetic field and to the velocity of the tracked object [18]. Other studies investigating the knee through DMRI achieved higher accuracy using higher intensities [15]. Nevertheless, the achieved accuracy is still enough to allow for the characterization of the physiological and pathological knee kinematics, while the low intensity of the magnetic field makes the analysis practically non-invasive and compatible, to some extent, with measures on patients with articular prostheses or other small medical devices. The registration algorithm proposed here is general and, thus, extendable to other DMR scanners, reasonably resulting in a higher accuracy.

The registration approach proved to be almost insensitive to the initial pose provided by the operator. In the few cases in which the algorithm did not converge on the reference motion, the results were evidently wrong and not physiological, thus allowing the easy identification of possible errors. Finally, the experimental procedure shows a good repeatability, allowing longitudinal investigations.

The reconstructed knee kinematics agree well with previous measurements [19,20]. In particular, the tibia internal rotation and the femur roll back associated with flexion are easily observable for all the volunteers. The comparison between dynamic and static evaluation of knee kinematics shows differences smaller than what was reported in the literature [7]. It is worth noting that static scans were collected in weight-bearing conditions and that dynamic scans were recorded at slow speed, possibly reducing the differences, although part of them could be ascribed to the different measuring conditions. In general, however, it is possible to observe a reduction in the maximum flexion reached during dynamic measurements, which is possibly associated with adduction of the pelvis during static scans. It is worth noting that the maximum flexion value was dictated by the possible stroke of the hydraulic piston in the rig, which was kept above a safety value for this investigation. Future tests will extend the maximum achievable flexion.

The clinical application of DMRI could provide complementary information to what is obtainable with traditional MRI. The latter provides very accurate yet static images of the joint structures; on the other side, DMRI allows for the observation of the interaction of the elements that participate in an articulation during its function, providing a new level of knowledge. For example, laxity tests could be performed in DMRI, making it possible to directly observe the load response of injured ligaments. In general, a quantification of the relative bone motion makes it possible to find the measure of quantities not directly observable in-vivo. For example, the amplitude and location of articular contact areas during knee flexion can be reconstructed from the tibio-femoral kinematics, providing data that may help to better understand the etiology and development of pathologies such as osteoarthritis.

Aside from the direct clinical applications, this procedure for the in-vivo quantification of knee joint kinematics has very interesting biomechanical applications. Indeed, the possibility to measure the individual joint kinematics non-invasively and in-vivo will help in the definition and validation of patient-specific joint and musculoskeletal models [21–25].

The work has limitations. Acquisitions on the two DMRI planes used for 2D/3D registration were performed in a series. It is thus possible that the two acquired motions differ, introducing some errors in the reconstructed motion. The same kind of approximation is, however, done with traditional cine-MRI, where a cyclic motion is reconstructed from successive scans taken at different times in subsequent cycles. Only three knees were analyzed in this investigation. A wider study will establish the performance of the proposed procedure.

Future work will test the presented algorithm on data from a 1.5 T MR scanner. Other anatomical compartments will be also investigated.

Author Contributions: Conceptualization, M.C., N.S. and V.P.-C.; methodology, M.C. and F.D.C., N.S. and G.M.; data collection, M.C., F.D.C., N.S. and G.M.; software, M.C. and M.B.; validation, M.C. and M.B.; formal analysis, M.C., M.B. and N.S.; writing—original draft preparation, M.C., M.B. and N.S.; writing—review and editing, M.C., F.D.C., M.B., N.S., V.P.-C. and G.M. All authors have read and agreed to the published version of the manuscript.

Funding: This research received no external funding.

Institutional Review Board Statement: Not applicable.

Informed Consent Statement: Informed consent was obtained from all subjects involved in the study.

Data Availability Statement: Not applicable.

Conflicts of Interest: The authors declare no conflict of interest.

References

1. Storheim, K.; Zwart, J.-A. Musculoskeletal disorders and the Global Burden of Disease study. *Ann. Rheum. Dis.* **2014**, *73*, 949–950. [CrossRef] [PubMed]
2. Vos, T.; Allen, C.; Arora, M.; Barber, R.M.; Bhutta, Z.A.; Brown, A.; Carter, A.; Casey, D.C.; Charlson, F.J.; Chen, A.Z.; et al. Global, regional, and national incidence, prevalence, and years lived with disability for 310 diseases and injuries, 1990–2015: A systematic analysis for the Global Burden of Disease Study 2015. *Lancet* **2016**, *388*, 1545–1602. [CrossRef] [PubMed]
3. Prieto-Alhambra, D.; Judge, A.; Javaid, M.K.; Cooper, C.; Diez-Perez, A.; Arden, N.K. Incidence and risk factors for clinically diagnosed knee, hip and hand osteoarthritis: Influences of age, gender and osteoarthritis affecting other joints. *Ann. Rheum. Dis.* **2014**, *73*, 1659–1664. [CrossRef] [PubMed]

4. Mathiessen, A.; Cimmino, M.A.; Hammer, H.B.; Haugen, I.K.; Iagnocco, A.; Conaghan, P.G. Imaging of osteoarthritis (OA): What is new? *Best Pract. Res. Clin. Rheumatol.* **2016**, *30*, 653–669. [CrossRef] [PubMed]
5. Wang, X.; Oo, W.M.; Linklater, J.M. What is the role of imaging in the clinical diagnosis of osteoarthritis and disease management? *Rheumatology* **2018**, *57*, iv51–iv60. [CrossRef] [PubMed]
6. Shapiro, L.M.; Gold, G.E. MRI of weight bearing and movement. *Osteoarthr. Cartil.* **2012**, *20*, 69–78. [CrossRef] [PubMed]
7. d'Entremont, A.G.; Nordmeyer-Massner, J.A.; Bos, C.; Wilson, D.R.; Pruessmann, K.P. Do dynamic-based MR knee kinematics methods produce the same results as static methods? *Magn. Reson. Med.* **2013**, *69*, 1634–1644. [CrossRef]
8. Draper, C.E.; Santos, J.M.; Kourtis, L.C.; Besier, T.F.; Fredericson, M.; Beaupre, G.S.; Gold, G.E.; Delp, S.L. Feasibility of using real-time MRI to measure joint kinematics in 1.5 T and open-bore 0.5 T systems. *J. Magn. Reson. Imaging* **2008**, *28*, 158–166. [CrossRef]
9. Shellock, F.G.; Mink, J.H.; Deutsch, A.L.; Foo, T.K.; Sullenberger, P. Patellofemoral joint: Identification of abnormalities with active-movement, "unloaded" versus "loaded" kinematic MR imaging techniques. *Radiology* **1993**, *188*, 575–578. [CrossRef]
10. McWalter, E.J.; Hunter, D.J.; Wilson, D.R. The effect of load magnitude on three-dimensional patellar kinematics in vivo. *J. Biomech.* **2010**, *43*, 1890–1897. [CrossRef]
11. Garetier, M.; Borotikar, B.; Makki, K.; Brochard, S.; Rousseau, F.; Salem, D.B. Dynamic MRI for articulating joint evaluation on 1.5 T and 3.0 T scanners: Setup, protocols, and real-time sequences. *Insights Imaging* **2020**, *11*, 66. [CrossRef] [PubMed]
12. Guillin, R.; Marchand, A.J.; Roux, A.; Niederberger, E.; Duvauferrier, R. Imaging of snapping phenomena. *Brit. J. Radiol.* **2012**, *85*, 1343–1353. [CrossRef] [PubMed]
13. Li, G.; Van de Velde, S.K.; Bingham, J.T. Validation of a non-invasive fluoroscopic imaging technique for the measurement of dynamic knee joint motion. *J. Biomech.* **2008**, *41*, 1616–1622. [CrossRef] [PubMed]
14. Teixeira, P.A.G.; Gervaise, A.; Louis, M.; Raymond, A.; Formery, A.-S.; Lecocq, S.; Blum, A. Musculoskeletal wide-detector CT kinematic evaluation: From motion to image. *Semin. Musculoskelet. Radiol.* **2015**, *19*, 456–462.
15. Borotikar, B.; Lempereur, M.; Lelievre, M.; Burdin, V.; Ben Salem, D.; Brochard, S. Dynamic MRI to quantify musculoskeletal motion: A systematic review of concurrent validity and reliability, and perspectives for evaluation of musculoskeletal disorders. *PLoS ONE* **2017**, *12*, e0189587. [CrossRef]
16. Tashman, S.; Anderst, W. In-vivo measurement of dynamic joint motion using high speed biplane radiography and CT: Application to canine ACL deficiency. *J. Biomech. Eng.* **2003**, *125*, 238–245. [CrossRef]
17. Grood, E.S.; Suntay, W.J. A joint coordinate system for the clinical description of three-dimensional motions: Application to the knee. *J. Biomech. Eng.* **1983**, *105*, 136–144. [CrossRef]
18. Draper, C.E.; Besier, T.F.; Fredericson, M.; Santos, J.M.; Beaupre, G.S.; Delp, S.L.; Gold, G.E. Differences in patellofemoral kinematics between weight-bearing and non-weight-bearing conditions in patients with patellofemoral pain. *J. Ortho. Res.* **2011**, *29*, 312–317. [CrossRef]
19. Gasparutto, X.; Moissenet, F.; Lafon, Y.; Cheze, L.; Dumas, R. Kinematics of the normal knee during dynamic activities: A synthesis of data from intracortical pins and biplane imaging. *Appl. Bionics. Biomech.* **2017**, *2017*, 1908618. [CrossRef]
20. Conconi, M.; Sancisi, N.; Parenti-Castelli, V. The geometrical arrangement of knee constraints that makes natural motion possible: Theoretical and experimental analysis. *J. Biomech. Eng.* **2019**, *141*, 051001. [CrossRef]
21. Conconi, M.; Sancisi, N.; Parenti-Castelli, V. Prediction of Individual Knee Kinematics From an MRI Representation of the Articular Surfaces. *IEEE Trans. Biomed. Eng.* **2020**, *68*, 1084–1092. [CrossRef] [PubMed]
22. Conconi, M.; Sancisi, N.; Parenti-Castelli, V. Exploiting Reciprocity Between Constraints and Instantaneous Motion to Reconstruct Individual Knee Kinematics. In *Advances in Robot Kinematics*; Springer: Cham, Switzerland, 2022.
23. Smale, K.B.; Conconi, M.; Sancisi, N.; Krogsgaard, M.; Alkjaer, T.; Parenti-Castelli, V.; Benoit, D.L. Effect of implementing magnetic resonance imaging for patient-specific OpenSim models on lower-body kinematics and knee ligament lengths. *J. Biomech.* **2019**, *83*, 9–15. [CrossRef] [PubMed]
24. Martelli, S.; Sancisi, N.; Conconi, M.; Pandy, M.G.; Kersh, M.E.; Parenti-Castelli, V.; Reynolds, K.J. The relationship between tibiofemoral geometry and musculoskeletal function during normal activity. *Gait Posture* **2020**, *80*, 374–382. [CrossRef]
25. Nardini, F.; Belvedere, C.; Sancisi, N.; Conconi, M.; Leardini, A.; Durante, S.; Parenti-Castelli, V. An anatomical-based subject-specific model of in-vivo knee joint 3D kinematics from medical imaging. *App. Sci.* **2020**, *10*, 2100. [CrossRef]

Disclaimer/Publisher's Note: The statements, opinions and data contained in all publications are solely those of the individual author(s) and contributor(s) and not of MDPI and/or the editor(s). MDPI and/or the editor(s) disclaim responsibility for any injury to people or property resulting from any ideas, methods, instructions or products referred to in the content.

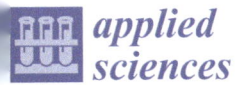

Perspective

Recent Innovations Brought about by Weight-Bearing CT Imaging in the Foot and Ankle: A Systematic Review of the Literature

François Lintz [1,*], Cesar de Cesar Netto [2], Claudio Belvedere [3], Alberto Leardini [3], Alessio Bernasconi [4] and on behalf of the International Weight-Bearing CT Society

1. Department of Foot and Ankle Surgery, Ramsay Healthcare Clinique de l'Union, 31240 Saint Jean, France
2. Department of Orthopedics, Duke University of Medicine, Durham, NC 27710, USA
3. Movement Analysis Laboratory, IRCCS Istituto Ortopedico Rizzoli, 40136 Bologna, Italy; alberto.leardini@ior.it (A.L.)
4. Department of Orthopedic Surgery, Federico II University Hospital, 80131 Napoli, Italy
* Correspondence: dr.f.lintz@gmail.com

Citation: Lintz, F.; de Cesar Netto, C.; Belvedere, C.; Leardini, A.; Bernasconi, A.; on behalf of the International Weight-bearing CT Society. Recent Innovations Brought about by Weight-Bearing CT Imaging in the Foot and Ankle: A Systematic Review of the Literature. *Appl. Sci.* 2024, 14, 5562. https://doi.org/10.3390/app14135562

Academic Editor: Roger Narayan

Received: 19 March 2024
Revised: 8 June 2024
Accepted: 21 June 2024
Published: 26 June 2024

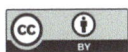

Copyright: © 2024 by the authors. Licensee MDPI, Basel, Switzerland. This article is an open access article distributed under the terms and conditions of the Creative Commons Attribution (CC BY) license (https://creativecommons.org/licenses/by/4.0/).

Abstract: The decade from 2010–2020 has seen the development of cone beam weight-bearing CT (WBCT) as a major innovation in the foot and ankle realm, becoming an important modality for bone and joint imaging. The ability to provide three-dimensional images of the naturally loaded skeleton has enabled several subsequent innovations to arise with aims to hasten image processing and to extend the clinical applications of WBCT. The objective of this work was to identify, categorize and explain those emerging techniques. We performed a structured review of the literature according to PRISMA standards, finally including 50 studies. We subsequently proposed a classification of these techniques. Segmentation and distance mapping were identified as key features. We conclude that although WBCT has already been adopted in a number of clinical communities with an immediate improvement in patient workflows, adoption of advanced techniques is yet to come. However, that relies mostly not on the technology itself, but on improvements in AI software allowing practitioners to quickly process images in daily practice and enabling the clinicians to obtain an accurate three-dimensional evaluation of the segment considered. Standardization will be paramount to amass large amounts of comparable data, which will fuel further innovations in a potentially virtuous circle.

Keywords: cone beam CT; weight-bearing CT; distance mapping; coverage maps; automatic segmentation; 3D biometrics; systematic review

1. Introduction

Among computed tomography (CT) techniques, cone beam CT (CBCT) provides three-plane tomography, radiography and 3D reconstructions in a single high-speed, versatile package which can image the entire human skeleton. As an identified technique, it was first published in the journal European Radiology in 1998 for use in the dental arena, following the works of a team led by P. Mozzo from the Department of Medical Physics at the University of Verona, Italy [1]. The dental field has since then become one of the most important uses of the technology, but it was not the first citation of cone beam in the literature, which dates back to 1979 [2], nor the first clinical application, which was in the vascular domain due to its ability to visualize highly contrasted material [3]. The technology is inspired by the mathematical concepts initiated by Hounsfield for parallel fan beam or multi-detector CT (MDCT) [4] using the Fourier and Radon transforms to produce spatially referenced slices of the anatomy. Later, in 1984, Feldkamp [5] described an algorithm based on convolution and back-projection designed to help with reconstruction of acquisitions with incomplete rotations, triggering the possibility of more practical and flexible gantry systems.

In orthopedics, the research around CBCT was initiated by Bab et al. [6] in 2001, for whom intended clinical uses were to be in orthopedic and chest applications. The first dedicated use in orthopedics was described in 2011 by Zbijewski et al. [7]. The first mention of a dedicated extremity CBCT device was by Muhit et al. in 2012 [8], and the first mention of weight-bearing CBCT (WBCT) in the lower limbs was in 2013 by Tuominen et al. [9]. The first mention of WBCT in the foot and ankle concerned the pes planovalgus [10], but that was simulated weight-bearing. The first publications on the use of true (i.e., under body weight) WBCT in the foot and ankle were in 2013 by Collan et al. [11] on the biomechanics of the first ray, followed by Richter in 2014 on the superiority of 3D WBCT measurements as compared to 2D or non-weight-bearing WBCT [12].

A quick look at the literature suggests that WBCT would allow clinicians to optimize acquisition speed, therefore reducing operating costs, with a smaller footprint compared to traditional two-dimensional radiography (2DXR) plus three-dimensional non weight-bearing fan beam MDCT in diverse areas [7,8,13–34]. This would enable clinicians to obtain marked improvements in the operative workflow [32,35]. Besides advantages for the clinicians, immediate advantages for patients are also huge time gains in their care pathway [32], more accurate diagnoses (i.e., increased chances of detecting injuries commonly missed through standard imaging) [12,30] and lower radiation doses [32,36,37] (Figure 1).

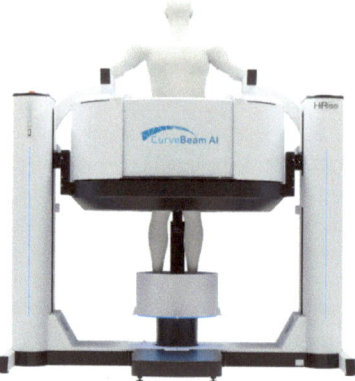

Figure 1. Example of a WBCT device with flexible gantry and ability to acquire the whole lower limb and the upper limb up to the elbow, including (HiRise™, image courtesy of CurvebeamAI, Hatfield, PA, USA).

However, it also seems that the advantages of CBCT are somewhat overshadowed by the weight-bearing side of the equation, since not many authors have focused on non-weight-bearing cone beam imaging so far [29,30,32,38]. Indeed, it is in the foot and ankle field that the industry has chosen to chase initial prospects, likely because this is where 3D combined with weight-bearing have shown the most evident improvements over the conventional 2DXR-MDCT sequence. In turn, this was due to the complex anatomy of the foot, including 28 bones with a variety of shapes and sizes, making it hard to correctly assess without 3D or without bearing weight [12]. A large body of literature preceding the WBCT period has already insisted on the importance of weight-bearing while imaging the foot and ankle, using custom devices to simulate weight-bearing with conventional prone MDCT protocols [10]. The advent of WBCT has since been seen as a step forward for clinicians and researchers specializing in the feet and ankles from the fields of orthopedics, biomechanics and engineering, soon reaching out to scientific societies and computer scientists [15], while new software companies have emerged to capitalize on the possibilities offered by WBCT. The vast majority of the innovations reported in this review are issued from a collaboration between the main stakeholders (WBCT manufacturers, clinicians and engineers) to solve problems regarding musculoskeletal pathology, for the ultimate benefit of patients. They are the result of the development of post-processing visualization (qualitative assessment) or measurement (quantitative assessment) software to make the best use of the available naturally 3D weight-bearing datasets.

In 2016, the International WBCT Study Group was formed on the initiative of pioneering researchers and officially institutionalized as an independent international non-profit scientific association based in Ghent, Belgium in 2017 and re-named the International WBCT Society (https://www.wbctsociety.org, accessed on 5 January 2024). It has since then, amongst other activities, been closely monitoring all relevant scientific publications on the subject, which has since seen an exponential growth. The object of the present review is to report, classify and explain the most recent innovations brought about by WBCT in the foot and ankle field, with a critical discussion of the evidence provided so far in terms of advantages, limitations and future areas of development.

2. Materials and Methods

This is a systematic review of the recent innovations brought by WBCT to the foot and ankle field. In order to specify the scope of the review, we defined 'recent' as after 2012, the year Muhit et al. [8] published the first paper on a dedicated extremity CBCT device. We defined innovative techniques as techniques which could not be performed using the conventional 2DXR-MDCT sequence (i.e., absence of concomitant 3D and natural weight-bearing). This would, in theory, include conventional measurements historically performed on weight-bearing 2DXR, performed on 3D WBCT datasets, for instance the first to second intermetatarsal angle [39] in the forefoot, or the Saltzman angle [14] in the hindfoot. In fact, most WBCT devices have the ability to produce digitally reconstructed radiographs (DRR) [40] to help with the user's learning curve in transitioning from the 2D to the 3D environment. This is possible because WBCT produces a digital clone of the patient's foot and ankle structure, which can in turn be virtually radiographed from multiple angles (Figure 2).

Classical measurements can therefore be performed in a standard way. However, this technique inevitably produces the same biases as conventional 2DXR. Otherwise, classical angles can be measured within the 3D dataset, using multiplanar reconstruction (MPR) views. In this case, a particular slice or slab must be chosen in order to perform the measurement, which requires multiple iterative changes in the orientation of the MPR, because the points which define the angles of interest are not necessarily on the same plane. For instance, the tibia longitudinal axis, the center of the ankle joint and the lowest weight-bearing point of the calcaneus do not belong to a single vertical plane. For the corresponding angle to be measured manually, a slice has to be found by tuning the orientation of the MPR dataset, but again, it is often not possible to find a slice which includes all three points. Another possibility is to select one segment of the angle (the tibia axis) on one plane and compare it to the other side (the calcaneal axis) using the available software, but measuring a single angle from different slices is not always an available function. A third method consists of manually recording 3D coordinates for the points of interest (in the present example, the tibia extremity and the center of the ankle joint's lowest calcaneal point) and calculating the angle using standard trigonometry. Whatever the solution or combination of solutions, this method is always time-consuming [41] and introduces a new kind of bias, which we may call 'slice' or 'slab' bias, materializing as we must choose a particular slice from which to take the measurements, based on surface landmarks which may vary, being dependent on the operator's habits or knowledge of the anatomy. Although these methods were and are still necessary to perform and describe throughout the process of standardization of measurement methods in WBCT research [15], they inevitably present practical disadvantages which prevent inclusion in the advanced methods review, for we aimed to describe here methods which actually improve the clinical workflow, not slow it down. Hence, articles describing such methods were not included for retrieval.

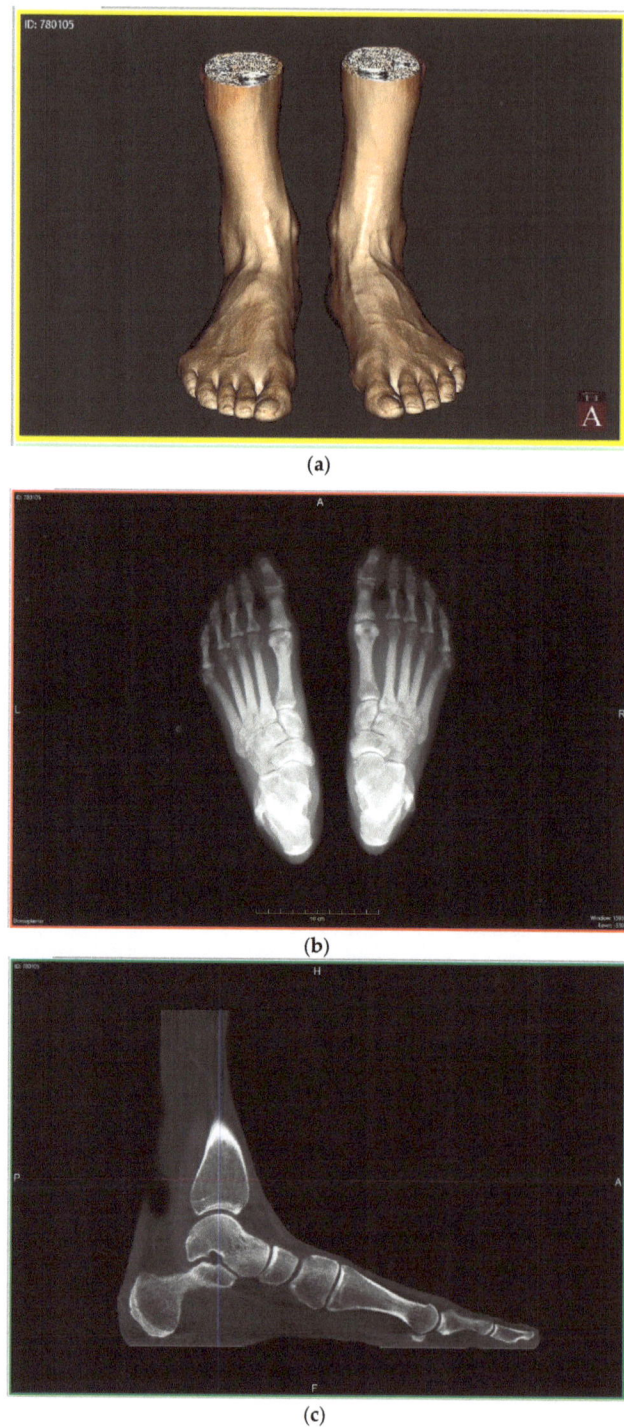

Figure 2. Example of a WBCT digital clone with skin rendering (**a**), digitally reconstructed dorsal-plantar radiograph (**b**) and saggital MPR view (**c**).

The PubMed database was used to identify relevant scientific references for the study. We included initially all references regarding CBCT and weight-bearing or WBCT, using the following key words: weightbearing, weight-bearing, standing, extremity, cone beam, CT, computed tomography, multiplanar, foot, ankle, ankle joint, ankle, joint, ankle joint, ankle. Filters were used to exclude references without an abstract or which were not available in English, French or German. Screening was then performed by two independent reviewers (FL and AB, both senior orthopedic foot and ankle consultants) at different places and times. No automated tool was used for this research. In cases of disagreement between the reviewers, inclusion or exclusion of the concerned references was resolved through discussion, and inclusion was retained only upon agreement by the two reviewers. Articles of interest were then retrieved for analysis.

Since this study describes innovative methods and does not report or meta-analyze numerical data from patients such as demographic or clinical data, no statistical method was applied. A review of the study protocol by our institutional review board was not deemed applicable.

3. Results

3.1. Pre-Screening

A total of 212 studies were initially identified. Five references were excluded at this stage due to returning results clearly outside of the scope of the study such as equine standing CT. At the end of the selection process, 50 studies were included as reported in the dedicated PRISMA-compliant (Preferred Reporting Items for Systematic Reviews and Meta-Analysis) flow chart [42] (Figure 3). The median and mean sample size were 31 and 59 cases, respectively (range from 1 to 500 cases).

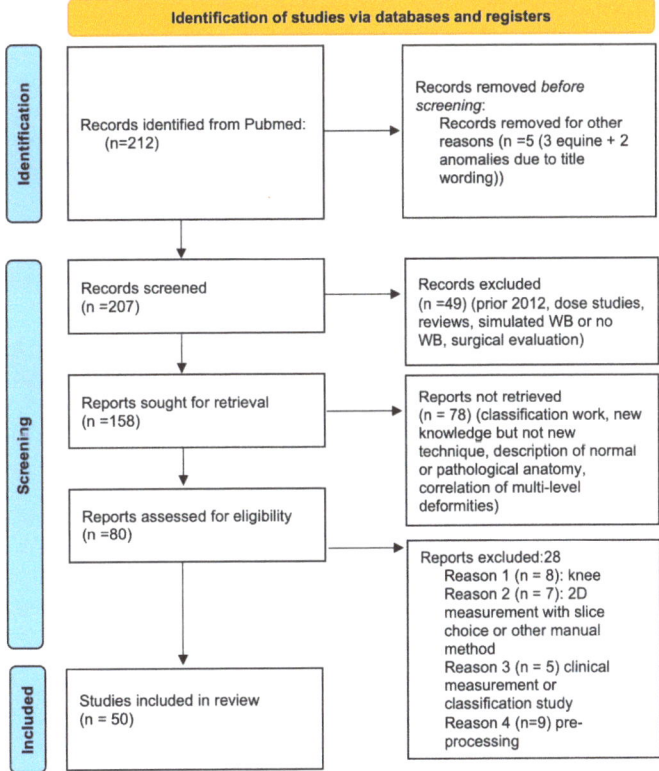

Figure 3. PRISMA type flow chart: all excluded studies were excluded by human intervention. No automated tool was used.

3.2. Screening

A total of 207 references were screened. Forty-nine studies were excluded based on the following criteria:
- Studies prior to 2012
- Studies of radiation dosage
- Simulated weight-bearing or absence thereof
- Use of WBCT for evaluation of surgical results without innovative methods

A total of 158 references were sought for retrieval. Seventy-eight further references were excluded based on the following criteria:
- WBCT classifications
- New knowledge but absence of an innovative technique
- Description of normal or pathological anatomy
- Multi-level biomechanical investigation

A total of 80 references were assessed for eligibility. A further 28 references were excluded based on the following criteria:
- Innovative WBCT techniques; study concerning the knee (8 studies)
- Two-dimensional method performed within 3D volume (7 studies)
- Clinical measurement or classification study (5 studies)
- Pre-processing techniques (9 studies)

3.3. Organization of the WBCT Workflow: Proposal for a Classification of Recent Innovations

A critical analysis of the 50 studies included enabled the authors to classify recent innovative techniques brought about by WBCT in the foot and ankle into categories. These categories are based on the nature of the innovations and on their positioning within the patient or image processing workflows. Some of these are identified in italic fonts below as hypotheses from the authors, based on the literature that was excluded from this specific work because it did not directly apply to our object, but which could in theory be applied to the foot and ankle field. For clarity, we included these in the classification, as well as pre-processing techniques in the initial exhaustive screening of the literature summarized and referenced hereunder.

- Techniques for image acquisition
  - Dynamic/augmented stress techniques
    - Ankle instability
      - Shod auto-varus [43]
      - Angled jigs/wedges [43]
    - Syndesmotic instability
      - Torque stress
    - Coleman block test [19]
  - Static techniques
    - Combination with pedography [44]
- Computerized techniques for image processing
  - Pre-processing (processing of the raw data before image rendering)
    - *Metal artifact reduction*
    - *Movement Artifact reduction*
  - Post-processing
    - 3D biometric techniques without segmentation
      - Manual
        - Linear HU assessment of joint space width [25]
        - Middle subtalar facet uncoverage [45]

- Automatic/semi-automatic:
  - Foot–ankle offset [19,44,46–48]
- 3D biometric techniques with segmentation (manual, semi-auto or auto)
  - Segmentation techniques
    - Statistical shape modelling (SSM) [49]
    - Mimics (materialization) [27,50,51]
    - CurvebeamAI [52]
    - Disior/Paragon [16,21,26,53–56]
  - Advanced techniques issued from segmentation (semi-automatic or fully automatic)
    - 3D bone absolute and relative relationships reporting [16,21,22,26,52–64]
    - 3D Joint space width (3D-JSW) mapping: distance mapping [65–69]
    - Coverage mapping [70]
    - Surface measurements
      - Syndesmosis [17]
      - Lisfranc [71]
    - Volumetric measurements
      - Syndesmosis [49,72–74]
      - Lisfranc [71]
    - Center of rotation assessment [75]
- Advanced clinical applications derived from computerized techniques
  - Customized/patient specific surgical jigs [76]
    - Supra malleolar osteotomy [18]
    - Total ankle replacement [77]
  - *Robotic surgical protocols*
  - Personalized risk assessment [47]

Following this exhaustive screening of the literature, the authors proposed a systematic classification of the WBCT computerized workflow to illustrate the role of each advanced technique associated with its development (Figure 4).

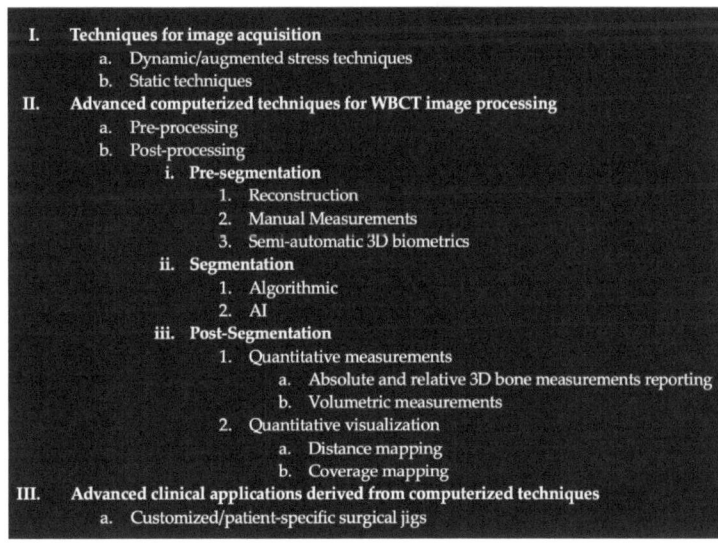

Figure 4. Proposed simplified classification of WBCT advanced technique workflow.

4. Discussion

The present systematic review found that recent innovations reported in WBCT literature are mostly post-segmentation techniques. The most reported tools aim to provide quantitative 3D bone positions, followed by visualization tools, the most frequently reported being joint space mapping or equivalents. Segmentation is not in itself an innovation, nor is it a clinically applicable method, but its implementation is an indispensable step in the development of innovations bearing the fruits of WBCT dissemination.

4.1. Limits

We acknowledge several limits in the present work. Firstly, the quality of a literature review is only scientifically as good as the quality of reviewed research, which is valid for every 'secondary' study. The level of evidence considered here being mostly level III (with the exception of a single level II study [41]), with level IV and V studies as well, our systematic review can be considered level V. However, given the research available on recent innovations in WBCT concerning imaging, most investigations can be performed ex vivo, rendering level II and level I research mostly superfluous. Furthermore, being at the diagnostic level for most (with the exception of patient-specific applications), the impact on treatment outcomes is still very difficult to assess, being a multifactorial problem with implications that spread out through a timescale that far exceeds the development of innovations that we chose to define as recent. Secondly, not all available research databases were assessed, as we limited the scope of this review to the records found on a single scientific database (PubMed). However, this method was chosen after a preliminary search of the most used other databases (Embase, Cochrane, Scopus, Web of Science) which did not lead to find any additional reference related to the development of WBCT. Thirdly, our classification of advanced techniques could be deemed arbitrary. However, we would like to emphasize that, to the best of our knowledge, no author so far has proposed any specific classification system in this area, so the present is intended as a proposal for a flexible benchmark to work from, not the immutable ground truth. The authors would be happy to revise or replace the proposed classification as progress is made, new methods arise and the technical landscape evolves in the future. Finally, we have only considered the foot and ankle field in the present work, but we fully acknowledge that WBCT devices already encompass the knee [20,65,78], with devices already available to image the pelvis and the upper limbs. There is no doubt that soon, devices able to image the full weight-bearing skeleton will be available. In this context, there is no doubt that, pending necessary adaptations locally, the recent innovations reported here will be disseminated to other joints, including the spine and the shoulders. One well-reported example is distance or 3D-JSW mapping, which has been reported on in the knees as well as the feet and ankles and should in the future become the gold standard for the evaluation of degenerative joint disease.

4.2. Literature Analysis

In light of the present systematic review, the most important fact to report is that segmentation is key to enabling the development of innovative techniques from WBCT datasets. Moreover, if these innovations are to be translated into clinically applicable solutions, it is paramount for fast and reproducible automatic segmentation methods to be available so that interpretation times remain possible within the clinical workflow. Furthermore, the push towards standardization of segmentation and measurement methods [15,60] initiated by scientific societies such as the International WBCT Society, the Orthopedic Research Society and the International Society of Biomechanics is of utmost importance if a disseminated acceptance of these innovative techniques and clinical solutions is to be achieved.

4.2.1. Description of Techniques for Image Acquisition

Within the WBCT workflow, techniques for image acquisition are used to dynamically position the patient under physiological load during acquisition to improve detection of designated pathologies. The most investigated one, syndesmotic instability [17,79,80], has cadaveric and clinical studies showing that, due to the configuration of the distal tibiofibular joint and the injury mechanism, external torque potentializes the diagnostic capabilities of WBCT. Without this stress test and if no post-processing is applied, WBCT does not appear to be superior to MDCT in diagnostic terms, although it already is in terms of radiation and time spent in the workflow. This occurs only if manual, one-dimensional measurements are taken. However, post-processing techniques such as distance mapping of the syndesmosis and surface or volumetric measurements described below have re-established this superiority.

The Coleman block test Is reported In a level IV study Investigating hindfoot alignment in cavovarus feet using clinical examination, radiographic views assessing the hindfoot angle and WBCT assessment of the foot–ankle offset [19], showing correlation between the 3 modalities.

In another level V report [43], the use of shod auto-varus is reported in the diagnosis of lateral ankle instability and suggests the use of standardized jigs to induce a normalized amount of varus or valgus depending on the target diagnosis (Figure 5).

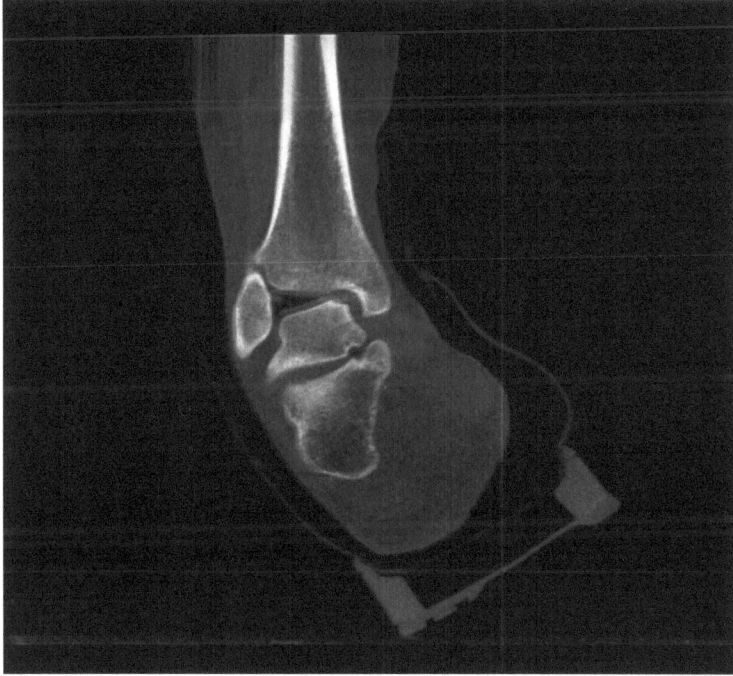

Figure 5. Example of a coronal plane MPR (multiplanar reconstruction) view following shod auto-varus in a case of lateral ankle instability with laxity.

Techniques for image acquisition also included static methods for acquiring more data. In a level III study, Richter et al. used a built-in pedography sensor [44] to assess the position of the center of pressure and compared it to the result of the foot–ankle offset (as anatomical foot center) in 90 patients (180 feet). They found an average distance between the two centers at 28.7 mm, being the anatomical foot center distal to the center of pressure in 175 feet and lateral to it in 112 feet. No significant medio-lateral differences were found. It could be anticipated that more sensors investigating weight or bone density could be used in the future to increase semeiology during WBCT acquisition. This could be useful in assessing bone health or pressure points in diabetic patients, for example, or more simply to standardize positioning of patients within the WBCT machine during acquisition. This issue has been taken into account by the industry, using specific gentry to standardize positioning, especially in the knee, but the reproducibility seems to remain questionable, as has been reported recently by a group of radiology researchers [15].

4.2.2. Description of Advanced Computerized Techniques for Image Processing

Pre-Processing

Pre-processing techniques involve the raw file that contains the patient dataset before it is processed to obtain interpretable multiplanar images. WBCT is a computerized tomography technique, meaning that the raw file is treated like a 3D stack of 2D slices. Unlike MDCT, in which it is the case because the acquisition requires 'slicing' up the anatomy with a 'flat', 0.5–0.8 mm-thick fan-shaped X-ray beam, WBCT acquisition results in a single raw file considered isotropic (the image definition is the same in all dimensions of space), due to the cone-shaped beam. Pre-processing has the single raw file as input and outputs a stack of 2D 0.2–0.4 mm slices in the form of DICOM files.

Other examples of pre-processing steps are metal artifact and movement reduction algorithms. They are based on highly specialized mathematical algorithms with the aim of improving the general quality of images and thus diagnostics.

Post-Processing

1. Pre-Segmentation
2. Reconstruction

The initial post-processing is performed by the WBCT device manufacturer's software (https://curvebeamai.com/products/cubevue-software/download-cubevue/, accessed on 5 January 2024) to obtain interpretable multiplanar images, usually presented in multiplanar reconstruction format, with three viewing windows corresponding to the three planes of space (two vertical planes, coronal and sagittal; and one horizontal, axial plane) sometimes including a fourth window with a 3D volume rendering view (Figure 6).

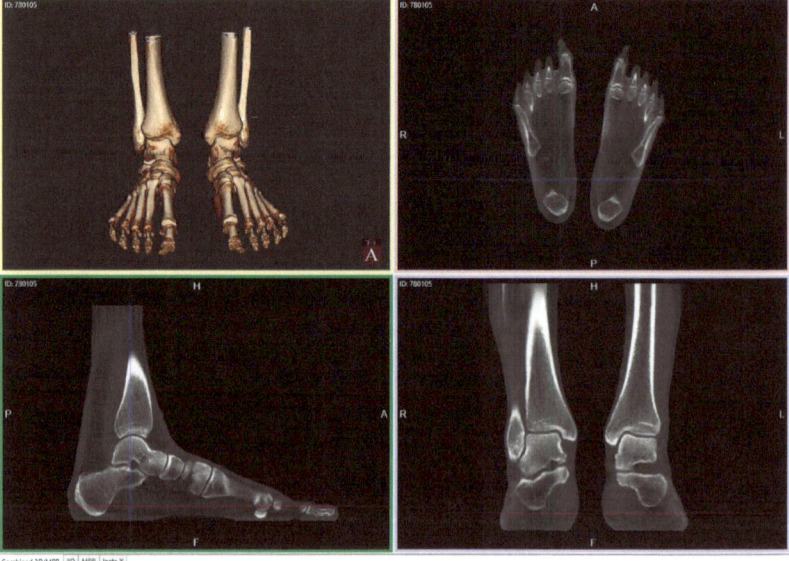

Figure 6. Example of a full MPR rendering with coronal, sagittal and axial views and a 3D fourth window.

After this process, advanced post-processing techniques are subsequently applied to provide recent innovations.

3. Manual Measurements

At this stage, classical measurements can be made manually, despite, as described earlier, inducing 'slice bias'. Innovative solutions for manual measurements include the measurement of middle facet uncoverage in progressive collapsing foot deformities and the measurement of joint space width in ankle osteoarthritis using variations in contrast (measured in Hounsfield units (Hus)) [25,45].

4. Semi-Automatic 3D Biometrics

The most reported post-processing, pre-segmentation semi-automatic tool is Cubeview Talas® (Curvebeam AI, Hatfield, PA, USA), which automatically gives the foot–ankle offset (FAO), a 3D biometric hindfoot alignment measurement, after manual identification of four anatomical landmarks: the weight-bearing points of M1 and M5, the calcaneus bones and the center of the ankle joint. Its result is given as a percentage offset of the foot length, which corresponds to the coronal offset between the center of the ankle joint and the bisector of the forefoot passing through the calcaneus weight-bearing point (Figure 7).

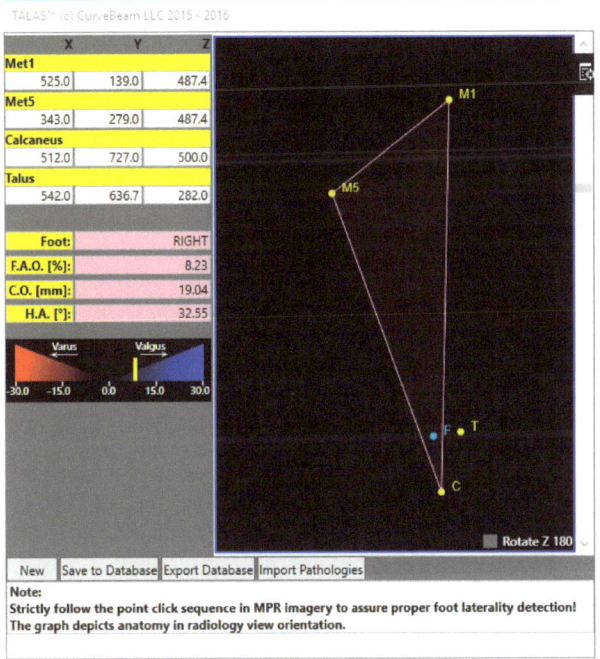

Figure 7. Example of a foot–ankle offset (FAO) measurement report using Talas® system (CurvebeamAI, Hatfield, PA, USA). FAO is a 3D biometric hindfoot alignment measurement which is calculated as a percentage after manual identification of four anatomical landmarks (the weight-bearing points of the first metatarsal (M1) and fifth metatarsal (M5), the calcaneus bones (C) and the center of the ankle joint (T)).

The FAO has proven to be an effective hindfoot alignment measurement [48], and from it originated the concept of 3D biometrics, in which a minimum of four points are required to obtain volumetric (3D) rather than surface, angular or linear measurements. Its intra- and interobserver reliability is improved compared to conventional 2D measurements [47,48] by levels nearing 100%, and its correlation with pathologies such as chronic lateral ankle instability [47] and PCFD has proven excellent. This is thought to be because the FAO takes into account the torsional effect of the forefoot on the hindfoot, unlike traditional measurements which only look at the alignment of the tibia versus the hindfoot. It may therefore be more sensitive in its ability to correlate with specific multidimensional pathologies like predicting the need for realignment osteotomies in total ankle replacement [81] or the risk of periprosthetic cysts [82]. However, it remains a measurement of hindfoot alignment and does not assess sub-level type deformities: it is not a diagnostic tool. Other techniques based on the traditional 2DXR-MDCT literature remain for now the only tools to allow for this [14,83].

5. Segmentation

We identified automatic segmentation techniques as the basis of other recent innovations [84,85]. It appears indispensable because the time required to perform manual segmentation is too much for clinical applications, confining potential innovations to the research area. The important word in 'automatic segmentation' is therefore 'segmentation', but this also turns out to be the most complicated to achieve.

Segmentation is the process by which individual bones are outlined and labelled. When segmentation is carried out manually, every single bone (28 in a single foot) must be manually outlined on every slice (up to 1000 per dataset), which amounts to 28,000 operations per foot, or 46,000 per bilateral scan. In practice, it generally takes 30 min to segment the hindfoot bones and 2 h to segment the whole foot and ankle [86]. It is therefore paramount that fast and reproducible automatic segmentation software become widely available. In that case, studies report that the same process can take a little as a few seconds [53]. The present review found four reported techniques or software solutions. These initially used automatic contouring based on contrast definition, evolving to more advanced techniques, ultimately aided by proprietary solutions. The two most reported in the literature are Bonelogics® (Disior Oy, then Paragon28) and Cubeview® (Curveabeam AI). Although much of their inner work remains undisclosed, the industry advertises that they rely on a combination of algorithms and artificial intelligence (AI) (i.e., to automatically identify bones, to reproduce surgical procedures such as osteotomies or arthroplasties and to run automatic measurements in order to anticipate which gestures are needed to obtain the desired alignment). Throughout the process, it is reported that some of the reasons for the failure of the automatic segmentation are the presence of metalwork; poor bone quality or the presence of arthritic joints leading to areas of contact between bones; and the misinterpretation of two touching bones as a single structure [52]. One important step in the segmentation process is the smoothing of bone contours. This is the equivalent of noise reduction in digital photography: smoothing reduces the risk of two touching bones being misinterpreted as a single one but results in a (marginal) reduction of the quantity of data. The AI training process helps in dealing with the aforementioned contouring issues as well as learning to correctly label the bones. It makes more sense from a practical and industrial standpoint to build a system that can label the anatomy and then produce all relevant measurements, rather than build multiple systems to perform each measurement. It transpires that large amounts of data are necessary to efficiently train these AIs, which will need to be scientifically evaluated by independent entities on a regular basis until satisfactory performance is reached. There is unequivocal agreement on this amongst authors and stakeholders [15,52,53].

Post-Segmentation

Once segmentation is achieved, a digital clone of the foot and ankle is created with all bones correctly labelled. Therefore, any measurement may be performed automatically, since all the spatial coordinates of all the voxels (the 3D equivalent of 2D pixels) are known, with all of them having been grouped into separated voxel clouds corresponding to the individual bones. Using these data and stepping up from classical measurements, new tools have been reported on in the literature to improve visualization and our comprehension of pathological processes. We present these below:

1. Absolute and Relative 3D Bone Measurement Reporting

Theoretically, an infinite number of measurements are possible, hence the diversity of measurements described in this area of the literature [16,21,22,26,52–64]. In more practical terms, considering there are on average 28 bones in the foot and ankle, each with a center of mass that has three spatial coordinates and three inertial vectors each, with each having three spatial coordinates, each bone may be described by a set of 12 'absolute' coordinates, which are calculated within the WBCT frame of reference (Figure 8).

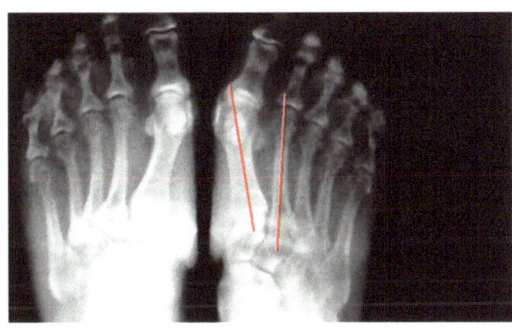

Figure 8. Example of a foot automatic measurement report (Disior OY/Paragon 28, Denver, CO, USA); (**a**) example of M1-M2 angle illustration; (**b**) example of forefoot measurement automated report.

This frame is referenced by the floor plane for the two vertical (sagittal and coronal) planes. There is no consensus on how to set the rotation in the axial plane, but the most commonly used is traditionally the second metatarsal or the bisector of the forefoot in 3D biometrics papers [48]. However, the possibility of relative measurements is remote, as any of the 12 absolute coordinates in each of the 28 bones can be described relative to any of the 12 absolute coordinates of the 27 other bones, which equates to 12^{27} possibilities. This huge number explains why there has always been a quest to discover new measurements in the realm of musculoskeletal research. Things were easier with 2D radiography, which results in dimensional reduction, thus reducing the possible number of measurements, albeit with a non-negligible loss of information. After the introduction of WBCT, a need has arisen to find and promote a standardized methodology for describing bone orientations in space, which is among the tasks of the International WBCT society mentioned above. However, the industry has anticipated this and is already proposing different off-the-shelf software solutions to provide systematic reporting of bone and joint angles, based on the historical literature, including such widely used angles as the M1-M2 angle for hallux valgus assessment, or the hindfoot alignment angle for deformity assessment. However, even these may be defined differently depending on the software provider, hence the importance and urgency of an international consensus on this matter so that reports may be comparable across all software platforms. There are many reasons for these differences, not the least being the absence of consensus in the existing literature. Other reasons pertain to computerized techniques used to obtain absolute measurements [60].

The 3 main techniques reported are as follows [87].

1—Principal component analysis (PCA) determines the center of mass and the three principal components or inertial axes of the bones through averaging the relative contributions of each spatial dimension, a rather common mathematical tool, but still complex to the layperson. Its advantage is that it can easily be made fully automatic. Its disadvantage is that it provides slightly different results depending on the volumetric shape of considered bones, which can be otherwise interpreted as increased variability in measuring anatomical axes depending on surface landmarks.

2—Statistical shape modelling averages a large number of real-life examples from pre-existing datasets of bones to create a library to which a given bone may then be compared. Once the bone has been recognized, its orientation can be derived from that of the library example. This technique is usually part of the segmentation process itself. Its disadvantages are that it depends on the existence of a large enough patient dataset library and it cannot consider a situation which is not already known within the library.

3—Fitting of geometric primitives averages the different parts of bones by fitting the closest 3D geometrical figure. For example, a long bone diaphysis may be approximated to a cylinder and its base and head to a truncated cone and a barrel shape, respectively. The orientation of the bone is then derived from the known geometry of the fitted primitives. The main disadvantage is that, unlike with a long bone such as a metatarsal, it is more difficult to apply this method to bones with a more complex shape such as the talus or calcaneus.

Depending on the proprietary mix of technologies used to obtain the 3D orientation of each bone, software can provide an automated report of chosen measurements, usually a set of basic metrics (such as the M1–M2 angle, sesamoid rotation angle (SRA) for the forefoot, sagittal and axial talus–M1 angle and hindfoot alignment angle or foot–ankle offset) and a customized set of measurements chosen by the user. Reports in the literature regarding the usefulness and efficiency of these systems agree on their celerity, resulting in important time gains compared to measurements by hand [52,53]. However, they also report that they differ from the latter, raising the question of which is the gold standard [53]. They also report a relevant number of failures or aberrant measurements, which are thought to be due to cases of low bone density, where the density of soft tissues is close to that of the bone, which can 'blur' the picture for the software, or the presence of metalwork or traumatic sequala, which are in any case unusual situations which can be misinterpreted by the software. Another explanation may be insufficient training when deep learning-based Ais are used. However, there is generally positive feedback regarding these new generation tools, with good reliability and excellent reproducibility [52,53,55,56,88].

2. Distance Mapping or 3D-JSW, surface and volume measurements

This is the advanced computerized method which has been the most reported on in the literature, to the best of our knowledge. This tool is based on analyzing the surface-to-surface distance map within any given weight-bearing joint. The sum of all these point-by-point distances adds up to a 3D joint space width map, which explains why it has been dubbed 'distance mapping' [66,67,69], '3D joint space width' [65,68,89,90] or a mix of both in the literature. Originally developed as way to visualize regions of bony approximation, authors presented ways to also use it as a quantification tool for such conditions as PCFD or cavovarus deformity, by averaging the distances in reproducible in pre-defined anatomical quadrants within the joints of interest (Figure 9).

Other than classical usage of this tool to quantify the evolution of osteoarthritic joints, authors have reported its ability to detect minute or more specific changes in the onset of hindfoot deformity, in PCFD [66] or cavovarus [67] configurations. This may lead in the future to early detection and preventive intervention in a wide range of foot and ankle pathologies. It is important to take into account that this technique does not enable the visualization of cartilage itself, but only the space in which the cartilage is to be found. It will therefore correctly depict an absence of cartilage, but not an area where cartilage is augmented, and an area where the joint is distracted may incorrectly be considered as cartilage augmentation. However, weight-bearing capacity largely eliminates these downsides, which in any event are also true of conventional 2DXR, while the analysis is not possible at all with conventional non-weight-bearing MDCT.

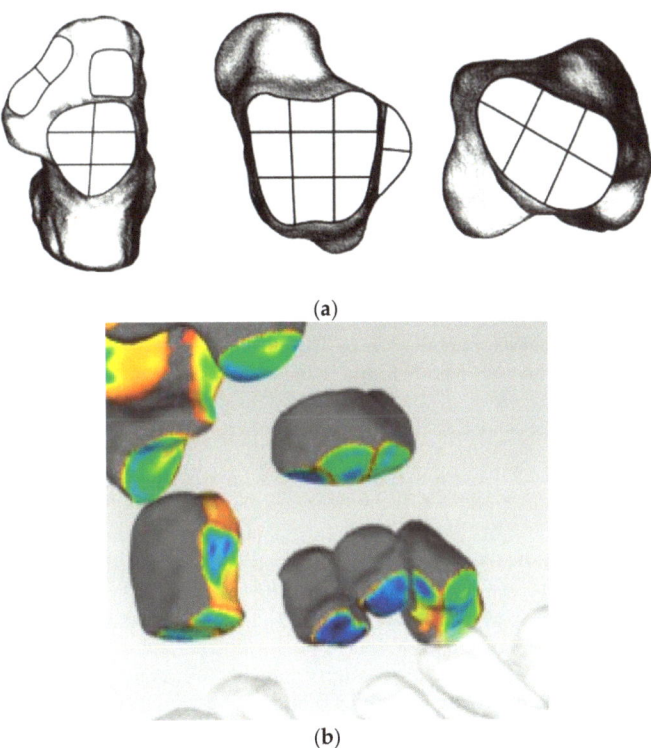

Figure 9. Distance mapping or 3D joint space width assessment (curtesy of Pr Sorin Siegler, Drexel University, Philadelphia, PA, USA); (**a**) example of quadrants in the talonavicular, tibiotalar and subtalar joints; (**b**) example of color-coded 3D distance map in the mid-tarsal joints.

3. Coverage Mapping

Coverage mapping has been investigated mostly in PCFD, to evaluate peritalar subluxation. Peritalar subluxation is thought to be the onset of PCFD pathology, while being extremely difficult to define and describe. Sangeorzean at al. [91,92] described it with the production of images showing overlap of the posterior subtalar facet and de Cesar Netto et al. have since then produced similar findings in the subtalar posterior and middle facets and reported a clinically significant correlation of coverage maps with patient reported outcome measures [70,93]. The technique involves digital reconstruction of the articular facets' borders. This concept in itself may be subject to variability depending on the computerized algorithm used because choices have to be made regarding multiple settings, such as where to define the limit between cartilage and bone when the cartilage cannot be seen. However, it is definitely a step forward in terms of diagnosis, which highlights again the importance of the standardization work [23] initiated by the international WBCT society.

4. Surface and Volumetric Measurements

As WBCT rose in the mid-2010s, it became apparent that traditional 2D measurements were not fit for the 3D environment, generating, as mentioned above, a new kind of so-called 'slice' bias. Also, performing a 2D measurement in a 3D environment is equivalent to a dimensional reduction, thus reducing the quantity of information available. New solutions had to be found, therefore, to make the best of the new technology. The syndesmotic distal tibiofibular joint is the best example of this evolution. In that case, single-dimensional measurements (distances like the medial clear space or angles) have often fallen short of demonstrating reliable diagnostic capabilities and must often be complemented by other modalities such as MRI [94]. Similarly to how the foot–ankle offset describes the use of four landmarks to redefine hindfoot alignment as a volume, authors have described first surface, then volumetric evaluation of the clear space between the distal tibia and fibula to assess syndesmotic instability [72–74,95,96]. The latter has offered unequaled diagnostic power, confirming that the 3D environment contains more diagnostic information which should be investigated where possible (i.e., when segmentation has been applied) using 3D measurements [97].

5. Centre of Rotation Assessment.

In a paper in Scientific Reports, Pena-Fernandez, Goldberg et al. used a method called digital volume correlation (DVC) to identify the center of rotation of the subtalar joint in a series of healthy volunteers. The subjects were placed in a PedCAT bilateral WBCT device (CurvebeamAI, Hatfield, PA, USA) and asked to perform inversion and eversion of their subtalar joints. The authors report that the center of rotation of the subtalar joint was consistently found in the middle of the subtalar joint [75]. The principles of DVC are to reference one of the implicated bones and to measure the displacement using a vector field associated to the other bone, between the two considered positions.

4.2.3. Description of Techniques for Advanced Clinical Applications Derived from WBCT Computerized Techniques

As mentioned before, segmentation is the key to identifying individual bone contours, and once that has been achieved, multiple new techniques can be applied. One of these is the externalized manufacturing of custom 3D-printed surgical guides for osteotomy [18] or total joint replacement [77], in this particular case ankle replacement. However, it is not clear, in the absence of dedicated literature, whether automatic segmentation software would be reliable enough to provide fully automatic surgical guide manufacturing. Indeed, human intervention by biomechanical engineers is still required to ensure the quality of the fit, according to the patient's specific bone surface characteristics and the quality of the alignment correction on the three planes of space. Therefore, whoever provides the segmentation software, implant manufacturers still must provide human resources to secure these steps, hence an increased cost to include customized bone cut guides, which may not be accessible to all patients, surgeons and healthcare systems. However, in the future, solutions should be found for widespread adoption, taking into account the multiple advantages of customized surgery, such as specific planning of the correction on natural stance WBCT datasets, faster learning curves, operative times and improved accuracy and reliability of axial corrections.

Although customized surgical guides existed before WBCT was implemented, it is important to distinguish what the added value of WBCT is in this case. Here, the segmentation and surface matching of the guide does not require weight-bearing; it is the planning for alignment correction that does. In that case, as mentioned earlier, the rapid acquisition of natural stance 3D-WBCT is definitely an improvement as compared to the traditional 2DXR-MDCT sequence. One often-heard argument here is that the correction is performed surgically on a patient who is lying down, so what is the point of planning on standing images? It is important to debunk this argument: first, planning is carried out standing because the alignment only makes sense standing. Also, even in the traditional sequence, the planning of corrections is made using standing 2D images (for total ankles, anterior–posterior and lateral 2DXR, including the knee), which are less reliable than 3D-WBCT. In that sequence, it is only the surface fitting of the guide which is performed using the MDCT: the cut itself and the corrections are planned using, again, the alignment measurement setup, in the former case, 2DXR.

Similarly, we anticipate that WBCT data will soon be implemented for use in robotic orthopedic surgery, although, to the best of our knowledge, no record of such a procedure has been recorded in the literature at the time this work is being written.

4.2.4. Current Limitations of the Technique

The cost of WBCT devices has often been discussed as potential limiting factor to the spread of the technology in clinical centers. While no cost-effectiveness studies have been published so far, in a population-based study led by Jacques T. et al. in 2021, two periods were compared in emergency setting: a 7-month period during which only a standard multi-detector CT was available and, one year later, an equivalent 7-month period during which a CBCT was also used [32]. The authors found a significant radiation dose and an accelerated turnover (23.6% faster) with CBCT in place. Based on this, and taking into account the need to reduce waiting lists in public hospitals in many Western countries, it could be hypothesized that the initial economical effort to buy the machine would soon be compensated for by the gain in terms of diagnostic workflow, as already discussed above.

On a different note, whether the management of WBCT devices should compete with radiologists (as it should be, given the nature of the device) or with orthopedic surgeons (which it does not, according to the literature discussed above) who, so far, have shown the greatest interest towards the technology given the clinical advantages in diagnosis and, even more, surgical three-dimensional planning, has also been a matter of debate. While, in an ideal setting, both specialties should collaborate and move in the same direction, the fact that this does not always happen and the lack of agreement felt by clinicians in daily practice is advocated as a further limitation to the acquisition and use of WBCT devices.

5. Conclusions

In conclusion, we have found that advanced computerized techniques developed using WBCT in the foot and ankle field can be classified. The most reported currently are standardized absolute and relative 3D relationship and joint distance mapping. Focus has to be made on the development of fast, reliable automatic segmentation software and international academic endeavors to scientifically validate such software. It is important to note that the techniques developed in the foot and ankle will be applicable to other fields, in particular the knees, hips, spine and shoulders and specialties: trauma and emergencies, pediatrics, sports medicine and rheumatology. We anticipate that, beyond measurements, further developments based on deep learning and artificial intelligence will lead to breakthroughs in diagnostics and prognostics.

However, as exciting as these perspectives might be, they remain somewhat distant, and therefore the advanced computer science should not overshadow the immediate clinical advantages of diminished radiation dose, improved diagnostics and slashed patient workflow delays observed with WBCT, which should make practitioners and researchers strive to realize its swift and widespread implementation in the musculoskeletal clinical realm.

Author Contributions: F.L.: concept, manuscript writing, submission. C.d.C.N.: review, text editing. A.B.: review, text editing. C.B.: review, text editing, invitation, concept. A.L.: review. IWBCTS: review, methods. All authors have read and agreed to the published version of the manuscript.

Funding: This research received no external funding.

Institutional Review Board Statement: Not applicable.

Informed Consent Statement: Not applicable.

Data Availability Statement: Not applicable.

Acknowledgments: The authors wish to thank the members and board of the International WBCT Society.

Conflicts of Interest: F.L.—CurvebeamAI: stock, consultancy; Paragon28/Disior: stock, consultancy; International WBCT Society: board. A.B.—CurvebeamAI: stock, consultancy; International WBCT Society: board. C.N.—CurvebeamAI: stock, consultancy; Paragon28/Disior: stock, consultancy; International WBCT Society: board.

References

1. Mozzo, P.; Procacci, C.; Tacconi, A.; Martini, P.T.; Andreis, I.A. A new volumetric CT machine for dental imaging based on the cone-beam technique: Preliminary results. *Eur. Radiol.* **1998**, *8*, 1558–1564. [CrossRef] [PubMed]
2. Minerbo, G. Maximum entropy reconstruction from cone-beam projection data. *Comput. Biol. Med.* **1979**, *9*, 29–37. [CrossRef] [PubMed]
3. Robert, N.; Peyrin, F.; Yaffe, M.J. Binary vascular reconstruction from a limited number of cone beam projections. *Med. Phys.* **1994**, *21*, 1839–1851. [CrossRef] [PubMed]
4. Ambrose, J.; Hounsfield, G. Computerized transverse axial tomography. *Br. J. Radiol.* **1973**, *46*, 148–149. [CrossRef]
5. Feldkamp, L.A.; Davis, L.C.; Kress, J.W. Practical cone-beam algorithms. *J. Opt. Soc. Am.* **1984**, *1*, 612–619. [CrossRef]
6. Bab, R.; Ueda, K.; Kuba, A.; Kohda, E.; Shiraga, N.; Sanmiya, T. Development of a subject-standing-type cone-beam computed tomography for chest and orthopedic imaging. *Front. Med. Biol. Eng.* **2001**, *11*, 177–189. [PubMed]
7. Zbijewski, W.; De Jean, P.; Prakash, P.; Ding, Y.; Stayman, J.W.; Packard, N.; Senn, R.; Yang, D.; Yorkston, J.; Machado, A.; et al. A dedicated cone-beam CT system for musculoskeletal extremities imaging: Design, optimization, and initial performance characterization. *Med. Phys.* **2011**, *38*, 4700–4713. [CrossRef] [PubMed]
8. Muhit, A.; Zbijewski, W.; Stayman, J.; Thawait, G.; Yorkston, J.; Foos, D.; Packard, N.; Yang, D.; Senn, R.; Carrino, J.; et al. WE-G-217BCD-04: Diagnostic Image Quality Evaluation of a Dedicated Extremity Cone-Beam CT Scanner: Pre-Clinical Studies and First Clinical Results. *Med. Phys.* **2012**, *39*, 3973. [CrossRef] [PubMed]
9. Tuominen, E.K.J.; Kankare, J.; Koskinen, S.K.; Mattila, K.T. Weight-bearing CT imaging of the lower extremity. *AJR Am. J. Roentgenol.* **2013**, *200*, 146–148. [CrossRef] [PubMed]
10. Ferri, M.; Scharfenberger, A.V.; Goplen, G.; Daniels, T.R.; Pearce, D. Weightbearing CT scan of severe flexible pes planus deformities. *Foot Ankle Int.* **2008**, *29*, 199–204. [CrossRef] [PubMed]
11. Collan, L.; Kankare, J.A.; Mattila, K. The biomechanics of the first metatarsal bone in hallux valgus: A preliminary study utilizing a weight bearing extremity CT. *Foot Ankle Surg.* **2013**, *19*, 155–161. [CrossRef]
12. Richter, M.; Seidl, B.; Zech, S.; Hahn, S. PedCAT for 3D-imaging in standing position allows for more accurate bone position (angle) measurement than radiographs or CT. *Foot Ankle Surg.* **2014**, *20*, 201–207. [CrossRef]
13. Alexander, N.B.; Sarfani, S.; Strickland, C.D.; Richardson, D.R.; Murphy, G.A.; Grear, B.J.; Bettin, C.C. Cost Analysis and Reimbursement of Weightbearing Computed Tomography. *Foot Ankle Orthop.* **2023**, *8*, 24730114231164143. [CrossRef]
14. Arena, C.B.; Sripanich, Y.; Leake, R.; Saltzman, C.L.; Barg, A. Assessment of Hindfoot Alignment Comparing Weightbearing Radiography to Weightbearing Computed Tomography. *Foot Ankle Int.* **2021**, *42*, 1482–1490. [CrossRef]
15. Brinch, S.; Wellenberg, R.H.H.; Boesen, M.P.; Maas, M.; Johannsen, F.E.; Nybing, J.U.; Turmezei, T.; Streekstra, G.J.; Hansen, P. Weight-bearing cone-beam CT: The need for standardised acquisition protocols and measurements to fulfill high expectations—A review of the literature. *Skeletal Radiol.* **2022**, *52*, 1073–1088. [CrossRef]
16. Broos, M.; Berardo, S.; Dobbe, J.G.G.; Maas, M.; Streekstra, G.J.; Wellenberg, R.H.H. Geometric 3D analyses of the foot and ankle using weight-bearing and non weight-bearing cone-beam CT images: The new standard? *Eur. J. Radiol.* **2021**, *138*, 109674. [CrossRef]
17. Campbell, T.; Mok, A.; Wolf, M.R.; Tarakemeh, A.; Everist, B.; Vopat, B.G. Augmented stress weightbearing CT for evaluation of subtle tibiofibular syndesmotic injuries in the elite athlete. *Skeletal Radiol.* **2023**, *52*, 1221–1227. [CrossRef]
18. Faict, S.; Burssens, A.; Van Oevelen, A.; Maeckelbergh, L.; Mertens, P.; Buedts, K. Correction of ankle varus deformity using patient-specific dome-shaped osteotomy guides designed on weight-bearing CT: A pilot study. *Arch. Orthop. Trauma Surg.* **2023**, *143*, 791–799. [CrossRef]
19. Foran, I.M.; Mehraban, N.; Jacobsen, S.K.; Bohl, D.D.; Lin, J.; Hamid, K.S.; Lee, S. Impact of Coleman Block Test on Adult Hindfoot Alignment Assessed by Clinical Examination, Radiography, and Weight-Bearing Computed Tomography. *Foot Ankle Orthop.* **2020**, *5*, 2473011420933264. [CrossRef]
20. Fritz, B.; Fritz, J.; Fucentese, S.F.; Pfirrmann, C.W.A.; Sutter, R. Three-dimensional analysis for quantification of knee joint space width with weight-bearing CT: Comparison with non-weight-bearing CT and weight-bearing radiography. *Osteoarthritis Cartilage* **2022**, *30*, 671–680. [CrossRef]
21. Kvarda, P.; Krähenbühl, N.; Susdorf, R.; Burssens, A.; Ruiz, R.; Barg, A.; Hintermann, B. High Reliability for Semiautomated 3D Measurements Based on Weightbearing CT Scans. *Foot Ankle Int.* **2022**, *43*, 91–95. [CrossRef]
22. Ortolani, M.; Leardini, A.; Pavani, C.; Scicolone, S.; Girolami, M.; Bevoni, R.; Lullini, G.; Durante, S.; Berti, L.; Belvedere, C. Angular and linear measurements of adult flexible flatfoot via weight-bearing CT scans and 3D bone reconstruction tools. *Sci. Rep.* **2021**, *11*, 16139. [CrossRef]
23. Pavani, C.; Belvedere, C.; Ortolani, M.; Girolami, M.; Durante, S.; Berti, L.; Leardini, A. 3D measurement techniques for the hindfoot alignment angle from weight-bearing CT in a clinical population. *Sci. Rep.* **2022**, *12*, 16900. [CrossRef]
24. Richter, M.; Zech, S.; Naef, I.; Duerr, F.; Schilke, R. Automatic software-based 3D-angular measurement for weight-bearing CT (WBCT) is valid. *Foot Ankle Surg.* **2024**. [CrossRef]
25. Tazegul, T.E.; Anderson, D.D.; Barbachan Mansur, N.S.; Kajimura Chinelati, R.M.; Iehl, C.; VandeLune, C.; Ahrenholz, S.; Lalevee, M.; de Cesar Netto, C. An Objective Computational Method to Quantify Ankle Osteoarthritis From Low-Dose Weight-bearing Computed Tomography. *Foot Ankle Orthop.* **2022**, *7*, 24730114221116805. [CrossRef]

26. Zaidi, R.; Sangoi, D.; Cullen, N.; Patel, S.; Welck, M.; Malhotra, K. Semi-automated 3-dimensional analysis of the normal foot and ankle using weight bearing CT—A report of normal values and bony relationships. *Foot Ankle Surg.* **2023**, *29*, 111–117. [CrossRef]
27. Zhong, Z.; Zhang, P.; Duan, H.; Yang, H.; Li, Q.; He, F. A Comparison Between X-ray Imaging and an Innovative Computer-aided Design Method Based on Weightbearing CT Scan Images for Assessing Hallux Valgus. *J. Foot Ankle Surg.* **2021**, *60*, 6–10. [CrossRef]
28. Mys, K.; Varga, P.; Stockmans, F.; Gueorguiev, B.; Neumann, V.; Vanovermeire, O.; Wyers, C.E.; van den Bergh, J.P.W.; van Lenthe, G.H. High-Resolution Cone-Beam Computed Tomography is a Fast and Promising Technique to Quantify Bone Microstructure and Mechanics of the Distal Radius. *Calcif. Tissue Int.* **2021**, *108*, 314–323. [CrossRef]
29. Hirschmann, A.; Pfirrmann, C.W.A.; Klammer, G.; Espinosa, N.; Buck, F.M. Upright cone CT of the hindfoot: Comparison of the non-weight-bearing with the upright weight-bearing position. *Eur. Radiol.* **2014**, *24*, 553–558. [CrossRef]
30. Borel, C.; Larbi, A.; Delclaux, S.; Lapegue, F.; Chiavassa-Gandois, H.; Sans, N.; Faruch-Bilfeld, M. Diagnostic value of cone beam computed tomography (CBCT) in occult scaphoid and wrist fractures. *Eur. J. Radiol.* **2017**, *97*, 59–64. [CrossRef]
31. Dartus, J.; Jacques, T.; Martinot, P.; Pasquier, G.; Cotten, A.; Migaud, H.; Morel, V.; Putman, S. The advantages of cone-beam computerised tomography (CT) in pain management following total knee arthroplasty, in comparison with conventional multi-detector CT. *Orthop. Traumatol. Surg. Res.* **2021**, *107*, 102874. [CrossRef]
32. Jacques, T.; Morel, V.; Dartus, J.; Badr, S.; Demondion, X.; Cotten, A. Impact of introducing extremity cone-beam CT in an emergency radiology department: A population-based study. *Orthop. Traumatol. Surg. Res.* **2021**, *107*, 102834. [CrossRef]
33. Ricci, P.M.; Boldini, M.; Bonfante, E.; Sambugaro, E.; Vecchini, E.; Schenal, G.; Magnan, B.; Montemezzi, S. Cone-beam computed tomography compared to X-ray in diagnosis of extremities bone fractures: A study of 198 cases. *Eur. J. Radiol. Open* **2019**, *6*, 119–121. [CrossRef]
34. Doan, M.K.; Long, J.R.; Verhey, E.; Wyse, A.; Patel, K.; Flug, J.A. Cone-Beam CT of the Extremities in Clinical Practice. *Radiographics* **2024**, *44*, e230143. [CrossRef]
35. Richter, M.; Lintz, F.; de Cesar Netto, C.; Barg, A.; Burssens, A. Results of more than 11,000 scans with weightbearing CT—Impact on costs, radiation exposure, and procedure time. *Foot Ankle Surg.* **2020**, *26*, 518–522. [CrossRef]
36. Koivisto, J.; Kiljunen, T.; Kadesjö, N.; Shi, X.Q.; Wolff, J. Effective radiation dose of a MSCT, two CBCT and one conventional radiography device in the ankle region. *J. Foot Ankle Res.* **2015**, *8*, 8. [CrossRef]
37. Mettler, F.A.; Huda, W.; Yoshizumi, T.T.; Mahesh, M. Effective doses in radiology and diagnostic nuclear medicine: A catalog. *Radiology* **2008**, *248*, 254–263. [CrossRef]
38. Pugmire, B.S.; Shailam, R.; Sagar, P.; Liu, B.; Li, X.; Palmer, W.E.; Huang, A.J. Initial Clinical Experience With Extremity Cone-Beam CT of the Foot and Ankle in Pediatric Patients. *AJR Am. J. Roentgenol.* **2016**, *206*, 431–435. [CrossRef]
39. Day, J.; de Cesar Netto, C.; Burssens, A.; Bernasconi, A.; Fernando, C.; Lintz, F. A Case-Control Study of 3D vs 2D Weightbearing CT Measurements of the M1-M2 Intermetatarsal Angle in Hallux Valgus. *Foot Ankle Int.* **2022**, *43*, 1049–1052. [CrossRef]
40. Moore, C.S.; Wood, T.J.; Saunderson, J.R.; Beavis, A.W. A method to incorporate the effect of beam quality on image noise in a digitally reconstructed radiograph (DRR) based computer simulation for optimisation of digital radiography. *Phys. Med. Biol.* **2017**, *62*, 7379–7393. [CrossRef]
41. de Cesar Netto, C.; Schon, L.C.; Thawait, G.K.; da Fonseca, L.F.; Chinanuvathana, A.; Zbijewski, W.B.; Siewerdsen, J.H.; Demehri, S. Flexible Adult Acquired Flatfoot Deformity: Comparison Between Weight-Bearing and Non-Weight-Bearing Measurements Using Cone-Beam Computed Tomography. *J. Bone Jt. Surg. Am.* **2017**, *99*, e98. [CrossRef]
42. Page, M.J.; McKenzie, J.E.; Bossuyt, P.M.; Boutron, I.; Hoffmann, T.C.; Mulrow, C.D.; Shamseer, L.; Tetzlaff, J.M.; Akl, E.A.; Brennan, S.E.; et al. The PRISMA 2020 statement: An updated guideline for reporting systematic reviews. *Syst. Rev.* **2021**, *10*, 89. [CrossRef]
43. Lintz, F.; Bernasconi, A.; Ferkel, E.I. Can Weight-Bearing Computed Tomography Be a Game-Changer in the Assessment of Ankle Sprain and Ankle Instability? *Foot Ankle Clin.* **2023**, *28*, 283–295. [CrossRef]
44. Richter, M.; Lintz, F.; Zech, S.; Meissner, S.A. Combination of PedCAT Weightbearing CT With Pedography Assessment of the Relationship Between Anatomy-Based Foot Center and Force/Pressure-Based Center of Gravity. *Foot Ankle Int.* **2018**, *39*, 361–368. [CrossRef]
45. de Cesar Netto, C.; Godoy-Santos, A.L.; Saito, G.H.; Lintz, F.; Siegler, S.; O'Malley, M.J.; Deland, J.T.; Ellis, S.J. Subluxation of the Middle Facet of the Subtalar Joint as a Marker of Peritalar Subluxation in Adult Acquired Flatfoot Deformity: A Case-Control Study. *J. Bone Jt. Surg. Am.* **2019**, *101*, 1838–1844. [CrossRef]
46. de Cesar Netto, C.; Myerson, M.S.; Day, J.; Ellis, S.J.; Hintermann, B.; Johnson, J.E.; Sangeorzan, B.J.; Schon, L.C.; Thordarson, D.B.; Deland, J.T. Consensus for the Use of Weightbearing CT in the Assessment of Progressive Collapsing Foot Deformity. *Foot Ankle Int.* **2020**, *41*, 1277–1282. [CrossRef]
47. Lintz, F.; Bernasconi, A.; Baschet, L.; Fernando, C.; Mehdi, N.; Weight Bearing CT International Study Group; de Cesar Netto, C. Relationship Between Chronic Lateral Ankle Instability and Hindfoot Varus Using Weight-Bearing Cone Beam Computed Tomography. *Foot Ankle Int.* **2019**, *40*, 1175–1181. [CrossRef]
48. Lintz, F.; Welck, M.; Bernasconi, A.; Thornton, J.; Cullen, N.P.; Singh, D.; Goldberg, A. 3D Biometrics for Hindfoot Alignment Using Weightbearing CT. *Foot Ankle Int.* **2017**, *38*, 684–689. [CrossRef]
49. Peiffer, M.; Burssens, A.; De Mits, S.; Heintz, T.; Van Waeyenberge, M.; Buedts, K.; Victor, J.; Audenaert, E. Statistical shape model-based tibiofibular assessment of syndesmotic ankle lesions using weight-bearing CT. *J. Orthop. Res.* **2022**, *40*, 2873–2884. [CrossRef]

50. Burssens, A.; Krähenbühl, N.; Lenz, A.L.; Howell, K.; Zhang, C.; Sripanich, Y.; Saltzman, C.L.; Barg, A. Interaction of loading and ligament injuries in subtalar joint instability quantified by 3D weightbearing computed tomography. *J. Orthop. Res.* **2022**, *40*, 933–944. [CrossRef]
51. Burssens, A.; Vermue, H.; Barg, A.; Krähenbühl, N.; Victor, J.; Buedts, K. Templating of Syndesmotic Ankle Lesions by Use of 3D Analysis in Weightbearing and Nonweightbearing CT. *Foot Ankle Int.* **2018**, *39*, 1487–1496. [CrossRef]
52. Day, J.; de Cesar Netto, C.; Richter, M.; Mansur, N.S.; Fernando, C.; Deland, J.T.; Ellis, S.J.; Lintz, F. Evaluation of a Weightbearing CT Artificial Intelligence-Based Automatic Measurement for the M1-M2 Intermetatarsal Angle in Hallux Valgus. *Foot Ankle Int.* **2021**, *42*, 1502–1509. [CrossRef]
53. Richter, M.; Duerr, F.; Schilke, R.; Zech, S.; Meissner, S.A.; Naef, I. Semi-automatic software-based 3D-angular measurement for Weight-Bearing CT (WBCT) in the foot provides different angles than measurement by hand. *Foot Ankle Surg.* **2022**, *28*, 919–927. [CrossRef]
54. Sangoi, D.; Ranjit, S.; Bernasconi, A.; Cullen, N.; Patel, S.; Welck, M.; Malhotra, K. 2D Manual vs 3D Automated Assessment of Alignment in Normal and Charcot-Marie-Tooth Cavovarus Feet Using Weightbearing CT. *Foot Ankle Int.* **2022**, *43*, 973–982. [CrossRef]
55. de Carvalho, K.A.M.; Walt, J.S.; Ehret, A.; Tazegul, T.E.; Dibbern, K.; Mansur, N.S.B.; Lalevée, M.; de Cesar Netto, C. Comparison between Weightbearing-CT semiautomatic and manual measurements in Hallux Valgus. *Foot Ankle Surg.* **2022**, *28*, 518–525. [CrossRef]
56. Krähenbühl, N.; Kvarda, P.; Susdorf, R.; Burssens, A.; Ruiz, R.; Barg, A.; Hintermann, B. Assessment of Progressive Collapsing Foot Deformity Using Semiautomated 3D Measurements Derived from Weightbearing CT Scans. *Foot Ankle Int.* **2022**, *43*, 363–370. [CrossRef]
57. Mens, M.A.; Bouman, C.M.B.; Dobbe, J.G.G.; Bus, S.A.; Nieuwdorp, M.; Maas, M.; Wellenberg, R.H.H.; Streekstra, G.J. Metatarsophalangeal and interphalangeal joint angle measurements on weight-bearing CT images. *Foot Ankle Surg.* **2023**, *29*, 538–543. [CrossRef]
58. Rowe, N.; Robertson, C.E.; Singh, S.; Campbell, J.T.; Jeng, C.L. Weightbearing CT Analysis of the Transverse Tarsal Joint During Eversion and Inversion. *Foot Ankle Int.* **2022**, *43*, 123–130. [CrossRef]
59. Bernasconi, A.; Cooper, L.; Lyle, S.; Patel, S.; Cullen, N.; Singh, D.; Welck, M. Pes cavovarus in Charcot-Marie-Tooth compared to the idiopathic cavovarus foot: A preliminary weightbearing CT analysis. *Foot Ankle Surg.* **2021**, *27*, 186–195. [CrossRef]
60. Carrara, C.; Belvedere, C.; Caravaggi, P.; Durante, S.; Leardini, A. Techniques for 3D foot bone orientation angles in weight-bearing from cone-beam computed tomography. *Foot Ankle Surg.* **2021**, *27*, 168–174. [CrossRef]
61. Sripanich, Y.; Weinberg, M.; Krähenbühl, N.; Rungprai, C.; Saltzman, C.L.; Barg, A. Change in the First Cuneiform-Second Metatarsal Distance After Simulated Ligamentous Lisfranc Injury Evaluated by Weightbearing CT Scans. *Foot Ankle Int.* **2020**, *41*, 1432–1441. [CrossRef]
62. Burssens, A.; Peeters, J.; Peiffer, M.; Marien, R.; Lenaerts, T.; WBCT ISG; Vandeputte, G.; Victor, J. Reliability and correlation analysis of computed methods to convert conventional 2D radiological hindfoot measurements to a 3D setting using weightbearing CT. *Int. J. Comput. Assist. Radiol. Surg.* **2018**, *13*, 1999–2008. [CrossRef]
63. Richter, M.; Zech, S.; Hahn, S.; Naef, I.; Merschin, D. Combination of pedCAT® for 3D Imaging in Standing Position With Pedography Shows No Statistical Correlation of Bone Position With Force/Pressure Distribution. *J. Foot Ankle Surg.* **2016**, *55*, 240–246. [CrossRef]
64. Kleipool, R.P.; Dahmen, J.; Vuurberg, G.; Oostra, R.J.; Blankevoort, L.; Knupp, M.; Stufkens, S.A.S. Study on the three-dimensional orientation of the posterior facet of the subtalar joint using simulated weight-bearing CT. *J. Orthop. Res.* **2019**, *37*, 197–204. [CrossRef]
65. Turmezei, T.D.; Malhotra, K.; MacKay, J.W.; Gee, A.H.; Treece, G.M.; Poole, K.E.S.; Welck, M.J. 3-D joint space mapping at the ankle from weight-bearing CT: Reproducibility, repeatability, and challenges for standardisation. *Eur. Radiol.* **2023**, *33*, 8333–8342. [CrossRef]
66. Bernasconi, A.; De Cesar Netto, C.; Siegler, S.; Jepsen, M.; Lintz, F.; International Weight-Bearing CT Society. Weightbearing CT assessment of foot and ankle joints in Pes Planovalgus using distance mapping. *Foot Ankle Surg.* **2022**, *28*, 775–784. [CrossRef]
67. Lintz, F.; Jepsen, M.; De Cesar Netto, C.; Bernasconi, A.; Ruiz, M.; Siegler, S.; International Weight-Bearing CT Society. Distance mapping of the foot and ankle joints using weightbearing CT: The cavovarus configuration. *Foot Ankle Surg.* **2021**, *27*, 412–420. [CrossRef]
68. Day, M.A.; Ho, M.; Dibbern, K.; Rao, K.; An, Q.; Anderson, D.D.; Marsh, J.L. Correlation of 3D Joint Space Width From Weightbearing CT With Outcomes After Intra-articular Calcaneal Fracture. *Foot Ankle Int.* **2020**, *41*, 1106–1116. [CrossRef]
69. Peiffer, M.; Ghandour, S.; Nassour, N.; Taseh, A.; Burssens, A.; Waryasz, G.; Bejarano-Pineda, L.; Audenaert, E.; Ashkani-Esfahani, S.; DiGiovanni, C.W. Normative contact mechanics of the ankle Joint: Quantitative assessment utilizing bilateral weightbearing CT. *J. Biomech.* **2024**, *168*, 112136. [CrossRef]
70. Behrens, A.; Dibbern, K.; Lalevée, M.; Alencar Mendes de Carvalho, K.; Lintz, F.; Barbachan Mansur, N.S.; de Cesar Netto, C. Coverage maps demonstrate 3D Chopart joint subluxation in weightbearing CT of progressive collapsing foot deformity. *Sci. Rep.* **2022**, *12*, 19367. [CrossRef]

71. Bhimani, R.; Sornsakrin, P.; Ashkani-Esfahani, S.; Lubberts, B.; Guss, D.; De Cesar Netto, C.; Waryasz, G.R.; Kerkhoffs, G.M.M.J.; DiGiovanni, C.W. Using area and volume measurement via weightbearing CT to detect Lisfranc instability. *J. Orthop. Res.* **2021**, *39*, 2497–2505. [CrossRef]
72. Ashkani Esfahani, S.; Bhimani, R.; Lubberts, B.; Kerkhoffs, G.M.; Waryasz, G.; DiGiovanni, C.W.; Guss, D. Volume measurements on weightbearing computed tomography can detect subtle syndesmotic instability. *J. Orthop. Res.* **2022**, *40*, 460–467. [CrossRef]
73. Bhimani, R.; Ashkani-Esfahani, S.; Lubberts, B.; Guss, D.; Hagemeijer, N.C.; Waryasz, G.; DiGiovanni, C.W. Utility of Volumetric Measurement via Weight-Bearing Computed Tomography Scan to Diagnose Syndesmotic Instability. *Foot Ankle Int.* **2020**, *41*, 859–865. [CrossRef]
74. Ashkani-Esfahani, S.; Lucchese, O.; Bhimani, R.; Taseh, A.; Waryasz, G.; Kerkhoffs, G.M.M.; Maas, M.; DiGiovanni, C.W.; Guss, D. Automation improves the efficiency of weightbearing CT scan 3D volumetric assessments of the syndesmosis. *Foot Ankle Surg.* **2024**, *in press*. [CrossRef]
75. Peña Fernández, M.; Hoxha, D.; Chan, O.; Mordecai, S.; Blunn, G.W.; Tozzi, G.; Goldberg, A. Centre of Rotation of the Human Subtalar Joint Using Weight-Bearing Clinical Computed Tomography. *Sci. Rep.* **2020**, *10*, 1035. [CrossRef]
76. Zeitlin, J.; Henry, J.; Ellis, S. Preoperative Guidance With Weight-Bearing Computed Tomography and Patient-Specific Instrumentation in Foot and Ankle Surgery. *HSS J.* **2021**, *17*, 326–332. [CrossRef]
77. Thompson, M.J.; Consul, D.; Umbel, B.D.; Berlet, G.C. Accuracy of Weightbearing CT Scans for Patient-Specific Instrumentation in Total Ankle Arthroplasty. *Foot Ankle Orthop.* **2021**, *6*, 24730114211061493. [CrossRef]
78. Segal, N.A.; Nevitt, M.C.; Lynch, J.A.; Niu, J.; Torner, J.C.; Guermazi, A. Diagnostic performance of 3D standing CT imaging for detection of knee osteoarthritis features. *Phys. Sportsmed.* **2015**, *43*, 213–220. [CrossRef]
79. Krähenbühl, N.; Bailey, T.L.; Weinberg, M.W.; Davidson, N.P.; Hintermann, B.; Presson, A.P.; Allen, C.M.; Henninger, H.B.; Saltzman, C.L.; Barg, A. Impact of Torque on Assessment of Syndesmotic Injuries Using Weightbearing Computed Tomography Scans. *Foot Ankle Int.* **2019**, *40*, 710–719. [CrossRef]
80. Krähenbühl, N.; Bailey, T.L.; Presson, A.P.; Allen, C.M.; Henninger, H.B.; Saltzman, C.L.; Barg, A. Torque application helps to diagnose incomplete syndesmotic injuries using weight-bearing computed tomography images. *Skeletal Radiol.* **2019**, *48*, 1367–1376. [CrossRef]
81. de Cesar Netto, C.; Day, J.; Godoy-Santos, A.L.; Roney, A.; Barbachan Mansur, N.S.; Lintz, F.; Ellis, S.J.; Demetracopoulos, C.A. The use of three-dimensional biometric Foot and Ankle Offset to predict additional realignment procedures in total ankle replacement. *Foot Ankle Surg.* **2022**, *28*, 1029–1034. [CrossRef]
82. Lintz, F.; Mast, J.; Bernasconi, A.; Mehdi, N.; de Cesar Netto, C.; Fernando, C.; International Weight-Bearing CT Society; Buedts, K. 3D, Weightbearing Topographical Study of Periprosthetic Cysts and Alignment in Total Ankle Replacement. *Foot Ankle Int.* **2020**, *41*, 1–9. [CrossRef]
83. Colin, F.; Horn Lang, T.; Zwicky, L.; Hintermann, B.; Knupp, M. Subtalar joint configuration on weightbearing CT scan. *Foot Ankle Int.* **2014**, *35*, 1057–1062. [CrossRef]
84. Sandberg, O.H.; Kärrholm, J.; Olivecrona, H.; Röhrl, S.M.; Sköldenberg, O.G.; Brodén, C. Computed tomography-based radiostereometric analysis in orthopedic research: Practical guidelines. *Acta Orthop.* **2023**, *94*, 373–378. [CrossRef]
85. Kaptein, B.L.; Pijls, B.; Koster, L.; Kärrholm, J.; Hull, M.; Niesen, A.; Heesterbeek, P.; Callary, S.; Teeter, M.; Gascoyne, T.; et al. Guideline for RSA and CT-RSA implant migration measurements: An update of standardizations and recommendations. *Acta Orthop.* **2024**, *95*, 256–267. [CrossRef]
86. Burssens, A.; Peeters, J.; Buedts, K.; Victor, J.; Vandeputte, G. Measuring hindfoot alignment in weight bearing CT: A novel clinical relevant measurement method. *Foot Ankle Surg.* **2016**, *22*, 233–238. [CrossRef]
87. Lenz, A.L.; Strobel, M.A.; Anderson, A.M.; Fial, A.V.; MacWilliams, B.A.; Krzak, J.J.; Kruger, K.M. Assignment of local coordinate systems and methods to calculate tibiotalar and subtalar kinematics: A systematic review. *J. Biomech.* **2021**, *120*, 110344. [CrossRef]
88. Bernasconi, A.; Cooper, L.; Lyle, S.; Patel, S.; Cullen, N.; Singh, D.; Welck, M. Intraobserver and interobserver reliability of cone beam weightbearing semi-automatic three-dimensional measurements in symptomatic pes cavovarus. *Foot Ankle Surg.* **2020**, *26*, 564–572. [CrossRef]
89. Turmezei, T.D.; Low, S.B.; Rupret, S.; Treece, G.M.; Gee, A.H.; MacKay, J.W.; Lynch, J.A.; Poole, K.E.; Segal, N.A. Multiparametric 3-D analysis of bone and joint space width at the knee from weight bearing computed tomography. *Osteoarthr. Imaging* **2022**, *2*, 100069. [CrossRef]
90. Kothari, M.D.; Rabe, K.G.; Anderson, D.D.; Nevitt, M.C.; Lynch, J.A.; Segal, N.A.; Franz, H. The Relationship of Three-Dimensional Joint Space Width on Weight Bearing CT With Pain and Physical Function. *J. Orthop. Res.* **2019**, *38*, 1333–1339. [CrossRef]
91. Probasco, W.; Haleem, A.M.; Yu, J.; Sangeorzan, B.J.; Deland, J.T.; Ellis, S.J. Assessment of coronal plane subtalar joint alignment in peritalar subluxation via weight-bearing multiplanar imaging. *Foot Ankle Int.* **2015**, *36*, 302–309. [CrossRef]
92. Ananthakrisnan, D.; Ching, R.; Tencer, A.; Hansen, S.T.J.; Sangeorzan, B.J. Subluxation of the talocalcaneal joint in adults who have symptomatic flatfoot. *J. Bone Jt. Surg. Am.* **1999**, *81*, 1147–1154. [CrossRef]
93. Dibbern, K.N.; Li, S.; Vivtcharenko, V.; Auch, E.; Lintz, F.; Ellis, S.J.; Femino, J.E.; de Cesar Netto, C. Three-Dimensional Distance and Coverage Maps in the Assessment of Peritalar Subluxation in Progressive Collapsing Foot Deformity. *Foot Ankle Int.* **2021**, *42*, 757–767. [CrossRef]

94. Krähenbühl, N.; Akkaya, M.; Dodd, A.E.; Hintermann, B.; Dutilh, G.; Lenz, A.L.; Barg, A.; International Weight Bearing CT Society. Impact of the rotational position of the hindfoot on measurements assessing the integrity of the distal tibio-fibular syndesmosis. *Foot Ankle Surg.* **2020**, *26*, 810–817. [CrossRef]
95. de Cesar Netto, C. CORR Insights®: Can Weightbearing Cone-beam CT Reliably Differentiate Between Stable and Unstable Syndesmotic Ankle Injuries? A Systematic Review and Meta-Analysis. *Clin. Orthop. Relat. Res.* **2022**, *480*, 1563–1565. [CrossRef]
96. Shakoor, D.; Osgood, G.M.; Brehler, M.; Zbijewski, W.B.; de Cesar Netto, C.; Shafiq, B.; Orapin, J.; Thawait, G.K.; Shon, L.C.; Demehri, S. Cone-beam CT measurements of distal tibio-fibular syndesmosis in asymptomatic uninjured ankles: Does weight-bearing matter? *Skeletal Radiol.* **2019**, *48*, 583–594. [CrossRef]
97. Auch, E.; Barbachan Mansur, N.S.; Alexandre Alves, T.; Cychosz, C.; Lintz, F.; Godoy-Santos, A.L.; Baumfeld, D.S.; de Cesar Netto, C. Distal Tibiofibular Syndesmotic Widening in Progressive Collapsing Foot Deformity. *Foot Ankle Int.* **2021**, *42*, 768–775. [CrossRef]

Disclaimer/Publisher's Note: The statements, opinions and data contained in all publications are solely those of the individual author(s) and contributor(s) and not of MDPI and/or the editor(s). MDPI and/or the editor(s) disclaim responsibility for any injury to people or property resulting from any ideas, methods, instructions or products referred to in the content.

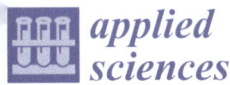

Review

Ins and Outs of the Ankle Syndesmosis from a 2D to 3D CT Perspective

Thibaut Dhont [1,†], Manu Huyghe [1,†], Matthias Peiffer [2,*], Noortje Hagemeijer [3], Bedri Karaismailoglu [4,5], Nicola Krahenbuhl [6], Emmanuel Audenaert [2] and Arne Burssens [2]

1. Faculty of Medicine and Health Sciences, Ghent University, 9000 Gent, Belgium
2. Department of Orthopedic Surgery and Traumatology, Ghent University Hospital, 9000 Ghent, Belgium
3. Department of Orthopedic Surgery, Amsterdam UMC, University of Amsterdam, Meibergdreef 9, 1105 AZ Amsterdam, The Netherlands
4. Department of Orthopedics and Traumatology, Istanbul University-Cerrahpasa, 34320 Istanbul, Turkey
5. CAST-Cerrahpasa Research, Simulation and Design Laboratory, Istanbul University-Cerrahpasa, 34320 Istanbul, Turkey
6. Department of Orthopedics and Traumatology, Universitätsspital Basel, 4031 Basel, Switzerland
* Correspondence: matthias.peiffer@ugent.be; Tel.: +32-9332-2251
† These authors contributed equally to this work.

Abstract: Despite various proposed measurement techniques for assessing syndesmosis integrity, a standardized protocol is lacking, and the existing literature reports inconsistent findings regarding normal and abnormal relationships between the fibula and tibia at the distal level. Therefore, this study aims to present an overview of two- (2D) and three-dimensional (3D) measurement methods utilized to evaluate syndesmosis integrity. A topical literature review was conducted, including studies employing 2D or 3D measurement techniques to quantify distal tibiofibular syndesmosis alignment on computed tomography (CT) or weight-bearing CT (WBCT) scans. A total of 49 eligible articles were included in this review. While most interclass correlation (ICC) values indicate favorable reliability, certain measurements involving multiple steps exhibited lower ICC values, potentially due to the learning curve associated with their implementation. Inconclusive results were obtained regarding the influence of age, sex, and height on syndesmotic measurements. No significant difference was observed between bilateral ankles, permitting the use of the opposite side as an internal control for comparison. There is a notable range of normal and pathological values, as evidenced by the standard deviation associated with each measurement. This review highlights the absence of a consensus on syndesmotic measurements for assessing integrity despite numerous CT scan studies. The diverse measurement techniques, complexity, and inconclusive findings present challenges in distinguishing between normal and pathological values in routine clinical practice. Promising advancements in novel 3D techniques offer potential for automated measurements and reduction of observer inaccuracies, but further validation is needed.

Keywords: ankle syndesmosis; weightbearing CT; 3D modelling; 2D measurements; sport injuries

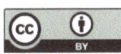

1. Introduction

The ankle syndesmosis entails a complex interplay of bony and ligamentous structures. The ankle ligaments play a crucial role in preventing tibiofibular displacement and maintaining a stable ankle mortise [1]. When this syndesmotic complex is impaired due to injury, whether high ankle sprains or fracture-associated, the normal mortise configuration is disrupted, leading to atypical biomechanics of the tibiotalar joint. This can result in an alteration of the contact area between the tibia and talus, leading to heightened pressure on the talar dome and tibial plafond [1,2]. The syndesmosis is injured in 4–24% of all ankle sprains and 10–45% of cases with concomitant ankle fractures [3–6]. Subgroups with more risk include athletes, females, children, adolescents, and patients with a history of ankle sprains [7].

The diagnosis of syndesmotic injuries is crucial as untreated or misdiagnosed lesions can lead to irreversible, long-term morbidity such as pain, poor function, mortise incongruence, early osteoarthritis, anterolateral soft tissue impingement, and local synovitis [4,8–10]. An accurate diagnosis can be obscured due to the low sensitivity and specificity of the clinical examination tests (i.e., ligament palpation tenderness, external rotation stress test according to Frick, squeeze test, cotton test, and fibula translation test) [11,12]. Consequently, advanced imaging modalities such as computed tomography (CT), magnetic resonance imaging (MRI), or arthroscopy are indispensable in current clinical practice [3,13,14]. Although arthroscopy is the most reliable method for diagnosis, it is hampered by its invasive nature, cost, and lack of native contralateral reference [9,10,13,14]. Therefore, non-invasive imaging modalities have been broadly described to visualize the syndesmosis and detect injury. However, their true value in diagnosing instability and integrity remains equivocal [8,14,15]. Radiographs are poorly sensitive and may be valuable only in cases of severe instability [8,9]. Furthermore, the position of the hindfoot during radiography affects the measurements subsequently [16]. Supine CT, on the other hand, has improved levels of sensitivity, but it underestimates the extent of subtle lesions due to its non-weight-bearing and non-dynamic nature [3,10]. While MRI is highly accurate in identifying ligamentous damage, its availability may be limited, and even when it detects such injury, it does not necessarily indicate the presence of instability [17,18]. Meanwhile, weight-bearing CT (WBCT) provides less radiation and allows for three-dimensional (3D) imaging of the weight-bearing dynamism, with the contralateral ankle serving as an internal control given the variable anatomy of the incisura [3,8,10].

Although several measurement techniques have been proposed to assess the syndesmosis, there is no established protocol, and the available literature shows inconsistent findings regarding the range of (ab)normal relationships between the fibula and tibia at the distal level. Therefore, the aim of this study is to provide an overview of the two-dimensional (2D) and 3D measurement methods for evaluating the integrity of the syndesmosis.

2. Methodology

2.1. Search Strategy

A topical literature review was conducted. Three major medical databases (PubMed, Web of Science, and Google Scholar) were searched through June 2023. The following search terms were used: (syndesmosis injury OR distal tibiofibular joint injury OR syndesmotic injury OR syndesmosis instability OR syndesmotic instability OR distal tibiofibular joint instability) and (CT OR computed tomography OR WBCT OR weight-bearing CT OR weight-bearing computed tomography). No limitations were held on the type of journal or publication date of the article.

2.2. Study Selection

The records were screened independently by two reviewers (T.D. and M.H.). Inclusion criteria were composed of studies involving 2D or 3D measurement methods to quantify the alignment of the distal tibiofibular syndesmosis on CT and WBCT imaging. Exclusion criteria consisted of case reports, review articles, different imaging modalities (i.e., ultrasound, MRI, or arthroscopy), studies involving patients < 18 years old, studies concerning post-operative alignment, and manuscripts in languages other than English. The additional literature was obtained by searching references in the manuscripts ("snowball method") [19].

2.3. Data Extraction

Mean values, normative reference values, pathological values, and interobserver reliability values (ICC) for the measurement methods were extracted from every record, if available. The weighted mean and standard deviation were calculated for every measurement method included in each record. The normative reference limit for these measurements was extracted, and the weighted mean was calculated if more than two reference limits were available for one measurement. Since weight-bearing has been reported to affect the kinematics of the syndesmosis [20], mean and reference values were established separately for WBCT and conventional CT studies. All calculations were computed using Microsoft® Excel (version 1808, 2019).

3. Results

3.1. Search Results

The aforementioned literature search generated 1716 articles. After the removal of duplicates, 1249 records remained and were consequently screened on the title, after which 262 were suitable for abstract assessment. After reviewing the abstracts, 53 articles met the inclusion criteria. The researchers assessed the final 53 records for eligibility. A total of 13 records were excluded based on the following criteria: case reports ($n = 2$), review articles ($n = 3$), other imaging modalities ($n = 6$), and studies including patients < 18 years old ($n = 2$). Moreover, nine additional studies were identified through the references cited in the selected manuscripts. Finally, 49 articles were included in the review (Figure 1).

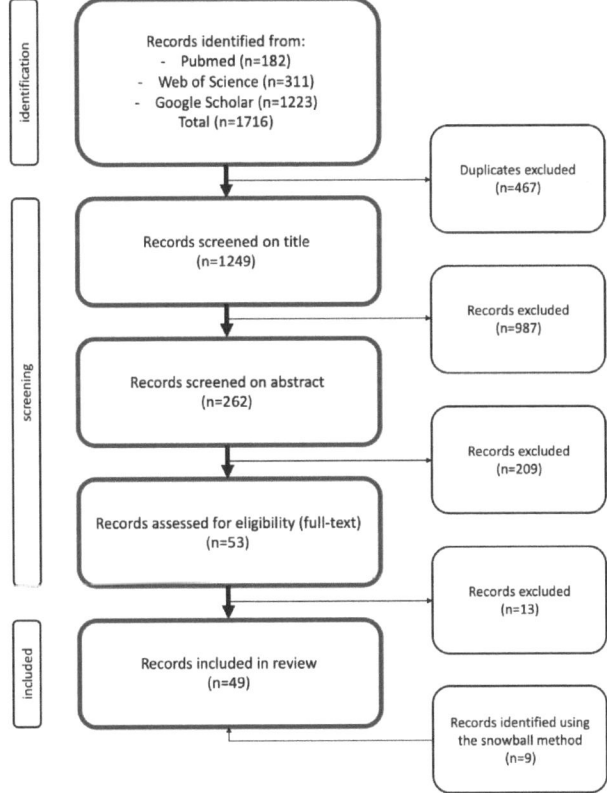

Figure 1. Flowchart illustrating the selection process of the included articles, according to the PRISMA guidelines [21].

3.2. Study Characteristics

Data were extracted from 29 of the 49 trials. The other trials were used to describe the measurements and their usefulness in daily practice but did not provide useful data.

Out of these, 13 (45%) articles utilized CT to assess the integrity of the syndesmosis, while 10 (35%) articles used WBCT, and 6 (20%) articles employed both methods. Furthermore, 8 studies analyzed both injured and healthy patients, while 1 study focused solely on injured patients, and 11 studies exclusively examined healthy individuals. Moreover, 1 article conducted its examination on cadaveric populations, whereas 19 articles conducted their examinations on in vivo populations. Additionally, out of the 13 measurements discussed in this review, only 1 measurement was performed at the talocrural level instead of 1 cm proximal to the tibia plafond. Ten articles were focused on novel (3D) imaging techniques.

3.3. Conventional 2D Measurements

In Table 1, a description of all 2D measurements is provided. Table 2 presents the mean, normative reference limit, and ICC per measurement, if available. Figures 2–4 depict the mediolateral translation measurements, fibular rotation measurements, and fibular translation measurements, respectively.

Table 1. Description of radiological measurements.

Measurement	Description	References
a. Mediolateral translation (diastasis)		
Anterior tibiofibular width (A)	The distance between the anterior tibial tubercle and the nearest fibular point.	[5,6,13,18,20,22–32]
Posterior tibiofibular width (B)	The distance between the posterior tibial tubercle and the nearest fibular point.	[5,6,13,20,22–24,26–29,31,32]
Middle tibiofibular width	The distance between the most central point of the incisura and the nearest fibular point.	[5,13,18,20,28,31–33]
Maximum tibiofibular width	The maximal distance between the tibia and fibula, regardless of the location	[32]
Minimum tibiofibular width	The minimal distance between the tibia and fibula, regardless of the location.	[26]
Syndesmotic area	The surface area, delineated by the medial cortex of the fibula and the lateral cortex of the tibial incisura, and two lines tangential to the anterior and posterior cortices of the tibia and fibula	[13,26,31,33–35]
b. Fibular rotation		
Fibular rotation by Dikos (α)	The angle between the fibular axis and the tangential line to the anterior and posterior tibial tubercles. A higher angle value indicates internal rotation of the fibula, while a lower angle value indicates external rotation.	[5,13,20,22,26,28,29,31,33,36]
Tang ratio	The ratio of distances from the tibial centroid to the most anterior fibular point and from the tibial centroid to the most posterior fibular point.	[23,26,29]
Ratio A/B	The ratio between the anterior tibiofibular width (A) and posterior tibiofibular width (B). The ratio increases as the fibula externally rotates.	[5,20,28]
Bimalleolar angle (β)	The angle between the tangential line to the medial cortex of the lateral malleolus and the tangential line to the lateral cortex of the medial malleolus, at the level of the talar dome or more distally.	[28,37]

Table 1. Cont.

Measurement	Description	References
c. Fibular translation		
Anteroposterior translational ratio by Nault	This is a three-step measurement. A line is drawn between the most anterior and most posterior points of the incisura. A perpendicular line is drawn in the middle of the first line. The distance between the anterior part of the fibula and the perpendicular line is the distance A. B is the distance between the posterior part of the fibula and the perpendicular line. The ratio A/B represents a description of the anteroposterior position.	[5,20,28]
Medial Phisitkul	A first reference line is established by drawing a tangential line along the most lateral aspect of the anterior and posterior tubercles of the fibular incisura. A second reference line is drawn perpendicular to this line at the anterior tubercle. The distance from the most medial point of the fibula to the first line represents the mediolateral position of the fibula. This measurement is positive if the fibula is lateral to the reference line and negative if the fibula is medial to the reference line.	[23,29,38]
Anterior Phisitkul	This distance is measured from the most anterior point of the fibula to the second reference line explained in the measurement above. If the fibula is anterior to the reference line, the value is negative; if the fibula is posterior to the reference line, the value is positive.	[5,13,20,23,26,28,29,38,39]

Table 2. Mean, definitive normative reference limit, and mean ICC per measurement.

Measurement	Mean ± SD	Definitive Normative Reference Limit	Mean ICC
a. Mediolateral translation (diastasis)			
Anterior tibiofibular width (in mm)	CT, normal: 2.71 ± 0.80 CT, injury: 3.50 ± 1.18 WBCT, normal: 3.51 ± 0.60 WBCT, injury: 3.77 ± 1.1	Cut-off max value, CT: 4 [32] Max normal difference with respect to contralateral ankle, CT: 0.7 [18]	CT: 0.834 WBCT: 0.758
Posterior tibiofibular width (in mm)	CT, normal: 4.74 ± 1.74 CT, injury: 4.92 ± 0.29 WBCT, normal: 5.97 ± 1.48 WBCT, injury: 7.38 ± 2.69	/	CT: 0.799 WBCT: 0.714
Middle tibiofibular width (in mm)	CT, normal: 3.58 ± 0.47 CT, injury: 4.25 ± 1.48 WBCT, normal: 4.28 ± 0.78 WBCT, injury: 5.05 ± 1.34	Cut-off max value, CT: 3.95 [32] Cut-off for the difference between injured and uninjured ankle, CT: 1.7 [18] Normative reference range, WBCT: 1.23–5.2 [5]	CT: 0.788 WBCT: 0.803
Maximum tibiofibular width (in mm)	CT, normal: 4.6 ± 1.4 CT, injury: 7.2 ± 2.96 WBCT, normal: / WBCT, injury: /	Cut-off max value, CT: 5.65 [32]	CT: 0.865
Minimum tibiofibular width (in mm)	CT, normal: 1.6 ± 0.2 CT, injury: 2.9 ± 0.3 WBCT, normal: 2.6 ± 0.2 WBCT, injury: 2.9 ± 0.3	/	CT: 0.899 WBCT: 0.875

Table 2. *Cont.*

Measurement	Mean ± SD	Definitive Normative Reference Limit	Mean ICC
Syndesmotic area (in mm^2)	CT, normal: 105.2 ± 22.6 CT, injury: 129.5 ± 31.3 WBCT, normal: 106.0 ± 16.9 WBCT, injury: 134.1 ± 28.2	/	CT: 0.96 WBCT: 0.93
b. Fibular rotation			
Fibular rotation Dikos (in degrees)	CT, normal: 13.6 ± 3.3 CT, injury: 15 ± 6.4 WBCT, normal: 12.3 ± 1.8 WBCT, injury: 7.39 ± 1.1	/	CT: 0.689 WBCT: 0.783
Tang ratio	CT, normal: 0.85 ± 0.05 CT, injury: / WBCT, normal: 0.85 ± 0.05 WBCT, injury: /	/	CT: 0.47 WBCT: 0.72
Ratio A/B	CT, normal: 0.55 ± 0.03 CT, injury: / WBCT, normal: 0.62 ± 0.03 WBCT, injury: /	Normative reference range, WBCT: 0.12–1.08 [5]	CT: 0.722 WBCT: 0.79
Bimalleolar angle (in degrees)	CT, normal: 7.67 ± 1.1 CT, injury: / WBCT, normal: / WBCT, injury: /	/	CT: 0.68 WBCT: /
c. Fibular translation			
Anteroposterior translational ratio by Nault	CT, normal: 1.54 ± 0.08 CT, injury: / WBCT, normal: 1.45 ± 0.00 WBCT, injury: /	Normative reference range, WBCT: 0.31–2.59 [5]	CT: 0.441 WBCT: 0.72
Medial Phisitkul (in mm)	/	/	CT: 0.86
Anterior Phisitkul (in mm)	CT, normal: 1.59 ± 0.50 CT, injury: 1.79 ± 1.55 WBCT, normal: 1.60 ± 0.14 WBCT, injury: 1.37 ± 0.27	Normative reference range, WBCT: −1.48–3.44 [5]	CT: 0.725 WBCT: 0.763

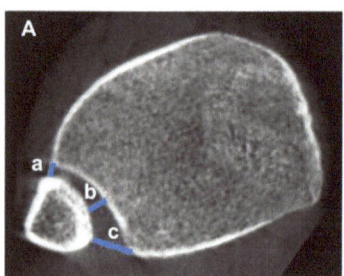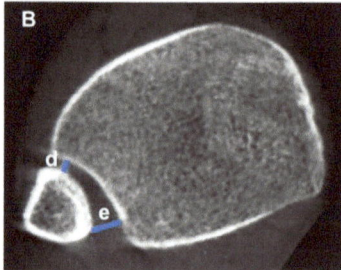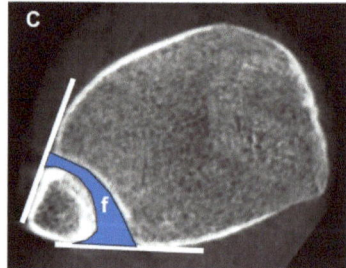

Figure 2. Mediolateral translation measurements on an axial CT image of an uninjured syndesmosis. (**A**) Anterior tibiofibular width (a), middle tibiofibular width (b), and posterior tibiofibular width (c). (**B**) Minimum tibiofibular width (d) and maximum tibiofibular width (e). (**C**) Syndesmotic area (blue area, f), based on the two lines tangential to the anterior and posterior cortices of the tibia and fibula (solid white lines).

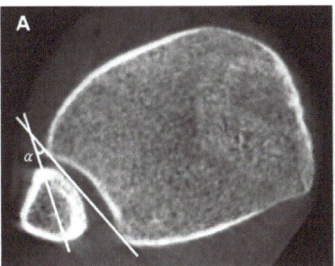 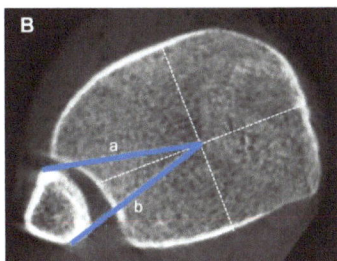 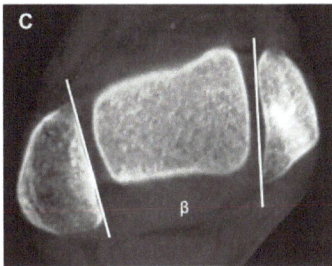

Figure 3. Fibular rotation measurements on an axial CT image of an uninjured syndesmosis and ankle. (**A**) Fibular rotation angle (α) by Dikos, The angle between the fibular axis and the tangential line to the anterior and posterior tibial tubercles (white lines) [36]. (**B**) Tang ratio of anterior (a) and posterior measurement (b), represented as the ratio of distances from the tibial centroid (white dashed lines) to the most anterior fibular point and the most posterior fibular point, respectively (blue solid lines). (**C**) Bimalleolar angle (β), calculated between the tangential line to the medial cortex of the lateral malleolus and the tangential line to the lateral cortex of the medial malleolus (solid white lines).

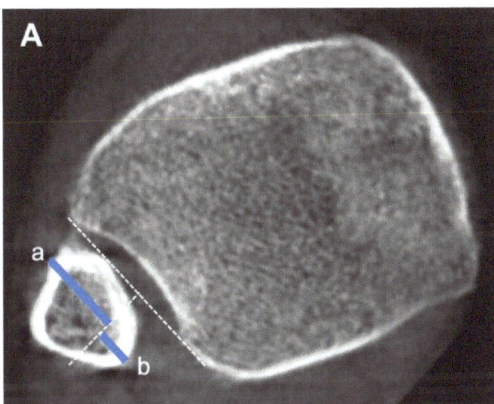 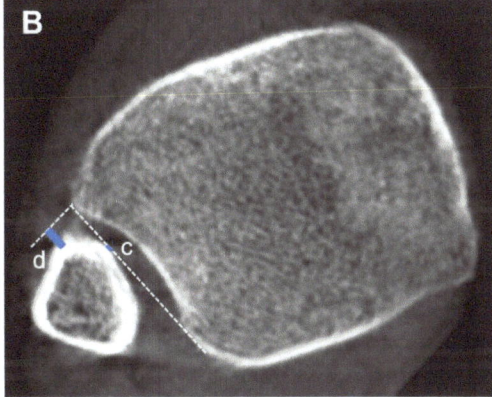

Figure 4. Fibular translation measurements on an axial CT image of an uninjured syndesmosis. (**A**) Anteroposterior translation ratio by Nault [28] of anterior distance (a) and posterior distance (b) (blue lines), calculated based from a perpendicular line, drawn from the middle of a line connecting the most anterior and posterior points of the incisura (white solid lines). (**B**) Medial (c) and anterior (d) Phisitkul measurement (blue lines), calculated from a line connecting the most anterior and posterior points of the incisura, and a perpendicular line perpendicular to the previous line at the level of the anterior tubercle (white dashed lines).

3.3.1. 2D Measurements Quantifying Tibiofibular Translation
Mediolateral Translation (Diastasis)

- Anterior, middle, posterior, maximum, and minimum tibiofibular width

First described by Gardner et al. [25], the anterior tibiofibular width (ATFW) and posterior tibiofibular width (PTFW) are the most commonly used measurements of the distal tibiofibular joint in the literature [5,6,13,18,20,22–32]. They serve as indicators of diastasis between the tibia and fibula [29]. Nault et al. introduced the middle tibiofibular width (MTFW) as an additional measurement for diastasis [28]. More recently, Yeung et al. and Ahn et al. introduced the maximum tibiofibular width (MxTFW) and minimum tibiofibular width (MnTFW), respectively [22,32]. These measurements are generally performed at the level of 1 cm proximal to the tibial plafond on axial images, as depicted in Figure 2A,B and described in Table 1 This level is consistently selected due to the prominent tibial tubercles and well-defined fibular incisura at this extent [6,13,22,24,25,27,28]. Most studies exhibit a wide standard deviation (SD), resulting in a broad normative range [28]. Furthermore, the reference values do not account for age and gender. Park et al. reported that the posterior width is significantly smaller in women ($p < 0.001$), and both ATFW and PTFW significantly decrease with age ($p < 0.001$) [6]. On the other hand, some studies showed no significant difference in AFTW and PFTW by age and gender [29,31]. However, there is no significant difference compared to the contralateral ankle, enabling bilateral comparison in the evaluation of syndesmotic injury [6,31]. No significant differences were observed in the ATFW, PTFW, and MTFW under both normal and weight-bearing conditions. [20,29]. Additionally, the interobserver reliability is excellent for the MnTFW and MxTFW and good for the ATFW, PTFW, and MTFW, indicating the reliability of these parameters.

A recent study compared the ATFW and MTFW of the injured ankle with the contralateral uninjured ankle in 68 patients under non-weight-bearing conditions [18]. The mean distances were 0.3 greater in injured ankles compared to uninjured for both measurements. Ideal cut-off values for instability assessing the difference between the injured and uninjured ankle were set at 0.7 and 1.7 for ATFW and MTFW, respectively. These values demonstrate low sensitivity (25%) but high specificity (97%) for ATFW. For MTFW, the value is primarily useful for ruling out syndesmotic injuries, with low sensitivity (0%) but high specificity (100%) [18]. Another study compared ATFW, MTFW, PTFW, and MxTFW in ankles that were assessed intraoperatively. The ankles were operated on due to ankle fractures, with syndesmotic integrity tests performed to differentiate between stable and unstable syndesmosis. There was a significant difference between the measurements for stable and unstable ankles for the ATFW, MTFW, PTFW, and MxTFW ($p < 0.001; p = 0.014; p = 0.042; p < 0.001$). Cut-off values were set at 4 (sens = 56.5, spec = 91.7) for ATFW, 3.95 (sens = 74.4, spec = 75) for MTFW, and 5.65 (sens = 74.4, spec = 78.9) for MxTFW. The authors recommended that the PTFW should not be used for diagnosis [32]. Hamard et al. conducted non-weight-bearing CT and WBCT scans on injured and uninjured ankles. The distance was significantly greater for the PTFW and MnTFW in both conditions, while the ATFW was only significantly larger in non-weight-bearing conditions [26]. Another study confirmed these findings specifically for ATFW and PTFW in non-weight-bearing conditions [22]. Under weight-bearing conditions, the MTFW is significantly greater in injured ankles [33].

Anteroposterior Translation

- Anteroposterior translation ratio by Nault

This ratio, first described by Nault et al., is a description of the anteroposterior position of the fibula in relation to the incisura and determines translation [28]. This ratio is obtained in three steps, as depicted in Figure 4A and described in Table 1. Due to the complexity of this measurement, the ICC varies in every study. Interestingly, more recent studies have better interobserver reliability than older studies, which could be explained by the learning curve of clinicians [5,20,28].

This measurement has only been documented in uninjured ankles [5,20,28]. In weight-bearing conditions, this ratio is significantly lower ($p = 0.007$) [20]. Injury may be suspected if values are outside the range of 0.31 to 2.59. No sensitivity or specificity is given for this range [5]. As no pathological values are known, these values cannot be compared with pathological values.

- Anterior and Medial Phisitkul

First described by Phisitkul et al., this translational parameter of the fibula has been used to assess syndesmosis reduction following ankle injury. Both measurements are depicted in Figure 4B and described in Table 1 [38]. Nowadays, the anterior Phisitkul is the most commonly used translational measurement [5,13,20,23,26,28,29,38,39].

Interobserver reliability is good for the anterior measurement and excellent for the medial measurement. No mean values could be obtained for the medial measurement.

Conflicting results have been found for differences between the sexes [5,29]. There is no significant difference between the two legs under normal conditions, indicating that the legs can be compared when assessing syndesmotic injury. Moreover, age has no influence on this measurement [5]. Weight-bearing conditions do not exert a substantial influence on both healthy and injured ankles [20]. The area under curve (AUC) values were 0.894 and 0.467 for CT and WBCT, respectively. Therefore, the authors stated that the anterior Phisitkul was excellent at differentiating between normal and injured syndesmosis using non-weight-bearing CT but less reliable in WBCT [26]. A normative reference range of −1.48 to 3.44 was obtained, but no sensitivity or specificity was reported [5].

3.3.1.3. The 2D Measurements Quantifying Tibiofibular Rotation

Assessment of fibular rotation plays a crucial role in evaluating the integrity of the syndesmotic joint. Injuries are generally characterized by diastasis and external rotation of the fibula [3,37]. The most cited method was initially described by Dikos et al., measuring fibular rotation relative to the tibial incisura, 1 cm proximal to the tibial plafond [5,13,20,22,26,28,29,31,33,36]. Alternative measurements are performed at the level of the talar dome or slightly distal therefrom, determining rotation along the medial and lateral malleolus [28,37]. However, some studies do not quantify rotation in degrees but rather use ratios, whereby an increase correlates with the external rotation of the fibula, e.g., the ratio of ATFW and PTFW [5,20,28]. An additional measurement ratio, defined by Tang, analyzes fibular rotation around the tibial centroid [23,26,29,40]. Measurements are depicted in Figure 3A–C and described in Table 1.

The orientation of the fibula within an uninjured syndesmosis has been described in relative detail in the currently available literature [5,13,20,22,28,29,31,33,36]. When imaged via CT, a mean internal rotation of 13.6° is observed in non-weight-bearing conditions, as opposed to 12.3° under weight-bearing conditions. Therefore, the fibula is exposed to an average 1.3° of external rotation when loaded. Fewer studies are available in the field of syndesmotic lesions. A mean external rotation of 7.61° was observed when comparing CT and WBCT. Furthermore, interobserver reliability was good in both non-weight-bearing (ICC = 0.689) and weight-bearing (ICC = 0.783) conditions. The reviewed studies reported no significant differences for age or sex, except for Wong et al., who noticed a naturally significant increase in internal rotation of 0.2° per year [31].

The bimalleolar angle was ascribed by two studies at different heights on axial CT images. Nault et al. measured the level of the talar dome, whereas Vetter et al. suggest that the ideal plane is located 4–6 mm more distal [28,37]. An average external rotation of 7.67° was achieved despite varying measurement heights. Good reliability was outlined by both authors (ICC = 0.68).

Just a handful of studies examined fibular rotation ratios, all within healthy syndesmosis populations [5,20,23,26,28,29]. A mean Tang ratio of 0.85 was found for both CT and WBCT. The corresponding ICC values are poor (ICC = 0.47) and good (ICC = 0.79), respectively. As for ratio A/B, a mean of 0.55 was found for CT and 0.62 for WBCT, thus resulting in a 0.07 increase of the external rotation when loaded. A good ICC was found in both CT (ICC = 0.72) and WBCT (ICC = 0.79).

3.3.2. The 2D Measurements Quantifying Syndesmotic Area

Despite numerous linear measurements, Malhotra et al. first described the area between the fibula and tibia 1 cm above the tibial plafond, i.e., the syndesmotic area, as depicted in Figure 2C and described in Table 1 [35]. Subsequently, this measure has been used increasingly. Multiple articles describe injured and uninjured syndesmoses in both non-weight-bearing and weight-bearing conditions [13,26,31,33–35].

Within healthy syndesmoses, a mean area of 105.2 mm^2 and 106 mm^2 was found for CT and WBCT, respectively. In the presence of lesions, the area increases to 129.5 mm^2 on CT and 134.1 mm^2 on WBCT. Therefore, injured syndesmoses are, on average, 24.3 mm^2 (CT) and 28.1 mm^2 (WBCT) larger compared to non-injured.

Hagemeijer et al. examined one cohort of unilateral injured and contralateral healthy syndesmoses in addition to a second cohort of bilateral uninjured ankles. Merely a mean difference of 0.41 mm^2 was detected between the left and right normal syndesmotic areas, in contrast to a difference of 46 mm^2 of unilateral injury. These findings support the use of contralateral, uninjured syndesmosis as an internal control for injury assessment [33].

A significantly greater area ($p < 0.001$) was identified on CT images in injured ankles relative to normal ones [26,34,35]. Similar significance ($p < 0.001$) was achieved for WBCT [26,34]. Del Rio et al. reported a mean increase in the syndesmotic area of 8.8% and 19.9% for CT and WBCT, respectively [34]. In addition, a larger area difference was detected between non-injured syndesmosis for men compared to women, which approached near significance for CT ($p = 0.069$) and WBCT ($p = 0.063$) [31,34]. Furthermore, weight-bearing induced a difference between normal and injured ankles that was significantly greater for men ($p = 0.04$) [34]. Wong et al. investigated the impact of a talocrural range of motion (ROM) on the syndesmotic area and found that the surface decreased on average by 26 mm^2 ($p < 0.001$) going from dorsiflexion to plantar flexion [31].

Excellent interobserver reliability was documented for syndesmotic area estimation for both CT (ICC = 0.96) and WBCT (ICC = 0.93).

3.4. Novel 3D Measurement Methods

Several studies have focused on transforming the aforementioned 2D measurements into a 3D framework. Several emerging 3D techniques have been found in the literature, which will be topically described below.

3.4.1. 3D Mirroring—Alignment Techniques

By mirroring the healthy and injured ankle in bilateral imaging, the contralateral ankle is used as internal control. After aligning both tibiae, the relative displacement of one fibula with respect to the control can be visualized and quantified (Figure 5). Ebinger et al. were the first to align both tibiae in a cadaveric study to quantify the 3D displacement of the fibula [23]. In their study, they have shown that 2D clinical measurements correlate poorly with the actual 3D displacement. Burssens et al. improved upon this using the contralateral healthy ankle as a template after mirroring the injured ankle to diagnose high ankle sprains and fracture-associated syndesmotic lesions [3]. In their study, the average mediolateral diastasis of both the sprained group (mean = 1.6 mm) and the fracture group (mean = 1.7 mm) exhibited significant differences compared to the control group ($p < 0.001$). Additionally, they found a significant difference in the average external rotation between the sprained group (mean = 4.7°) and the fracture group (mean = 7.0°) when compared to the control group ($p < 0.05$). Peiffer et al. refined the examination of subtle syndesmotic lesions using external torque during WBCT [41]. Significance was proven for ATFW and alpha angle computed on patient-specific 3D models.

3.4.2. The 3D Distance Mapping

Recently, the calculation of 3D distance maps has been introduced in ankle syndesmosis. These maps assess the relative position between two surfaces at each point, plotted on the bony contour. They are defined and calculated as the shortest surface-to-surface distance between each point of the 3D model and the opposing surface. Dibbern et al. were the first to apply these distance maps to the clinical entity of the syndesmosis [42]. The benefit of this technique is that it allows for an accurate and straightforward interpretation of the 3D tibiofibular diastasis in one image. In Figure 6, we have presented an example of distance mapping in a patient with a syndesmotic injury.

3.4.3. The 3D Volume Measurements

Several authors have investigated the use of volumetric measurements of the distal tibiofibular articulation. In this technique, the total interosseous volume is calculated, extending from the level of the tibial plafond up to a height of 1, 3, 5, or 10 cm proximally (Figure 7). These 3D volume measurements were introduced by Taser et al. in their cadaveric experiment, showing a 43% (441 mm^3) increase in syndesmotic volume after 1 mm diastasis and an additional 20% increase for each extra 1 mm [43]. Ten years later, Kocadal et al. described the use of volume measurements to compare the post-operative syndesmotic reduction between screw fixation and suture-button techniques, unveiling a significant increase of 8% (118.5 mm^3) in suture-button fixation [44]. Additionally, they found an intra-observer reliability of 0.882 and an interobserver reliability of 0.861 for their measurement technique. Bhimani et al. and Ashkani-Esfahani et al. recently popularized these 3D volume measurements, showing high sensitivity (95.8%) and specificity (83.3%) for the detection of syndesmotic instability [8,9]. Moreover, they stated a cut-off value of 11.6 cm^3 (or 25.4% increase in volume) at the level of 5 cm above the tibial plafond, which reported an excellent ICC of 0.93.

3.4.4. The 3D Statistical Shape Model—Based Techniques

Peiffer et al. focused on using statistical shape models and ligament modeling techniques to model the path and quantify the predicted length of the syndesmotic ligaments in patients with high ankle sprains and asymptomatic controls [17]. They reported a statistically significant difference in anterior tibiofibular ligament length between ankles with syndesmotic lesions and healthy controls (p = 0.017). They also found a significant correlation between the presence of syndesmotic injury and the positional alignment between the distal tibia and fibula (r = 0.873, p < 0.001). More specifically, they described an "anterior open-book injury" of the ankle syndesmosis as a result of anterior inferior tibiofibular ligament elongation/rupture (Figure 8).

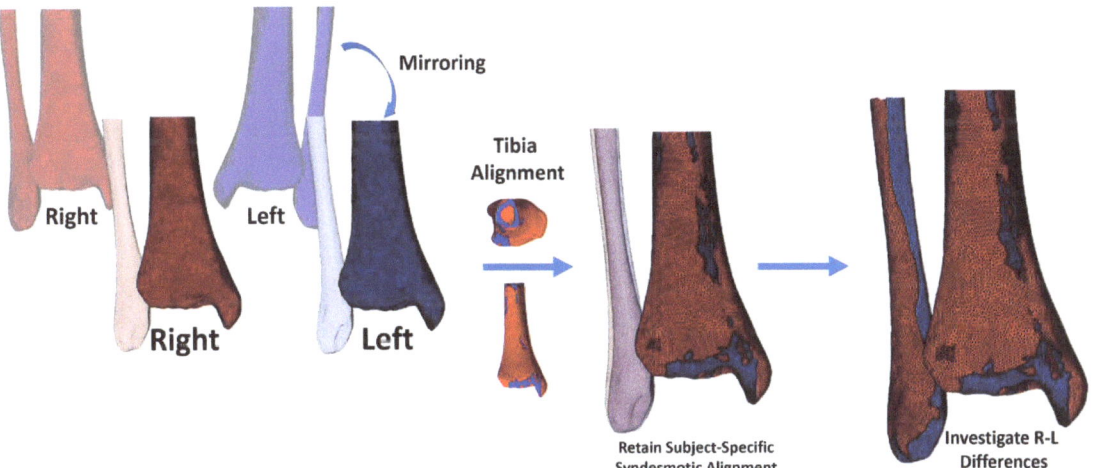

Figure 5. Mirroring and alignment of the right (red) and left (blue) ankle. The left ankle tibia is mirrored and rigidly registered to the right tibia. By aligning both tibiae, the side-specific anatomical configuration of the ankle syndesmosis is retained, and the relative displacement of the fibula can be visualized.

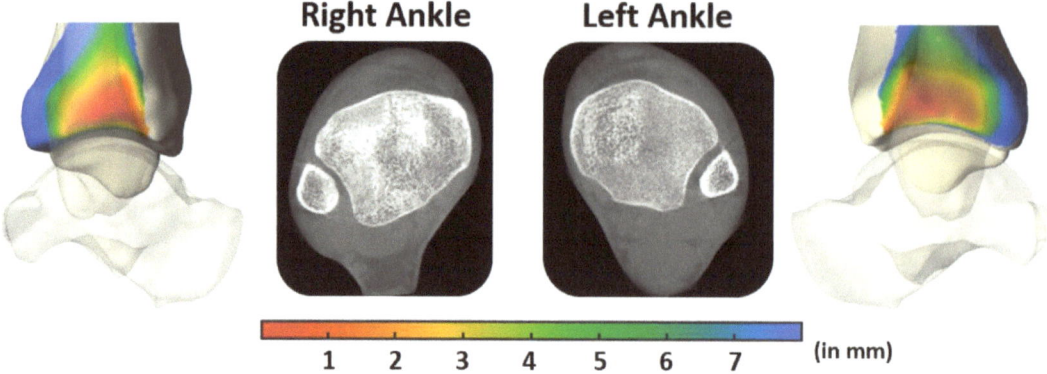

Figure 6. Example of distance map analysis. Weight-bearing CT images in a patient with a syndesmotic injury in the left ankle. A corresponding 3D distance mapping is presented, which reveals an increased tibiofibular clear space on the left side.

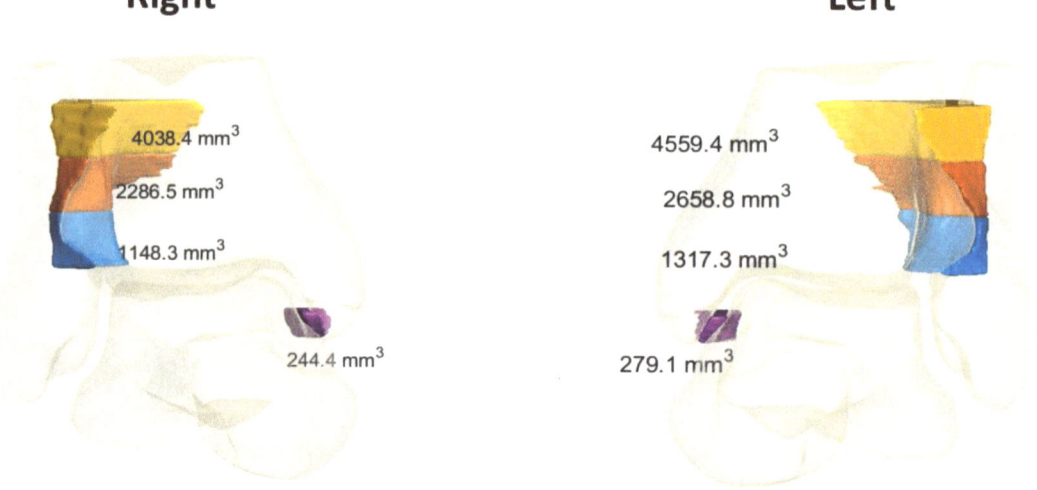

Figure 7. Volumetric measurements of the **right** and **left** distal tibiofibular joint (up to 1, 2, and 3 cm) and medial gutter in a patient with **left** Weber-B fracture using Disior™ (Paragon 28®, Bonelogic F&A).

3.4.5. Other Novel Measurement Techniques

More recently, a study explored the use of dual-energy CT post-processing algorithms [45]. More specifically, they looked at the accuracy of collagen mapping technology compared to grayscale CT analysis in the assessment of syndesmotic integrity. The results showed that collagen mapping significantly enhanced sensitivity, specificity, positive predictive value, negative predictive value, and overall accuracy for detecting distal tibiofibular syndesmosis injuries. Additionally, collagen mapping achieved higher diagnostic confidence, image quality, and noise scores compared to grayscale CT.

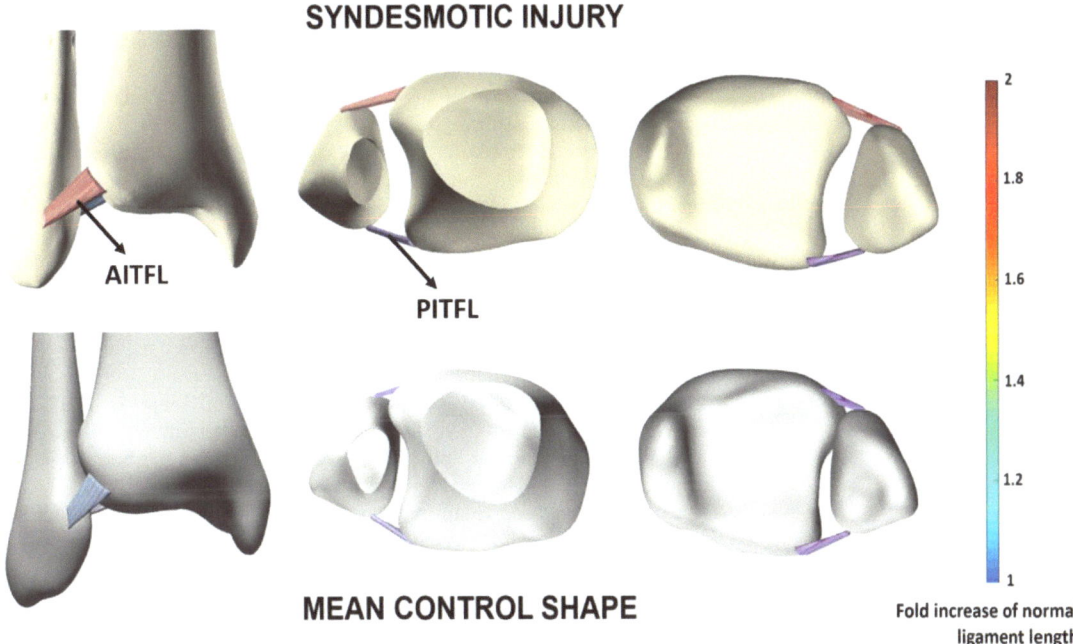

Figure 8. Distal tibiofibular joint anatomy in a documented syndesmotic lesion (**top**) versus the mean control distal tibiofibular joint anatomy, derived from a statistical shape model (**bottom**). The statistical shape model-based ligament modeling framework was able to detect an increase of anterior inferior tibiofibular ligament distance by 170%, resulting in an anterior "open-book" injury.

4. Discussion

A broad set of measurements exists to evaluate syndesmotic integrity [46]. However, these measurements are scattered across the literature. Therefore, this topical review compiled the current evidence available in the literature, with the aim of providing a comprehensive overview of which 2D/3D measurements are at hand. No systematic review was obtained because of the heterogeneity of the trials. This made it difficult to compare the results of the trials. Secondly, the aim was to look at newer and emerging techniques. These are usually described in individual trials, so a systematic review was not possible. Although the majority of ICC values for 2D measurements indicate high reliability, specific measurements that involve multiple steps show lower ICC values, likely due to the learning curve. The 3D measurement techniques are emerging as promising alternatives and could replace 2D measurements in the future, but they have not yet been integrated into daily clinical practice.

Regarding 2D measurements, there are several techniques to quantify mediolateral translation, anteroposterior translation, rotation, and area. The mediolateral tibiofibular translation measurements were the most commonly used [5,6,13,18,20,22–32]. Interobserver reliability was good to excellent for all measurements. There was also no significant difference between bilateral ankles, which can be compared to assess syndesmotic integrity [6,31]. No studies have shown a significant increase in width between non-weight-bearing and weight-bearing conditions, but the average of the means was greater in weight-bearing conditions for each measurement [20,29]. Greater distances have been shown for each measurement when comparing normal and injured ankles in non-weight-bearing conditions. In weight-bearing conditions, only a significant difference has been shown for one mediolateral translation measurement: MTFW [22,26,32,33,47]. Studies have reported cut-off values for ATFW, MTFW, and MxTFW with varying sensitivity and specificity [5,18,32]. For each measure, there are studies that demonstrate that the measure is adequate to discriminate between normal and injured ankles, but more research is needed to formulate a consensus on cut-off values.

The anteroposterior translation of the fibula relative to the tibia can be assessed using two commonly used measurements [5,28,38]. The anterior Phisitkul is the most commonly used translational parameter [5,13,20,23,26,28,29,38,39]. Unfortunately, most studies only include normal ankles, and just one study evaluated injured ankles in both non-weight-bearing and weight-bearing conditions [39]. An excellent AUC value was achieved in non-weight-bearing conditions (0.894), suggesting that the anterior Phisitkul could be an excellent parameter in the diagnosis of syndesmotic injuries [26]. Nault's translational parameter is an interesting method but is only used in three studies with normal ankles [5,20,28]. Comparative studies are needed to assess whether this parameter can be used in the diagnosis of syndesmotic injury. Other studies have also described measurements of anteroposterior translation, but as these measurements were rarely used and lacked validation, they were not discussed in this review [26,27,33].

The main rotation measurements were the fibular rotation parameter by Dikos et al. [34]. With respect to this measurement, our findings suggest that the mean rotation of the fibula under weight-bearing conditions was 12.3° internal rotation, as compared to 7.39° in the presence of lesions. A lesser-used rotational parameter, the bimalleolar angle, has been suggested by Vetter et al. as a valid alternative, given its simpler methodology with clear anatomical landmarks. The measurement is made at a talocrural level, which could potentially be advantageous in the evaluation of fractures and dislocations [37]. Moreover, ratios describing the fibular rotations have been infrequently reported. A possible explanation could be the complexity and inherent errors associated with these measurements [5].

The syndesmotic area exhibited a significant increase in injured syndesmoses, as observed in both CT and WBCT scans, in comparison to non-injured cases [13,26,31,33–35]. The difference in the area under weight-bearing conditions was notably larger, with an additional 3.8 mm^2 [31,34]. Notably, the syndesmotic area demonstrated particularly high ICC values of 0.96 for CT and 0.93 for WBCT, surpassing other measurements. These findings emphasize the validity of the syndesmotic area as the currently most reliable parameter available.

Regarding 3D Measurements, we found a broad set of novel techniques to circumvent the flaws of 2D measurement techniques. Particularly, distance mapping and volumetric analysis have shown great potential to increase the inter- and intra-observer reliability and automate the measurement process. The ICC of these volume measurements has increased up to 0.93, while distance mapping measurements have been performed fully automated, eliminating all observer inaccuracies [8,9,42–44].

This review demonstrates that despite the existence of numerous studies investigating syndesmotic measurements on CT scans, a definitive consensus regarding the appropriate measurements for assessing syndesmotic integrity is still lacking. Multiple measurements have been described, each varying in complexity, which creates difficulty in discerning the most reliable approaches. While most ICC values indicate good to excellent reliability, certain measurements involving multiple steps exhibit lower ICC values, likely due to the learning curve associated with their implementation. Findings regarding the influence of age, sex, and height on syndesmotic measurements are inconclusive, but there is no significant difference observed between bilateral ankles, allowing for the comparison to the opposite side as an internal control. There is a considerable range of normal and pathological values, as evidenced by the standard deviation associated with each measurement. Taken together, these factors contribute to the challenge of distinguishing between normal and pathological values in routine clinical practice.

Several limitations should be noted in this review. Firstly, many studies have small sample sizes. In addition, this review includes a diverse group of studies, and not all studies include patients with a syndesmotic injury. Additionally, it was difficult to make direct comparisons between every injury group due to variations in the nature of the injuries.

Furthermore, it is difficult to draw conclusions about the diagnostic accuracy of CT and WBCT as most of the studies looked at normal syndesmotic anatomy. As a result, it is evidently difficult to establish cut-off values. Studies with larger sample sizes, including more patients with syndesmotic injuries, could further clarify the remaining questions about the diagnostic accuracy of CT and WBCT measurements.

Future Perspectives

Future studies should continue to examine the merits of WBCT over CT to diagnose (subtle) syndesmotic lesions, preferably in a (semi-)automated manner [48]. Larger populations of injured versus healthy individuals should be analyzed. The implementation of external rotation stress during WBCT needs to be validated as a potential enhancer for the detection of lesions. The emergence of 3D techniques requires further exploration, whether in terms of distance, area, or volume measures. In clinical practice, cut-off values for both 2D and 3D measurements are necessary to improve lesion diagnosis and correlate these with therapy strategies.

5. Conclusions

In this review, we have topically described the available 2D and 3D measurements to assess and quantify syndesmotic integrity. While most ICC values of 2D measurements indicate good to excellent reliability, certain measurements involving multiple steps exhibit lower ICC values, likely due to the learning curve. The 3D measurement techniques are emerging as encouraging alternatives but are not implemented yet in daily clinical practice.

Author Contributions: Conceptualization, M.P. and A.B.; methodology, T.D. and M.H.; software, T.D. and M.H.; formal analysis, T.D. and M.H.; investigation, T.D., M.H. and M.P.; resources, T.D. and M.H.; data curation, T.D. and M.H.; writing—original draft preparation, T.D. and M.H.; writing—review and editing, M.P., B.K., N.H., N.K. and E.A.; visualization, T.D., M.H. and M.P.; supervision, E.A. and A.B.; project administration, M.P. All authors have read and agreed to the published version of the manuscript.

Funding: This research received no external funding.

Institutional Review Board Statement: Not applicable.

Informed Consent Statement: Not applicable.

Data Availability Statement: Data sharing not applicable. No new data were created or analyzed in this study. Data sharing is not applicable to this article.

Conflicts of Interest: The authors declare no conflict of interest.

References

1. Campbell, S.E.; Warner, M. MR Imaging of Ankle Inversion Injuries. *Magn. Reson. Imaging Clin. N. Am.* **2008**, *16*, 1–18. [CrossRef] [PubMed]
2. Chans-Veres, J.; Vallejo-Márquez, M.; Galhoum, A.E.; Tejero, S. Analysis of the uninjured tibiofibular syndesmosis using conventional CT-imaging and axial force in different foot positions. *Foot Ankle Surg.* **2022**, *28*, 650–656. [CrossRef] [PubMed]
3. Burssens, A.; Vermue, H.; Barg, A.; Krähenbühl, N.; Victor, J.; Buedts, K. Templating of Syndesmotic Ankle Lesions by Use of 3D Analysis in Weightbearing and Nonweightbearing CT. *Foot Ankle Int.* **2018**, *39*, 1487–1496. [CrossRef] [PubMed]
4. Chun, D.-I.; Cho, J.-H.; Min, T.-H.; Yi, Y.; Park, S.Y.; Kim, K.-H.; Kim, J.H.; Won, S.H. Diagnostic accuracy of radiologic methods for ankle syndesmosis injury: A systematic review and meta-analysis. *J. Clin. Med.* **2019**, *8*, 968. [CrossRef] [PubMed]
5. Patel, S.; Malhotra, K.; Cullen, N.P.; Singh, D.; Goldberg, A.J.; Welck, M.J. Defining reference values for the normal tibiofibular syndesmosis in adults using weight-bearing CT. *Bone Jt. J.* **2019**, *101-B*, 348–352. [CrossRef] [PubMed]
6. Park, C.H.; Kim, G.B. Tibiofibular relationships of the normal syndesmosis differ by age on axial computed tomography—Anterior fibular translation with age. *Injury* **2019**, *50*, 1256–1260. [CrossRef] [PubMed]
7. Ng, N.; Onggo, J.R.; Nambiar, M.; Maingard, J.T.; Ng, D.; Gupta, G.; Nandurkar, D.; Babazadeh, S.; Bedi, H. Which test is the best? An updated literature review of imaging modalities for acute ankle diastasis injuries. *J. Med. Radiat. Sci.* **2022**, *69*, 382–393. [CrossRef]
8. Esfahani, S.A.; Bhimani, R.; Lubberts, B.; Kerkhoffs, G.M.; Waryasz, G.; DiGiovanni, C.W.; Guss, D. Volume measurements on weightbearing computed tomography can detect subtle syndesmotic instability. *J. Orthop. Res.* **2022**, *40*, 460–467. [CrossRef]

9. Bhimani, R.; Ashkani-Esfahani, S.; Lubberts, B.; Guss, D.; Hagemeijer, N.C.; Waryasz, G.; DiGiovanni, C.W. Utility of Volumetric Measurement via Weight-Bearing Computed Tomography Scan to Diagnose Syndesmotic Instability. *Foot Ankle Int.* **2020**, *41*, 859–865. [CrossRef]
10. Campbell, T.; Mok, A.; Wolf, M.R.; Tarakemeh, A.; Everist, B.; Vopat, B.G. Augmented stress weightbearing CT for evaluation of subtle tibiofibular syndesmotic injuries in the elite athlete. *Skelet. Radiol.* **2022**, *52*, 1221–1227. [CrossRef]
11. Sman, A.D.; Hiller, C.E.; Rae, K.; Linklater, J.; Black, D.A.; Nicholson, L.L.; Burns, J.; Refshauge, K.M. Diagnostic accuracy of clinical tests for ankle syndesmosis injury. *Br. J. Sports Med.* **2015**, *49*, 323–329. [CrossRef] [PubMed]
12. Baltes, T.P.A.; Al Sayrafi, O.; Arnáiz, J.; Al-Naimi, M.R.; Geertsema, C.; Geertsema, L.; Holtzhausen, L.; D'hooghe, P.; Kerkhoffs, G.M.M.J.; Tol, J.L. Acute clinical evaluation for syndesmosis injury has high diagnostic value. *Knee Surg. Sports Traumatol. Arthrosc.* **2022**, *30*, 3871–3880. [CrossRef] [PubMed]
13. Abdelaziz, M.E.; Hagemeijer, N.; Guss, D.; El-Hawary, A.; El-Mowafi, H.; DiGiovanni, C.W. Evaluation of Syndesmosis Reduction on CT Scan. *Foot Ankle Int.* **2019**, *40*, 1087–1093. [CrossRef] [PubMed]
14. Anand Prakash, D.A. Syndesmotic stability: Is there a radiological normal?—A systematic review. *Foot Ankle Surg.* **2018**, *24*, 174–184. [CrossRef] [PubMed]
15. Chang, A.L.; Mandell, J.C. Syndesmotic Ligaments of the Ankle: Anatomy, Multimodality Imaging, and Patterns of Injury. *Curr. Probl. Diagn. Radiol.* **2020**, *49*, 452–459. [CrossRef] [PubMed]
16. Krähenbühl, N.; Akkaya, M.; Dodd, A.E.; Hintermann, B.; Dutilh, G.; Lenz, A.L.; Barg, A. Impact of the rotational position of the hindfoot on measurements assessing the integrity of the distal tibio-fibular syndesmosis. *Foot Ankle Surg.* **2020**, *26*, 810–817. [CrossRef] [PubMed]
17. Peiffer, M.; Burssens, A.; De Mits, S.; Heintz, T.; Van Waeyenberge, M.; Buedts, K.; Victor, J.; Audenaert, E. Statistical shape model-based tibiofibular assessment of syndesmotic ankle lesions using weight-bearing CT. *J. Orthop. Res.* **2022**, *40*, 2873–2884. [CrossRef]
18. Rodrigues, J.C.; do Amaral e Castro, A.; Rosemberg, L.A.; de Cesar Netto, C.; Godoy-Santos, A.L. Diagnostic Accuracy of Conventional Ankle CT Scan with External Rotation and Dorsiflexion in Patients with Acute Isolated Syndesmotic Instability. *Am. J. Sports Med.* **2023**, *51*, 985–996. [CrossRef]
19. Wohlin, C. Guidelines for snowballing in systematic literature studies and a replication in software engineering. In Proceedings of the 18th International Conference on Evaluation and Assessment in Software Engineering, London, UK, 13–14 May 2014; ACM: New York, NY, USA, 2014; pp. 1–10. [CrossRef]
20. Malhotra, K.; Welck, M.; Cullen, N.; Singh, D.; Goldberg, A.J. The effects of weight bearing on the distal tibiofibular syndesmosis: A study comparing weight bearing-CT with conventional CT. *Foot Ankle Surg.* **2019**, *25*, 511–516. [CrossRef]
21. Page, M.J.; McKenzie, J.E.; Bossuyt, P.M.; Boutron, I.; Hoffmann, T.C.; Mulrow, C.D.; Shamseer, L.; Tetzlaff, J.M.; Akl, E.A.; Brennan, S.E.; et al. The PRISMA 2020 statement: An updated guideline for reporting systematic reviews. *BMJ* **2021**, *372*, n71. [CrossRef]
22. Ahn, T.K.; Choi, S.M.; Kim, J.Y.; Lee, W.C. Isolated Syndesmosis Diastasis: Computed Tomography Scan Assessment with Arthroscopic Correlation. *Arthrosc. J. Arthrosc. Relat. Surg.* **2017**, *33*, 828–834. [CrossRef] [PubMed]
23. Ebinger, T.; Goetz, J.; Dolan, L.; Phisitkul, P. 3D Model analysis of existing CT syndesmosis measurements. *Iowa Orthop. J.* **2013**, *33*, 40–46. [PubMed]
24. Elgafy, H.; Semaan, H.B.; Blessinger, B.; Wassef, A.; Ebraheim, N.A. Computed tomography of normal distal tibiofibular syndesmosis. *Skelet. Radiol.* **2010**, *39*, 559–564. [CrossRef] [PubMed]
25. Gardner, M.J.; Demetrakopoulos, D.; Briggs, S.M.; Helfet, D.L.; Lorich, D.G. Malreduction of the Tibiofibular Syndesmosis in Ankle Fractures. *Foot Ankle Int.* **2006**, *27*, 788–792. [CrossRef] [PubMed]
26. Hamard, M.; Neroladaki, A.; Bagetakos, I.; Dubois-Ferrière, V.; Montet, X.; Boudabbous, S. Accuracy of cone-beam computed tomography for syndesmosis injury diagnosis compared to conventional computed tomography. *Foot Ankle Surg.* **2020**, *26*, 265–272. [CrossRef] [PubMed]
27. Lepojärvi, S.; Niinimäki, J.; Pakarinen, H.; Leskelä, H.V. Rotational Dynamics of the Normal Distal Tibiofibular Joint with Weight-Bearing Computed Tomography. *Foot Ankle Int.* **2016**, *37*, 627–635. [CrossRef] [PubMed]
28. Nault, M.-L.; Hébert-Davies, J.; Laflamme, G.-Y.; Leduc, S. CT Scan Assessment of the Syndesmosis: A New Reproducible Method. *J. Orthop. Trauma.* **2013**, *27*, 638–641. [CrossRef]
29. Shakoor, D.; Osgood, G.M.; Brehler, M.; Zbijewski, W.B.; Netto, C.d.C.; Shafiq, B.; Orapin, J.; Thawait, G.K.; Shon, L.C.; Demehri, S. Cone-beam CT measurements of distal tibio-fibular syndesmosis in asymptomatic uninjured ankles: Does weight-bearing matter? *Skelet. Radiol.* **2019**, *48*, 583–594. [CrossRef]
30. Wong, F.; Mills, R.; Mushtaq, N.; Walker, R.; Singh, S.K.; Abbasian, A. Correlation and comparison of syndesmosis dimension on CT and MRI. *Foot* **2016**, *28*, 36–41. [CrossRef]
31. Wong, M.T.; Wiens, C.; Lamothe, J.; Edwards, W.B.; Schneider, P.S. Four-Dimensional CT Analysis of Normal Syndesmotic Motion. *Foot Ankle Int.* **2021**, *42*, 1491–1501. [CrossRef]
32. Yeung, T.W.; Chan, C.Y.G.; Chan, W.C.S.; Yeung, Y.N.; Yuen, M.K. Can pre-operative axial CT imaging predict syndesmosis instability in patients sustaining ankle fractures? Seven years' experience in a tertiary trauma center. *Skelet. Radiol.* **2015**, *44*, 823–829. [CrossRef] [PubMed]

33. Hagemeijer, N.C.; Chang, S.H.; Abdelaziz, M.E.; Casey, J.C.; Waryasz, G.R.; Guss, D.; DiGiovanni, C.W. Range of Normal and Abnormal Syndesmotic Measurements Using Weightbearing CT. *Foot Ankle Int.* **2019**, *40*, 1430–1437. [CrossRef] [PubMed]
34. del Rio, A.; Bewsher, S.M.; Roshan-Zamir, S.; Tate, J.; Eden, M.; Gotmaker, R.; Wang, O.; Bedi, H.S.; Rotstein, A.H. Weightbearing Cone-Beam Computed Tomography of Acute Ankle Syndesmosis Injuries. *J. Foot Ankle Surg.* **2020**, *59*, 258–263. [CrossRef] [PubMed]
35. Malhotra, G.; Cameron, J.; Toolan, B.C. Diagnosing chronic diastasis of the syndesmosis: A novel measurement using computed tomography. *Foot Ankle Int.* **2014**, *35*, 483–488. [CrossRef] [PubMed]
36. Dikos, G.D.; Heisler, J.; Choplin, R.H.; Weber, T.G. Normal Tibiofibular Relationships at the Syndesmosis on Axial CT Imaging. *J. Orthop. Trauma.* **2012**, *26*, 433–438. [CrossRef] [PubMed]
37. Vetter, S.Y.; Gassauer, M.; Uhlmann, L.; Swartman, B.; Schnetzke, M.; Keil, H.; Franke, J.; Grützner, P.A.; Beisemann, N. A standardised computed tomography measurement method for distal fibular rotation. *Eur. J. Trauma. Emerg. Surg.* **2021**, *47*, 891–896. [CrossRef] [PubMed]
38. Phisitkul, P.; Ebinger, T.; Goetz, J.; Vaseenon, T.; Marsh, J.L. Forceps reduction of the syndesmosis in rotational ankle fractures: A cadaveric study. *J. Bone Joint Surg. Am.* **2012**, *94*, 2256–2261. [CrossRef] [PubMed]
39. Osgood, G.M.; Shakoor, D.; Orapin, J.; Qin, J.; Khodarahmi, I.; Thawait, G.K.; Ficke, J.R.; Schon, L.C.; Demehri, S. Reliability of distal tibio-fibular syndesmotic instability measurements using weightbearing and non-weightbearing cone-beam CT. *Foot Ankle Surg.* **2019**, *25*, 771–781. [CrossRef]
40. Tang, C.W.; Roidis, N.; Vaishnav, S.; Patel, A.; Thordarson, D.B. Position of the Distal Fibular Fragment in Pronation and Supination Ankle Fractures: A CT Evaluation. *Foot Ankle Int.* **2003**, *24*, 561–566. [CrossRef]
41. Peiffer, M.; Dhont, T.; Cuigniez, F.; Tampere, T.; Ashkani-Esfahani, S.; D'hooghe, P.; Audenaert, E.; Burssens, A. Application of external torque enhances the detection of subtle syndesmotic ankle instability in a weight-bearing CT. *Knee Surg. Sports Traumatol. Arthrosc*, 2023; *Online ahead of print.* [CrossRef]
42. Dibbern, K.; Vivtcharenko, V.; Mansur, N.S.B.; Lalevée, M.; de Carvalho, K.A.M.; Lintz, F.; Barg, A.; Goldberg, A.J.; Netto, C.d.C. Distance mapping and volumetric assessment of the ankle and syndesmotic joints in progressive collapsing foot deformity. *Sci. Rep.* **2023**, *13*, 4801. [CrossRef]
43. Taser, F.; Shafiq, Q.; Ebraheim, N.A. Three-dimensional volume rendering of tibiofibular joint space and quantitative analysis of change in volume due to tibiofibular syndesmosis diastases. *Skelet. Radiol.* **2006**, *35*, 935–941. [CrossRef] [PubMed]
44. Kocadal, O.; Yucel, M.; Pepe, M.; Aksahin, E.; Aktekin, C.N. Evaluation of Reduction Accuracy of Suture-Button and Screw Fixation Techniques for Syndesmotic Injuries. *Foot Ankle Int.* **2016**, *37*, 1317–1325. [CrossRef] [PubMed]
45. Gruenewald, L.D.; Leitner, D.H.; Koch, V.; Martin, S.S.; Yel, I.; Mahmoudi, S.; Bernatz, S.; Eichler, K.; Gruber-Rouh, T.; Dos Santos, D.P.; et al. Diagnostic Value of DECT-Based Collagen Mapping for Assessing the Distal Tibiofibular Syndesmosis in Patients with Acute Trauma. *Diagnostics* **2023**, *13*, 533. [CrossRef] [PubMed]
46. Krähenbühl, N.; Weinberg, M.W.; Davidson, N.P.; Mills, M.K.; Hintermann, B.; Saltzman, C.L.; Barg, A. Imaging in syndesmotic injury: A systematic literature review. *Skelet. Radiol.* **2018**, *47*, 631–648. [CrossRef] [PubMed]
47. Rodrigues, J.C.; Santos, A.L.G.; Prado, M.P.; Alloza, J.F.M.; Masagão, R.A.; Rosemberg, L.A.; Barros, D.D.C.S.; e Castro, A.D.A.; Demange, M.K.; Lenza, M.; et al. Comparative CT with stress manoeuvres for diagnosing distal isolated tibiofibular syndesmotic injury in acute ankle sprain: A protocol for an accuracy-test prospective study. *BMJ Open* **2020**, *10*, e037239. [CrossRef] [PubMed]
48. Peiffer, M.; Van Den Borre, I.; Segers, T.; Ashkani-Esfahani, S.; Guss, D.; De Cesar Netto, C.; DiGiovanni, C.W.; Victor, J.; Audenaert, E. Implementing automated 3D measurements to quantify reference values and side-to-side differences in the ankle syndesmosis. *Sci. Rep.* **2023**, *13*, 13774. [CrossRef]

Disclaimer/Publisher's Note: The statements, opinions and data contained in all publications are solely those of the individual author(s) and contributor(s) and not of MDPI and/or the editor(s). MDPI and/or the editor(s) disclaim responsibility for any injury to people or property resulting from any ideas, methods, instructions or products referred to in the content.

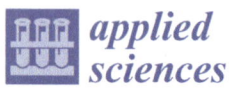

Article

Aging Alters Cervical Vertebral Bone Density Distribution: A Cross-Sectional Study

Eun-Sang Moon [1], Seora Kim [1], Nathan Kim [1], Minjoung Jang [1], Toru Deguchi [1], Fengyuan Zheng [2], Damian J. Lee [2] and Do-Gyoon Kim [1,*]

[1] Division of Orthodontics, College of Dentistry, The Ohio State University, Columbus, OH 43210, USA; moon.200@buckeyemail.osu.edu (E.-S.M.); kim.4226@buckeyemail.osu.edu (S.K.); kim.6417@buckeyemail.osu.edu (N.K.); mj9@illinois.edu (M.J.); deguchi.4@osu.edu (T.D.)

[2] Division of Restorative and Prosthodontics Dentistry, College of Dentistry, The Ohio State University, Columbus, OH 43210, USA; fyzheng@gmail.com (F.Z.); lee.6221@osu.edu (D.J.L.)

* Correspondence: kim.2508@osu.edu; Tel.: +614-247-8089; Fax: +614-688-3077

Abstract: Osteoporosis reduces bone mineral density (BMD) with aging. The incidence of cervical vertebral injuries for the elderly has increased in the last decade. Thus, the objective of the current study was to examine whether dental cone beam computed tomography (CBCT) can identify age and sex effects on volumetric BMD and morphology of human cervical vertebrae. A total of 136 clinical CBCT images were obtained from 63 male and 73 female patients (20 to 69 years of age). Three-dimensional images of cervical vertebral bodies (C2 and C3) were digitally isolated. A gray level, which is proportional to BMD, was obtained and its distribution was analyzed in each image. Morphology, including volume, heights, widths, and concavities, was also measured. Most of the gray level parameters had significantly higher values of C2 and C3 in females than in males for all age groups ($p < 0.039$). The female 60-age group had significant lower values of Mean and Low5 of C2 and C3 than both female 40- and 50-age groups ($p < 0.03$). The reduced BMD of the female 60-age group likely resulted from postmenopausal demineralization of bone. Current findings suggest that dental CBCT can detect age-dependent changes of cervical vertebral BMD, providing baseline information to develop an alternative tool to diagnose osteoporosis.

Keywords: CBCT; cervical vertebra; clinical assessment; diagnosis; postmenopause

1. Introduction

Osteoporosis is an age-dependent systematic disease that results in bone loss, increasing the risk of fracture [1–3]. The vertebra is one of the most common anatomical sites where osteoporotic fractures were observed [4,5]. While thoracic and lumbar fractures have been frequently reported, recent clinical observations indicated that fall-induced severe cervical vertebral injuries steeply rose more than eight times for elderly population over the 47 years [6]. However, relatively limited studies have focused on osteoporosis of cervical spine.

Bone mineral density (BMD) is a primary parameter assessed to diagnose osteoporosis [7–9]. The World Health Organization (WHO) defined an osteoporotic patient as someone who has BMD with 2.5 standard deviation lower than young healthy women [10,11]. Dual energy X-ray absorptiometry (DEXA) has been used as a standard technique to diagnose BMD [7,11,12]. However, DEXA is used at low radiation doses but produces a low resolution with approximately 500 μm of two-dimensional (2D) image that only provides areal BMD [11,13] (Table 1). On the other hand, three-dimensional (3D) quantitative computed tomography (QCT) was applied to measure BMD and related parameters of cervical and lumbar vertebrae [7–9]. However, the QCT was limited due to its relatively high radiation dose and rough resolutions at the range of in-plane pixel size of 0.29 to 0.68 mm and slice thickness of 1.25 to 2.5 mm.

Table 1. Descriptive summary of X-ray based technologies [11].

Technologies	Voxel Size (μm)	Effective Radiation Dose (μSv)	Scan Time (Second)
DXA	500	1–20	~120
MDCT	156–500	100–8000	<30
CBCT	130–400	6.3–2100	10–40 (Rotation) 1.92–7.2 (Exposure)
Micro-CT	0.3–100	NA	>600

Cone beam computed tomography (CBCT) has been widely used in a dental clinical setting [14–18]. Cervical spine, especially C2 and C3, is captured during a routine CBCT scan used in dentistry. This technique uses moderate radiation doses and provides higher resolutions (0.2 to 0.4 mm) of 3D images [17]. While it was indicated that there has been scarcity of studies that examine capability of CBCT to screen patients' BMD [19], a few studies showed that CBCT images of cervical vertebra can be used to detect osteoporosis of patients [20–22]. However, these studies are limited by using 2D region of interest that provides the relative measures of areal BMD. On the other hand, we successfully calibrated 3D CBCT images by showing the strong positive correlations between hydroxyapatite phantoms with three different densities (1000, 1250, and 1750 mg/cm^3) and gray levels scanned using three different resolutions (200, 300, and 400 μm) at full field of view (FOV) of CBCT (Figure 1) [11]. Thus, the objective of the current study is to examine whether dental CBCT can identify age and sex effects on volumetric BMD and morphology of human cervical vertebrae.

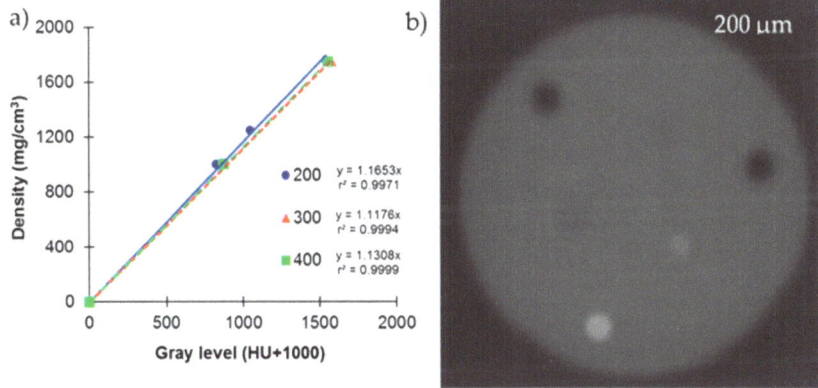

Figure 1. (a) Strong positive correlations in the calibration curves of gray values for (b) phantoms of bone materials (hydroxyapatite) with three different densities (1000, 1250, and 1750 mg/cm^3) scanned using three different resolutions (200, 300, and 400 μm) of CBCT (Reprinted with unrestricted permission for non-commercial use) [11].

2. Materials and Methods

The protocol used in the current study was approved by institutional review board at The Ohio State University (Protocol no. 2011H0128). A total of 136 CBCT images was randomly selected from records on routine dental patients (63 images for male and 73 images for female) at The Ohio State University, College of Dentistry. Those 3D images were taken by a CBCT machine (iCAT, Imaging Science International, Hatfield, PA, USA) with resolutions of 0.25 mm for four images, 0.3 mm for 127 images, and 0.4 mm for five images under the same scanning energy (120 kV and 5 mA) with full field of view (FOV) at different scanning times (26.9 s, 8.9 s, and 8.9 s for images with 0.25 mm, 0.3 mm, and 0.4 mm voxel sizes, respectively). These scanning conditions are routinely used in clinical practices. The exclusion criteria for the CBCT images were craniofacial anomalies, vertebral anomalies (fusions and major vertebral asymmetries), orthognathic patients with bone plates, and limited field of view images without second and third cervical vertebrae. Three age groups including 40-age group (20 to 49 years old, 36.61 ± 11 years), 50-age group (50 to 59 years old, 54.55 ± 2.94 years), and 60-age group (older than 60 years old, 64.81 ± 2.82 years) were assigned for male (21 images for each age group) and female (29 images for 40-age group, 24 images for 50-age group, and 20 images for 60-age group). The sample size was determined using a previous clinical observation that showed the significant changes of CBCT based cervical vertebral mean gray levels with aging (1948.31 ± 81.87 vs. 1997.26 ± 50.03) [18]. Fifteen CBCT images turned out to provide the minimum number of samples needed to obtain significant results ($p < 0.05$) with 80% statistical power. Therefore, the current number of CBCT images used for each age group was assumed to be sufficient to satisfy the power of statistical analysis.

The 3D CBCT images were imported to image-analysis software (ImageJ, NIH) (Figure 2a), and two cervical vertebrae (C2 and C3) were digitally cropped and saved to individual image files. Non-bone voxels outside of vertebra were removed using semi-automatic heuristic algorithm [16,18,23]. Posterior and lateral processes were cut from 10 voxels away from the endplates of vertebral body producing an integral volume of vertebral body. A gray level of each voxel, which is proportional to BMD, was obtained (Figure 2e) and collected for its histogram of C2 and C3 (Figure 2f,g). The values of Mean, standard deviation (SD), and low and high gray levels at the 5th and the 95th percentiles (Low$_5$ and High$_5$) of voxel counts in the histogram were determined (Figure 2f).

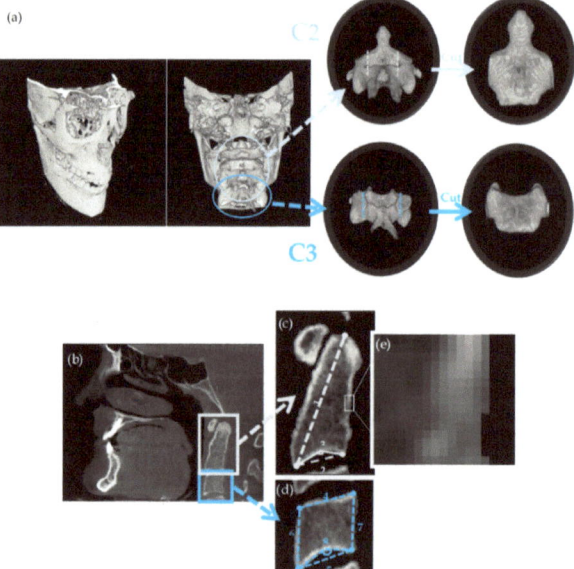

Figure 2. *Cont.*

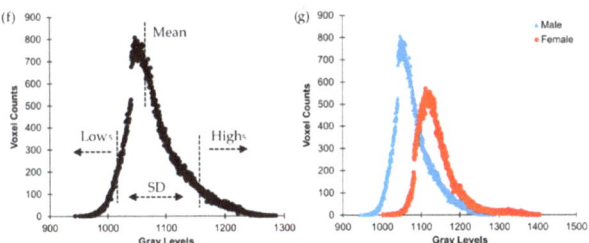

Figure 2. (**a**) Digital isolating process of C2 and C3 in 3D CBCT images for (**b**) the mid-sagittal CBCT slide views for (**c**) C2 and (**d**) C3 to measure (1) C2 height, (2) C2 width, (3) C2 concavity, (4) C3 top width, (5) C3 bottom width, (6) C3 anterior height, (7) C3 posterior height, and (8) C3 concavity. (**e**) Heterogeneity of gray levels, (**f**) a typical gray level histogram with gray level parameters, and (**g**) a comparison of the histograms between male and female. Male had higher voxel counts (i.e., volume) and female had higher gray levels (i.e., BMD parameters).

Morphology of C2 and C3 were measured at a single mid-sagittal CBCT slide. The CBCT images were aligned at the orientation of the cervical vertebrae using imaging software (Dataviewer, Bruker, Kontich, Belgium). The aligning process consisted of the following: (1) odontoid process of second cervical vertebrate should coincide with the mid-sagittal plane of the head, (2) transverse process of the second cervical vertebrae should be coplanar, and (3) posterior surface of the odontoid process should be aligned with the coronal plane of the head. Then, a mid-sagittal slide that bisects the odontoid process of C2 was selected (Figure 2b) and reference points on the vertebra were placed following a protocol modified from a previous study [24]. The reference points were placed at the most convex areas. The morphological parameters including C2 height, C2 width, C2 concavity, C3 top width, C3 bottom width, C3 anterior height, C3 posterior height, and C3 concavity were measured using ImageJ (Figure 2c,d).

3. Statistical Analyses

Reliability tests for measurements of all parameters (five samples each) were made using intra- and inter-rater agreements with intra-class correlation coefficient (ICC). Pearson correlations were tested between all parameters. Analysis of variance (ANOVA) followed by Tukey HSD (honestly significant difference) post hoc testing was also utilized to compare all of the parameters between age and sex groups for C2 and C3. The significant level is set at $p < 0.05$.

4. Results

The ICCs for all of BMD parameters were higher than 0.997 for both intra- and inter-rater agreements ($p < 0.001$) and those for the morphological parameters were higher than 0.763 ($p < 0.039$).

The C2 had significantly higher values of SD, volume, and height but significantly lower values of Mean, Low_5, and concavity than the C3 ($p < 0.014$). The width of the C2 was measured significantly wider than the top of the C3 but significantly narrower than the bottom of the C3 ($p < 0.001$). The value of $High_5$ was not significantly different between C2 and C3 ($p = 0.433$). Most of values of the gray level and morphological parameters were significantly correlated between C2 and C3 ($p < 0.001$) except concavity in male ($p = 0.116$). In particular, the values of Mean and volume had strong positive correlations between C2 and C3 ($r > 0.837$, $p < 0.001$) (Figure 3a,b).

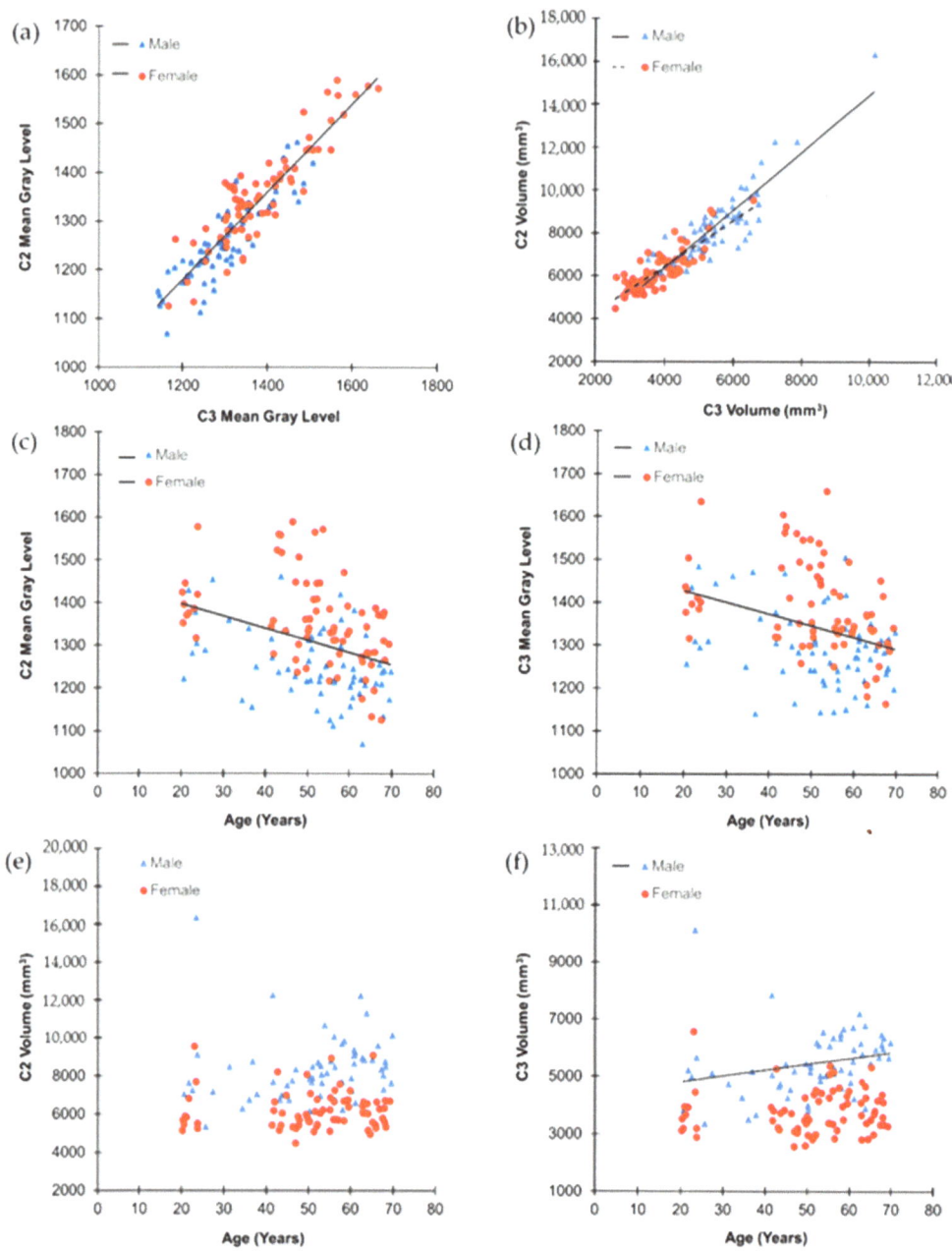

Figure 3. Correlations between C2 and C3 for (**a**) Mean gray level and (**b**) volume, and those of age with (**c**) C2 and (**d**) C3 Mean gray levels, and (**e**) C2 and (**f**) C3 volumes. The trend lines indicate a significant correlation ($p < 0.05$). A significant interaction of sex on the correlation of volume between C2 and C3 ($p = 0.033$) but not all other significant correlations ($p > 0.118$).

The values of Mean and volume had significant positive correlations with most of other gray level and morphological parameters of C2 and C3 in both male and female, respectively ($p < 0.01$).

Most of the gray level parameters had significantly higher values of C2 and C3 in female than in male for all age groups ($p < 0.039$) except Mean and Low_5 values of C3 for 60-age group between male and female ($p > 0.055$) (Figures 2g, 3 and 4). On the other hand, most of the morphological parameters had significantly higher values of C2 and C3 in male than in female for all age groups ($p < 0.035$) except concavity of C2 for all age groups and C3 for 40- and 50-age groups between male and female ($p > 0.131$) (Figure 4).

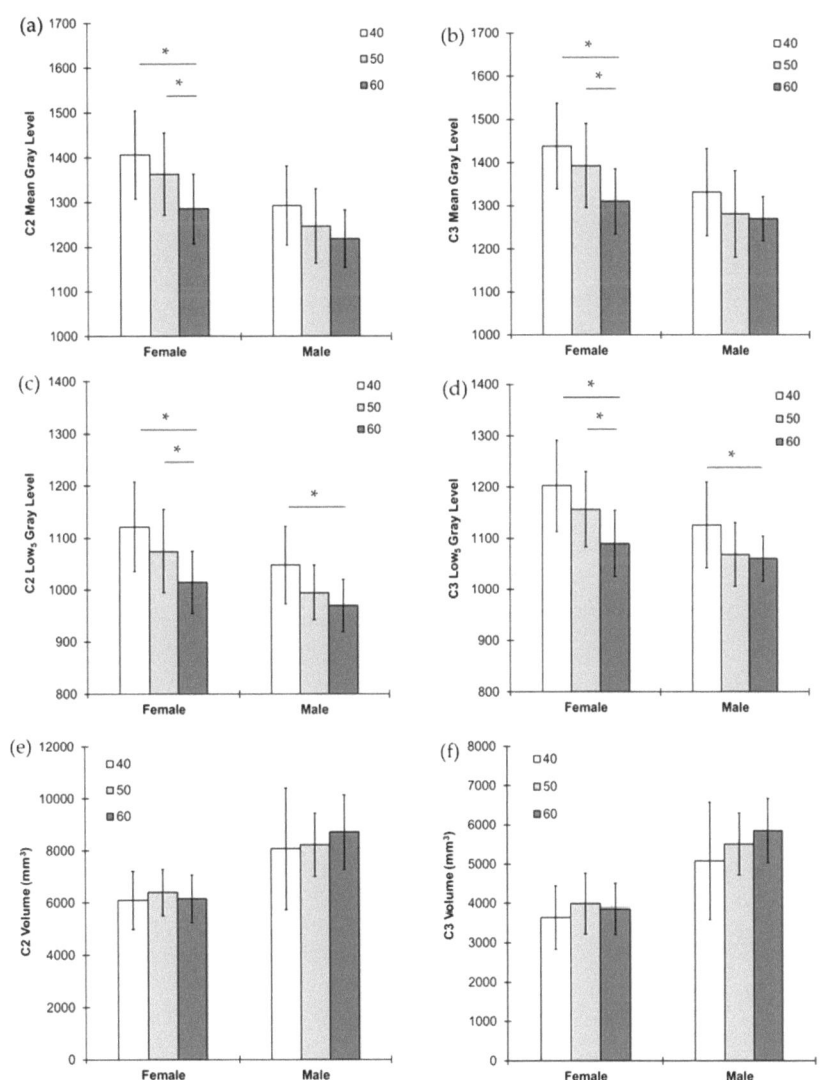

Figure 4. Comparisons between age groups of younger than 50 (40), 50s (50), and older than 50 (60) years in each female and male for (**a**) C2 and (**b**) C3 Mean gray levels, (**c**) C2 and (**d**) C3 Low5 gray levels, and (**e**) C2 and (**f**) C3 volumes. * $p < 0.05$.

Age had significant negative correlations with the values of Mean, Low_5, and $High_5$ of C2 and C3 in both male and female ($p < 0.05$) (Figure 4c,d). Males had significant positive correlations of age with volume and width of C2 and C3 ($p < 0.05$) while females had a negative correlation with height of C2 ($p = 0.04$). The female 60-age group had significantly lower values of Mean and Low$_5$ of C2 and C3 than both the female 40- and 50-age groups ($p < 0.03$) (Figure 4). The values of High$_5$ of C2 and C3 were significantly lower for the female 60-age group than the female 40-age group and both female 40- and 50-age groups, respectively ($p < 0.015$). The values of these parameters were not significantly different between the female 40- and 50-age groups ($p > 0.34$). The male 60-age group had significantly lower values of Low$_5$ and width of C2 and C3 than the male 40-age groups ($p < 0.05$) (Figure 4). All other comparisons and correlations were not significant ($p > 0.05$).

5. Discussion

The current study found that the female cervical vertebrae (C2 and C3) had higher bone mineral density (BMD) but smaller size than the male C2 and C3, respectively. The cervical vertebral BMD substantially decreases in the female 60-age group, that is likely in postmenopause, while their size was maintained the same between age groups. On the other hand, the male age groups showed no changes of BMD and size between age groups. These results were consistent with previous clinical studies using QCT for human cervical and lumbar vertebrae [7,8]. As such, it is suggested that the current dental CBCT based analyses of the cervical vertebral BMD distribution and size can provide useful information to diagnose osteoporosis.

5.1. Evaluation of Methodology

It has been a long-standing debate about whether the CBCT can assess BMD. The main issue stemmed from the reliability and consistency to assess the X-ray attenuation using Hounsfield unit (HU) [25–27]. However, the current CBCT machine is successfully calibrated with the strong positive correlations between hydroxyapatite phantoms and gray levels (Figure 1) [11]. The current study used the gray levels without converting them to BMD because the absolute BMD values are different between CBCT machines depending on their calibration tools [17]. If the gray levels are converted using the equation in Figure 1, the Mean gray level values of C3 female 40- and 60-age groups are corresponding to BMD values of 1600.41 ± 115.7 mg/cm^3 and 1458.36 ± 86.14 mg/cm^3, respectively. Those values are at comparable range of integral volumetric BMD for human lumbar vertebrae measured by 3D QCT [7].

As BMD has significant correlations with mechanical properties of vertebrae, it has been considered as an important surrogate to estimate the risk of bone fracture due to osteoporosis [2,7–9,28]. In addition to BMD, the current study investigated more parameters including its distribution and morphology of the cervical vertebrae. The heterogeneous distribution of BMD in the vertebra is resulted from bone remodeling that occurs at different time points. In particular, estrogen deficiency at menopause triggers active bone resorption followed by formation [3]. As bone resorption outbalances bone formation, a net bone loss occurs in postmenopausal osteoporosis [2,3]. As a result, more mineralized pre-existing bone tissues are resorbed, and less mineralized newly formed bone tissues are formed producing reduction of overall BMD. The gray level histogram in the current study reflects on this biological change of minerals in bone (Figure 2). Resorption of the pre-existing bone tissues decreases the value of High$_5$ while formation of new bone tissues decreases the value of Low$_5$ [23]. The value of Mean gray level is determined in association with those of High$_5$ and Low$_5$ as accounted for their strong positive correlations.

5.2. Clinical Application

Consistent with the current findings, volumetric BMDs of human C2 and C3 showed a strong positive correlation in the previous study using QCT [9]. Furthermore, many QCT based human studies have observed that females have higher BMD and smaller size of cervical and lumbar vertebrae than males [7,8]. These observations support reliability of the current dental CBCT based BMD and morphological analysis. The bigger cross sectional area and volume of male lumber vertebra has an advantage to bear more axial static loading due to body weight [7,29]. In contrast, it is indicated that incidence of fall-induced cervical vertebral injury is more in males than females [6,30]. These results provide an insight that higher BMD in female cervical vertebra may provide more resistance to fall-induced impact loading than bigger size of male cervical vertebra. Further studies are needed to clarify the relationships between functional demands and characteristics at different anatomical sites of spine.

While both males and females had the similar reducing trend of gray level parameters with advancing age, females showed significant rapid reduction between 50- and 60-age groups, which was not observed in males. These findings suggest that the altered gray level parameters of female 60-age group likely results from rapid decrease in BMD due to menopause while males experience progressive decrease in BMD due to senile osteoporosis as observed in other anatomical sites [1].

The gray level parameters and volume of cervical vertebrae were computed based on 3D images. The volume had significant correlations with other morphological parameters that changed slightly with ages. These findings indicate that the structure of cervical vertebrae was maintained with ages in adult patients examined in the current study. In addition, the SD of gray level, which represents heterogeneity of BMD and changes by adding or losing bone tissues, was also consistent with age, indicating that the absolute values of BMD decreased without bone loss.

A limitation of the current study is that cross-sectional analysis was performed using the existing patients' CBCT images. A longitudinal study for individual patients at different time periods of age is expected to provide more significant results for progressively developing osteoporosis with aging. However, multiple radiographic scanning for the same patient is limited due to potential accumulation of radiation dose. Another limitation may arise from that the current CBCT images were investigated retrospectively. The current findings would be more informative if they are compared with those from other anatomical sites using the standard BMD measurement with DEXA and the same methodologies used in the current study. However, it is not available to rescan the same patients. Instead, we found a previous study showing that a radiographic density obtained from a 2D slide of CBCT image for the cervical vertebrae had significant correlations with DEXA based osteoporotic scores at lumbar and femoral neck [31]. Moreover, 3D QCT based BMD of C2 and C3 showed significant correlations with those of thoracic and lumbar vertebrae [9]. These results suggest further studies that can be designed to compare BMD and morphology of cervical vertebrae using dental CBCT and those of other vertebrae using medical CT.

In conclusion, this is the first study that examined capability of dental CBCT to assess the integral volume BMD of human cervical vertebrae. The current study provided evidence that CBCT based analysis may suggest additional information to detect the rapid BMD reduction of C2 and C3 at the postmenopausal age. As the CBCT is widely used for routine dentistry including dental implant planning, visualization of abnormal teeth, evaluation of the jaws and face, cleft palate assessment, diagnosis of dental caries, endodontic diagnosis, and diagnosis of dental trauma as indicated by FDA (Food & Drug Administration) [32], it is an easily accessible tool to provide additional health information to patients who have taken CBCT for other dental treatments. As such, the strength of the current study is to produce a baseline data that can be used to develop CBCT technique to be a future diagnostic tool of osteoporosis. The knowledge of cervical vertebral BMD and morphology is also helpful for surgeons to obtain a better treatment plan of cervical vertebral degeneration and osteoporotic fracture. It was indicated that cervical spine is more vulnerable to fracture than lumbar spine [33] and elderly patients can have cervical spine damage with a minor trauma to head and neck sites [29]. Further studies need to investigate relationships of the CBCT based BMD and risk assessment of cervical spine with existing knowledge based on lumbar spine.

Author Contributions: Conceptualization, D.-G.K. and E.-S.M.; methodology, D.-G.K., E.-S.M., S.K., N.K. and M.J.; software, D.-G.K., E.-S.M., S.K., N.K. and M.J.; validation, D.-G.K. and E.-S.M.; formal analysis, D.-G.K. and E.-S.M.; investigation, D.-G.K. and E.-S.M.; resources, D.-G.K., T.D., F.Z. and D.J.L.; data curation, D.-G.K. and E.-S.M.; writing—original draft preparation, D.-G.K. and E.-S.M.; writing—review and editing, D.-G.K., T.D., F.Z. and D.J.L.; visualization, E.-S.M., S.K., N.K. and M.J.; supervision, D.-G.K.; project administration, D.-G.K.; funding acquisition, D.-G.K. and E.-S.M. All authors have read and agreed to the published version of the manuscript.

Funding: This study was, in part, supported by student research program, College of Dentistry, The Ohio State University.

Institutional Review Board Statement: The protocol used in the current study was approved by institutional review board at Ohio State University (Protocol no. 2011H0128).

Informed Consent Statement: Informed consent was obtained from all subjects involved in the study.

Data Availability Statement: Not applicable.

Acknowledgments: We thank Jie Liu and Keiichiro Watanabe for helping with data collection.

Conflicts of Interest: The authors declare no conflict of interest.

References

1. Seeman, E. Reduced bone formation and increased bone resorption: Rational targets for the treatment of osteoporosis. *Osteoporos. Int.* **2003**, *14* (Suppl. 3), S2–S8. [CrossRef] [PubMed]
2. Seeman, E. Pathogenesis of osteoporosis. *J. Appl. Physiol.* **2003**, *95*, 2142–2151. [CrossRef] [PubMed]
3. Eastell, R.; O'Neill, T.W.; Hofbauer, L.C.; Langdahl, B.; Reid, I.R.; Gold, D.T.; Cummings, S.R. Postmenopausal osteoporosis. *Nat. Rev. Dis. Primers* **2016**, *2*, 16069. [CrossRef] [PubMed]
4. Lems, W.F.; Paccou, J.; Zhang, J.; Fuggle, N.R.; Chandran, M.; Harvey, N.C.; Cooper, C.; Javaid, K.; Ferrari, S.; Akesson, K.E. Vertebral fracture: Epidemiology, impact and use of DXA vertebral fracture assessment in fracture liaison services. *Osteoporos. Int.* **2021**, *32*, 399–411. [CrossRef] [PubMed]
5. Robinson, W.A.; Carlson, B.C.; Poppendeck, H.; Wanderman, N.R.; Bunta, A.D.; Murphy, S.; Sietsema, D.L.; Daffner, S.D.; Edwards, B.J.; Watts, N.B.; et al. Osteoporosis-related Vertebral Fragility Fractures: A Review and Analysis of the American Orthopaedic Association's Own the Bone Database. *Spine* **2020**, *45*, E430–E438. [CrossRef] [PubMed]
6. Kannus, P.; Niemi, S.; Parkkari, J.; Mattila, V.M. Sharp Rise in Fall-Induced Cervical Spine Injuries Among Older Adults Between 1970 and 2017. *J. Gerontol. A-Biol.* **2019**, *75*, 2015–2019. [CrossRef] [PubMed]
7. Bruno, A.G.; Broe, K.E.; Zhang, X.; Samelson, E.J.; Meng, C.A.; Manoharan, R.; D'Agostino, J.; Cupples, L.; Kiel, D.P.; Bouxsein, M.L. Vertebral size, bone density, and strength in men and women matched for age and areal spine BMD. *J. Bone Miner. Res.* **2014**, *29*, 562–569. [CrossRef] [PubMed]
8. Anderst, W.J.; West, T.; Donaldson, W.F.; Lee, J.Y. Cervical spine bone density in young healthy adults as a function of sex, vertebral level and anatomic location. *Eur. Spine J.* **2017**, *26*, 2281–2289. [CrossRef] [PubMed]
9. Yoganandan, N.; Pintar, F.A.; Stemper, B.D.; Baisden, J.L.; Aktay, R.; Shender, B.S.; Paskoff, G.; Laud, P. Trabecular bone density of male human cervical and lumbar vertebrae. *Bone* **2006**, *39*, 336–344. [CrossRef] [PubMed]
10. Genant, H.K.; Cooper, C.; Poor, G.; Reid, I.; Ehrlich, G. Interim report and recommendations of the World Health Organization task-force for osteoporosis. *Osteoporos. Int.* **1999**, *10*, 259–264. [CrossRef] [PubMed]
11. Kim, D.G. Can dental cone beam computed tomography assess bone mineral density? *J. Bone Metab.* **2014**, *21*, 117–126. [CrossRef] [PubMed]
12. Genant, H.K.; Engelke, K.; Prevrhal, S. Advanced CT bone imaging in osteoporosis. *Rheumatology* **2008**, *47* (Suppl. 4), 9–16. [CrossRef] [PubMed]
13. Guermazi, A.; Mohr, A.; Grigorian, M.; Taouli, B.; Genant, H.K. Identification of Vertebral Fractures in Osteoporosis. *Semin. Musculoskelet. Radiol.* **2002**, *6*, 241–252. [CrossRef] [PubMed]
14. Scarfe, W.C.; Farman, A.G. What is cone-beam CT and how does it work? *Dent. Clin. N. Am.* **2008**, *52*, 707–730. [CrossRef] [PubMed]
15. Scarfe, W.C.; Farman, A.G.; Sukovic, P. Clinical applications of cone-beam computed tomography in dental practice. *J. Can. Dent. Assoc.* **2006**, *72*, 75–80. [PubMed]
16. Taylor, T.; Gans, S.; Jones, E.; Firestone, A.R.; Johnston, W.M.; Kim, D.G. Comparison of micro-CT and cone beam CT-based assessments for relative difference of gray level distribution in a human mandible. *Dentomaxillofac. Radiol.* **2013**, *42*, 25117764. [CrossRef] [PubMed]
17. England, G.M.; Moon, E.-S.; Roth, J.; Deguchi, T.; Firestone, A.R.; Beck, F.M.; Kim, D.G. Conditions and calibration to obtain comparable gray values between different clinical cone beam computed tomography scanners. *Dentomaxillofac. Radiol.* **2017**, *46*, 20160322. [CrossRef] [PubMed]

18. Crawford, B.; Kim, D.G.; Moon, E.S.; Johnson, E.; Fields, H.W.; Palomo, J.M.; Johnston, W.M. Cervical vertebral bone mineral density changes in adolescents during orthodontic treatment. *Am. J. Orthod. Dentofacial. Orthop.* **2014**, *146*, 183–189. [CrossRef] [PubMed]
19. Guerra, E.N.S.; Almeida, F.T.; Bezerra, F.V.; Figueiredo, P.T.D.S.; Silva, M.A.G.; De Luca, C.G.; Pachêco-Pereira, C.; Leite, A.F. Capability of CBCT to identify patients with low bone mineral density: A systematic review. *Dentomaxillofac. Radiol.* **2017**, *46*, 20160475. [CrossRef] [PubMed]
20. Payahoo, S.; Jabbari, G. The Ability of Cone Beam Computed Tomography to Predict Osteopenia and Osteoporosis via Radiographic Density Derived from Cervical Vertebrae. *Int. J. Sci. Res. Dent. Med. Sci.* **2019**, *1*, 18–22.
21. Slaidina, A.; Nikitina, E.; Abeltins, A.; Soboleva, U.; Lejnieks, A. Gray values of the cervical vertebrae detected by cone beam computed tomography for the identification of osteoporosis and osteopenia in postmenopausal women. *Oral Surg. Oral Med. Oral Pathol. Oral Radiol.* **2022**, *133*, 100–109. [CrossRef]
22. Carvalho, B.F.; de Castro, J.G.K.; de Melo, N.S.; Figueiredo, P.T.S.; Moreira-Mesquita, C.R.; de Paula, A.P.; Sindeaux, R.; Leite, A.F. Fractal dimension analysis on CBCT scans for detecting low bone mineral density in postmenopausal women. *Imaging Sci. Dent.* **2022**, *52*, 20210172. [CrossRef]
23. Kim, D.G.; Navalgund, A.R.; Tee, B.C.; Noble, G.J.; Hart, R.T.; Lee, H.R. Increased variability of bone tissue mineral density resulting from estrogen deficiency influences creep behavior in a rat vertebral body. *Bone* **2012**, *51*, 868–875. [CrossRef] [PubMed]
24. Altan, M.; Nebioglu, D.O.; Iseri, H. Growth of the cervical vertebrae in girls from 8 to 17 years. A longitudinal study. *Eur. J. Orthod.* **2012**, *34*, 327–334. [CrossRef] [PubMed]
25. Molteni, R. Prospects and challenges of rendering tissue density in Hounsfield units for cone beam computed tomography. *Oral Surg. Oral Med. Oral Pathol. Oral Radiol.* **2013**, *116*, 105–119. [CrossRef]
26. Katsumata, A.; Hirukawa, A.; Okumura, S.; Naitoh, M.; Fujishita, M.; Ariji, E.; Langlais, R.P. Relationship between density variability and imaging volume size in cone-beam computerized tomographic scanning of the maxillofacial region: An in vitro study. *Oral Surg. Oral Med. Oral Pathol. Oral Radiol. Endod.* **2009**, *107*, 420–425. [CrossRef]
27. Schulze, R.; Heil, U.; Gross, D.; Bruellmann, D.D.; Dranischnikow, E.; Schwanecke, U.; Schoemer, E. Artefacts in CBCT: A review. *Dentomaxillofac. Radiol.* **2011**, *40*, 265–273. [CrossRef]
28. Berlemann, U.; Heini, P.F. Cervical Spine Fractures and Osteoporosis. In *Management of Fractures in Severely Osteoporotic Bone*; Obrant, K., Ed.; Springer: London, UK, 2000.
29. Korhonen, N.; Kannus, P.; Niemi, S.; Parkkari, J.; Sievänen, H. Rapid increase in fall-induced cervical spine injuries among older Finnish adults between 1970 and 2011. *Age Ageing* **2014**, *43*, 567–571. [CrossRef]
30. Genant, H.; Engelke, K.; Fuerst, T.; Glüer, C.C.; Grampp, S.; Harris, S.T.; Jergas, M.; Lang, T.; Lu, Y.; Majumdar, S.; et al. Noninvasive assessment of bone mineral and structure: State of the Art. *J. Bone Miner. Res.* **1996**, *11*, 707–730. [CrossRef]
31. Barngkgei, I.; Joury, E.; Jawad, A. An innovative approach in osteoporosis opportunistic screening by the dental practitioner: The use of cervical vertebrae and cone beam computed tomography with its viewer program. *Oral Surg. Oral Med. Oral Pathol. Oral Radiol.* **2015**, *120*, 651–659. [CrossRef]
32. FDA. Dental Cone-Beam Computed Tomography. Available online: https://www.fda.gov/radiation-emitting-products/medical-x-ray-imaging/dental-cone-beam-computed-tomography (accessed on 14 September 2021).
33. Przybyla, A.S.; Skrzypiec, D.; Pollintine, P.; Dolan, P.; Adams, M.A. Strength of the cervical spine in compression and bending. *Spine* **2007**, *32*, 1612–1620. [CrossRef] [PubMed]

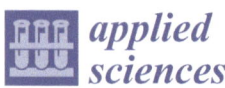

Article

Numerical Analysis Applying the Finite Element Method by Developing a Complex Three-Dimensional Biomodel of the Biological Tissues of the Elbow Joint Using Computerized Axial Tomography

Daniel Maya-Anaya *, Guillermo Urriolagoitia-Sosa *, Beatriz Romero-Ángeles, Miguel Martinez-Mondragon, Jesús Manuel German-Carcaño, Martin Ivan Correa-Corona, Alfonso Trejo-Enríquez, Arturo Sánchez-Cervantes, Alejandro Urriolagoitia-Luna and Guillermo Manuel Urriolagoitia-Calderón

Instituto Politécnico Nacional, Escuela Superior de Ingeniería Mecánica y Eléctrica, Sección de Estudios de Posgrado e Investigación, Unidad Profesional Adolfo López Mateos Zacatenco, Lindavista, Ciudad de México 07320, Mexico; bromeroa@ipn.mx (B.R.-Á.); miguemgon@gmail.com (M.M.-M.); german_17jun@hotmail.com (J.M.G.-C.); mcorreac1000@alumno.ipn.mx (M.I.C.-C.); atrejoe1201@alumno.ipn.mx (A.T.-E.); artursc4@hotmail.com (A.S.-C.); alex_ul56@hotmail.com (A.U.-L.); urrio332@hotmail.com (G.M.U.-C.)
* Correspondence: danmaa02@gmail.com (D.M.-A.); guiurri@hotmail.com (G.U.-S.)

Abstract: Numerical analysis computational programs are applied to the research of biological tissues, which have complex forms. Continuous technological advance has facilitated the development of biomodels to evaluate biological tissues of different human body systems using computerized axial tomography to produce complex three-dimensional models that represent the morphological and physiological characteristics of the real tissues. Biomodels are applied to numerical analysis using the Finite Element Method and provide a perspective of the mechanical behavior in the system. In this study, a numerical evaluation was performed by developing a biomodel of the humerus, radius, and ulna (the elbow joint, composed of cortical bone, trabecular bone, and cartilage). Also introduced to the biomodel were the ligaments of the capsule joint, collateral ligaments of the ulna, and collateral ligaments of the radius. The biomodel was imported into a computer program to perform a numerical analysis considering the mechanical properties of cortical and trabecular bone (including elasticity modulus, shear modulus, Poisson relation, and density). The embedding conditions were defined to restrict displacements and rotations in the proximal zone of the humerus, applying a compression load to the other end of the biomodel at the distal area of the radius and ulna. The results are the direct consequence of how boundary conditions and external agents are applied to the structure to be analyzed, and the data obtained show how the behavior of the force applied through the component produces stresses and strains as a whole, as well as for each of the components. These stresses and strains can indicate zones with structural problems and the detection areas causing pain (assisting in a better diagnosis).

Keywords: computer tomography; finite element method; numerical analysis; biomodel; biological tissue

1. Introduction

Elbow injuries are very diverse, with varied degrees of severity, and are caused by different factors derived from several activities that a person performs in their daily life. They also occur due to the deterioration of bone structure caused by aging. The symptoms are usually joint or upper arm pain. In activities such as tennis or golf, it is common to suffer elbow injuries. For example, tendonitis is frequently caused by this kind of sports activity, producing inflammation in the tendons. Also, an adequate diagnosis and optimal rehabilitation treatment for elbow injuries are difficult. In this sense, the use of

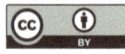

numerical simulations (the Finite Element Method) to assess this type of injury can be a great healing tool. The Finite Element Method makes it possible to produce numerical analyses to develop complex biomodels from computerized axial tomography [1]. The Finite Element Method divides the continuum (structure, body, or biological tissue) and characterizes the physical behavior of the problem to be investigated [2]. The continuum is mathematically characterized by several finite elements (discretization) distinguished by a series of unions through nodes. Each node represents a matrix solution [3]. The results are the data obtained as displacements, strains, stresses, and the vectorial distribution of the load. Currently, the use of computer programs is an effective alternative for the development of research because it is convenient for performing numerical evaluations through the structural model in digital form [4] due to the implementation of different CAD (Computer-Aided Design and Drafting) design methodologies for the representation of geometries, structures, and biological tissues in a three-dimensional space. The human body is considered a structure constituted by bones, which support the body, where each element is linked by connections formed by ligaments, which together form the skeletal system [5–7]. Computer programs have advanced considerably, providing the opportunity to develop biomodels with morphological characteristics (almost identical to the real ones) with the assurance of not compromising the patient's physical integrity. In this research project, a complete biomodel of the elbow joint was carried out, composed of four types of biological tissues (cortical bone, trabecular bone, ligament, and cartilage) [8,9]. We developed a numerical analysis using a computer program that implements a mathematical solution by the Finite Element Method [10–12]. These biomodels can be taken as measurement points, which indicate an approximation of how the bone structure's biological tissues deteriorate, indicate the severity of the injury, help propose recovery treatments, etc. This numerical analysis was performed on a healthy subject but could be applied to an injured patient to generate a biomodel with a malformation, such as blunt trauma to the joint or wear on the ligaments, tendons, and cartilage. This new methodology is an alternative to prosthesis fabrication since the biomodels of any system of the human body that presents some condition can be reproduced in a personalized manner (without compromising the patient's physical integrity). Even applying this new methodology preceding reconstructive surgical procedures can improve the surgical process and rehabilitation. For example, physiotherapeutic treatments that use resources, such as massage therapy techniques, electrical stimuli, and thermal means, among others, can apply the numerical evaluation to determine the amount of force that could produce an injury.

2. Methodology

The methodology to develop a biomodel derives from a series of steps that involve computerized tomography in the DICOM format. For this study case, a computerized tomography scan of half of the patient's torso was performed, where the working area to be characterized was enclosed (Figure 1) and included the elbow bones (humerus–radius–ulna), cartilage, and ligaments (Figure 2) [13]. Initially, the files obtained were imported into a computer program that can read the format. Next, a workspace was opened, consisting of four views (coronal, sagittal, axial, and total visualization of the model) where the slices that make up the tomography could be seen (Figure 3). It is possible to delimit the working area, and the software can automatically differentiate biological tissues. For this biomodel, a density mask range selection had a minimum value of 226 and a maximum value of 3071. The computational program can delimit the contour of the area of interest (Figure 4) without exceeding the established thickness (in this case, the cortical bone of the humerus, radius, and ulna). For trabecular bone, the density mask range was produced by an automatic procedure (cavity fill command), which identifies the cavity in the cortical bone and fills the space with soft material. However, the ligaments cannot be seen in computerized tomography, so ligaments were introduced in the biomodel by filling material in the space where the biological tissue is missing, which must be carried out manually (although the ligaments may present structural contact mismatch due to the complex shape or thickness of the structure) (Figure 5). Biomodel errors or mismatches are modified using reduction and smoothing commands for the component until the desired biological shape is correct. When generating contact between cortical bone and ligament, the most common thing that occurs is elements overlapping, which is resolved by performing a Boolean operation (removing the excess in material) and generating a uniformly smooth contact. Once the process has finished for each of the layers, the biomodel is operational and can be observed in the design window (Figure 6).

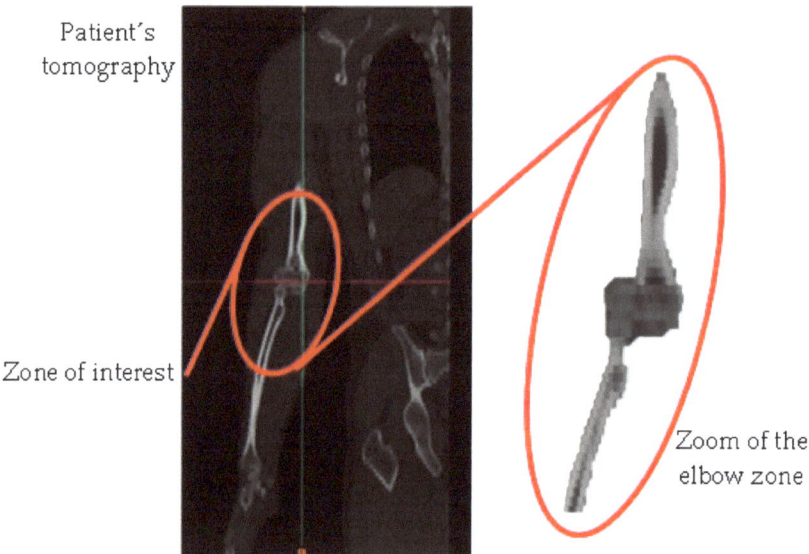

Figure 1. Patient's tomography.

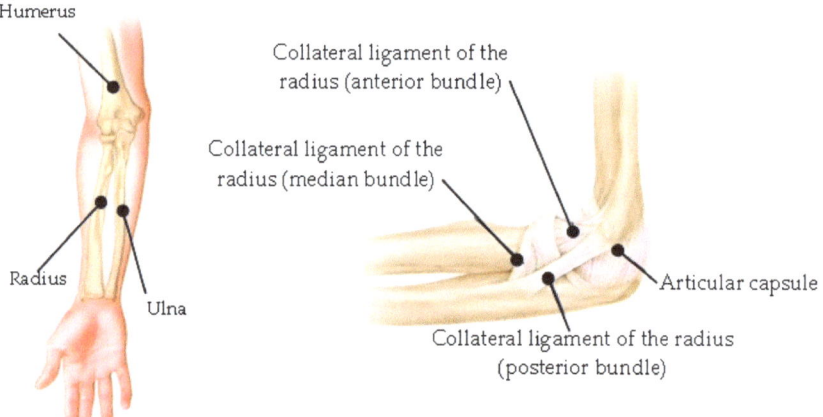

Figure 2. Arm components.

After the construction of the model, it was necessary to perform smoothing on the surface of each element. The procedure was completed by importing the model into another design software and producing a solid component (volume). The component elements were generated from discretization procedures of similar sizes and shapes. The model file was saved in an STL format, and the biomodel was exported to the Finite Element Method software and retained the same characteristics developed from the previous program because it was discretized as a solid mesh (which does not interfere with the defining time construction in the FEM discretization). The final biomodel was composed of different geometries—the cortical–trabecular bone, the cartilage (radius–ulna–humerus), and the elbow ligaments (capsule joint–collateral ligament and annular ligament of the radius–collateral ligament of the ulna)—which are assembled (representing the elbow joint) (Figure 6).

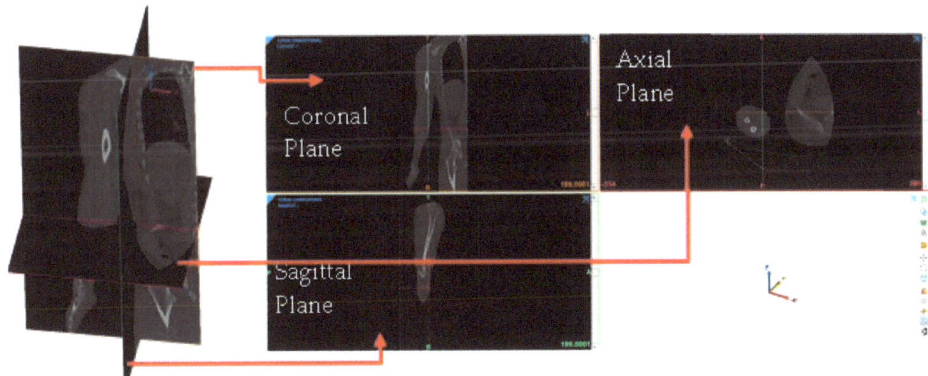

Figure 3. View of the work areas for the biomodel design.

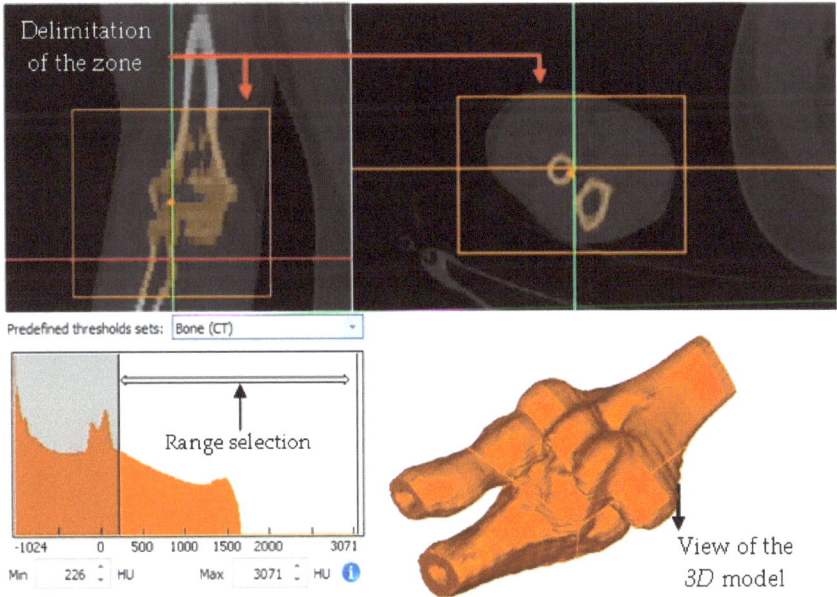

Figure 4. Delimitation of the working area.

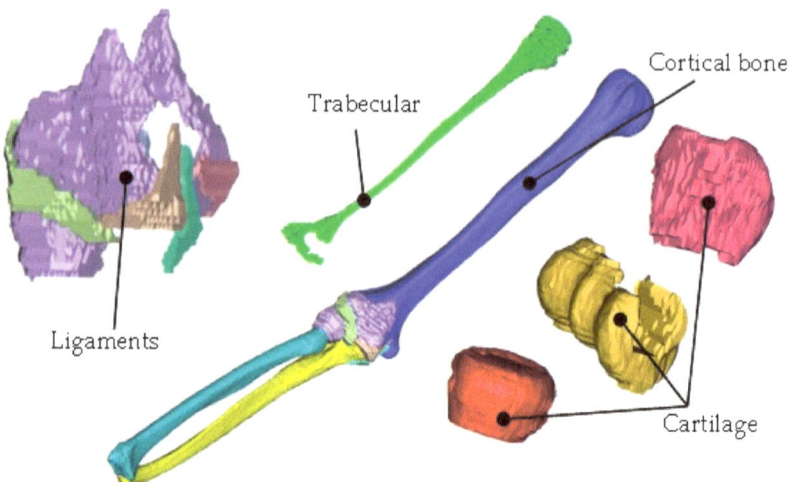

Figure 5. Initial biomodel.

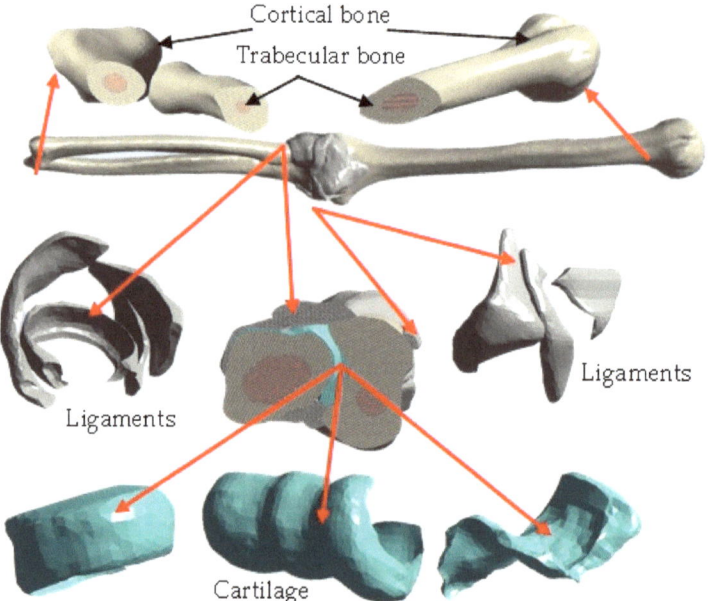

Figure 6. Solid model geometry.

The development of the biomodeling of the elbow articulation (arm bones, ligaments, and cartilage) was performed as follows [14,15]:

- Obtaining of the computerized axial tomography (upper limb).
- Development of images in DICOM format.
- Image importation into the Materialise Mimics® computer program.
- Delimitation of the area of interest for the development of the biomodel (elbow).
- Application of masks in the work area where the bones (cortical and trabecular) and cartilage will be represented.

- Development of the capsule joint, implementing the mask around the contour between the bones that make up the elbow joint (humerus, radius, and ulna).
- Development of ligaments through a mask that fills the gaps between the bones.
- Application of smoothing to the surface of the biomodel.
- Export of the biomodel to the 3-Matic Medical® program for the application of a mesh to obtain elements of similar size.
- Solidification of the biomodel through re-meshing.
- Exportation of the biomodel to a format with an extension compatible with the Ansys Workbench® program, which implements the Finite Element Method, for the development of numerical analysis.

3. Numerical Analysis

The execution of the numerical analysis was carried out in a computer program, Ansys Workbench® R1 2021, which applied a solution produced by the Finite Element Method using the previous numerical biomodel (representation of the biological tissue assembly). A structural static analysis was performed considering linear elastic behavior and orthotopic mechanical properties. Tables 1–3 show the mechanical properties characterizing the biological tissues (cortical bone, trabecular bone, ligaments, and cartilage) [16–18]. Figure 7 shows the loading and boundary condition configuration (free body diagram). Figure 8 shows the commands and the windows where the data in the tables are introduced. For discretization, high-order elements were selected, and the total assembly of the biomodel was composed of 17 solids, consisting of 857,746 nodes and 485,731 elements (Figure 9). The boundary conditions were given by the characteristics of an embedding, where the degrees of freedom were limited for the X, Y, and Z axes. Also, we restricted rotations in the XY, YZ, and XZ planes. In the humeral head part (Figure 10, yellow area), the load was applied on the distal part of the radius and ulna (on the longitudinal axis), which corresponds to the X axis (Figure 10, red area), as if the human being were standing on their hands. An individual weighing 78 kg was selected, and the weight was divided between the two arms on which the individual stood (conversion to Newtons was performed). The external agent was applied to the individual's head (in the longitudinal axis), and the axial load applied was approximately 382.6 N.

Table 1. Mechanical properties assigned to the computational biomodel of cortical bone.

Young's Modulus (MPa)	Shear Modulus (MPa)	Poisson Ratio
$E_1 = 16{,}000$	$G_{12} = 3200$	$v_{12} = 0.30$
$E_2 = 6880$	$G_{23} = 3600$	$v_{23} = 0.45$
$E_3 = 6300$	$G_{13} = 3300$	$v_{13} = 0.30$

Table 2. Mechanical properties assigned to the computational biomodel of trabecular bone.

Young's Modulus (MPa)	Shear Modulus (MPa)	Poisson Ratio
$E_1 = 1352$	$G_{12} = 292$	$v_{12} = 0.30$
$E_2 = 968$	$G_{23} = 370$	$v_{23} = 0.30$
$E_3 = 676$	$G_{13} = 505$	$v_{13} = 0.30$

Table 3. Mechanical properties assigned to the computational biomodel.

Component	Young's Modulus	Poisson Ratio
Ligament	6100 MPa	0.45
Cartilage	0.8 MPa	0.07

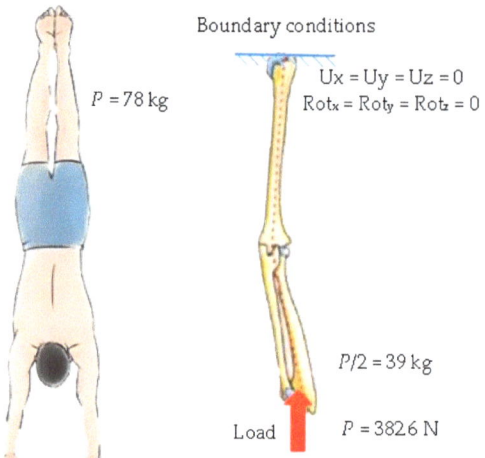

Figure 7. Loading free body diagram.

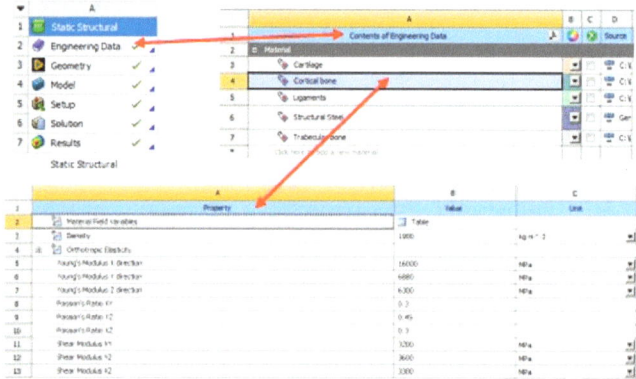

Figure 8. Data windows in Ansys Workbench®.

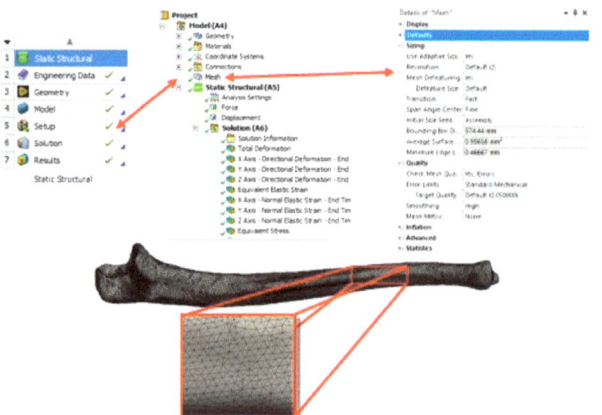

Figure 9. Commands to generate the discretization in the model.

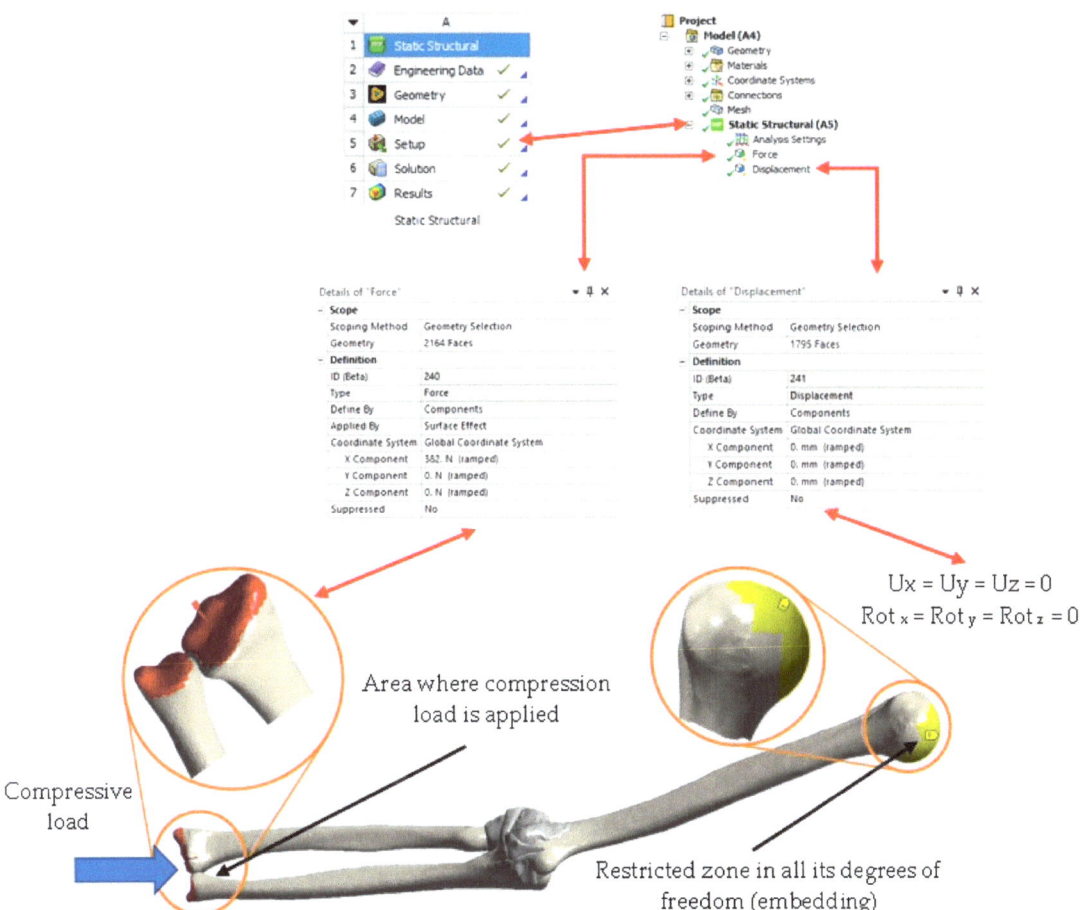

Figure 10. Application of boundary and load conditions to the model.

4. Results

The numerical simulation results concerning the compressive load (along the longitudinal axis of the biomodel) show significant effects represented by the total displacement, general strains, and von Mises stress. Nevertheless, more results could be presented in the form of stresses, strains, and displacements to distinguish different effects, but for this study the above data show the highlighted consequences. Also, the results can be seen as a biomodel assembly conjunction or viewed individually for each element that makes up the biomodel (Figures 11–21).

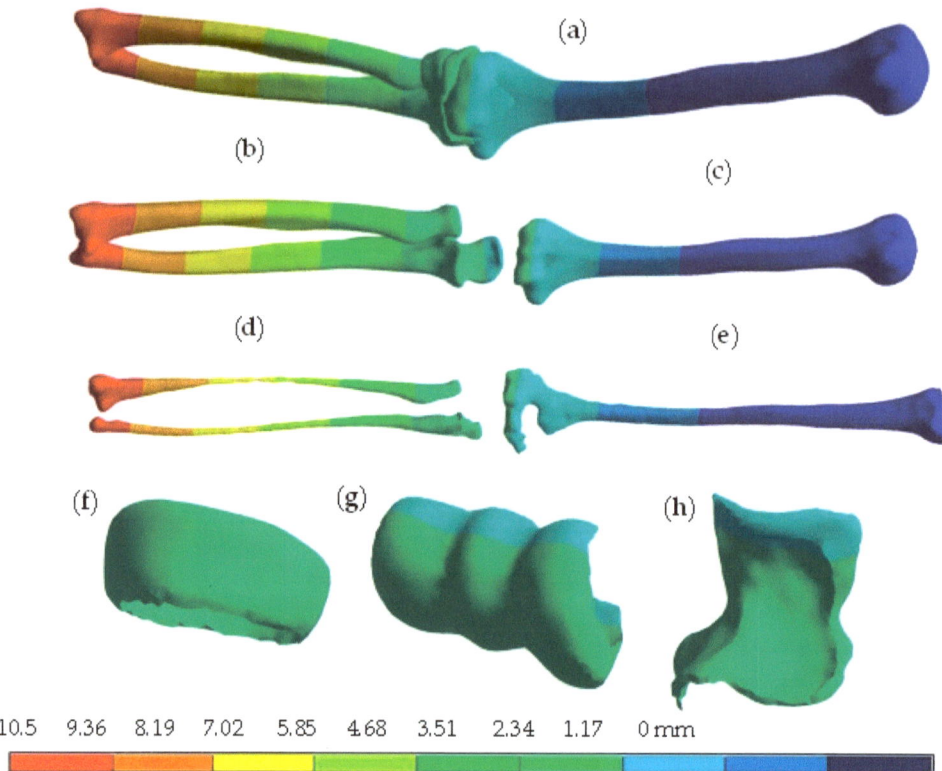

Figure 11. Total displacement results. (**a**) Complete model of the elbow joint. (**b**) Radius–ulna (cortical bone). (**c**) Humerus cortical bone. (**d**) Radius–ulna (trabecular bone). (**e**) Humerus trabecular bone. (**f**) Radius cartilage. (**g**) Cartilage of the humerus. (**h**) Ulna cartilage.

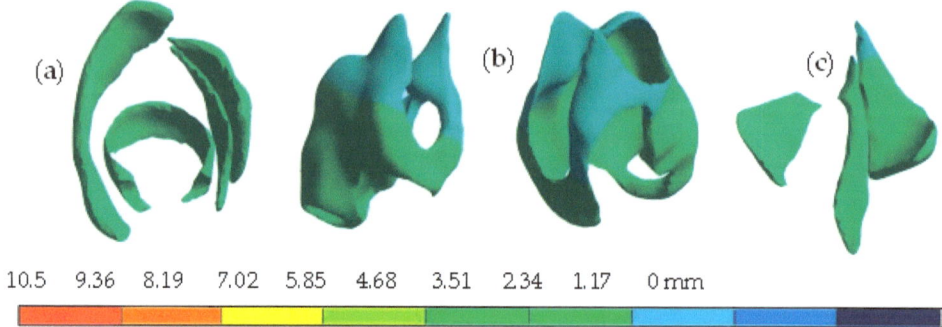

Figure 12. Total displacement results. (**a**) Collateral and annular ligaments of the radius. (**b**) Elbow joint capsule (front–rear view). (**c**) Collateral ligaments of the ulna.

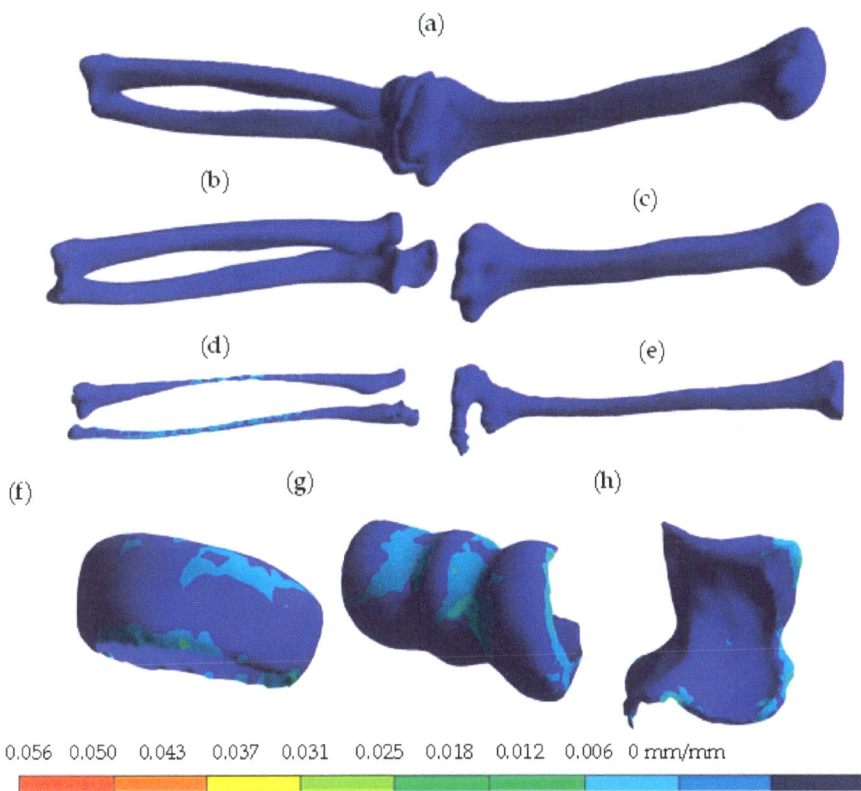

Figure 13. Total elastic strain results. (**a**) Complete model of the elbow joint. (**b**) Radius–ulna (cortical bone). (**c**) Humerus cortical bone. (**d**) Radius–ulna (trabecular bone). (**e**) Humerus trabecular bone. (**f**) Radius cartilage. (**g**) Cartilage of the humerus. (**h**) Ulna cartilage.

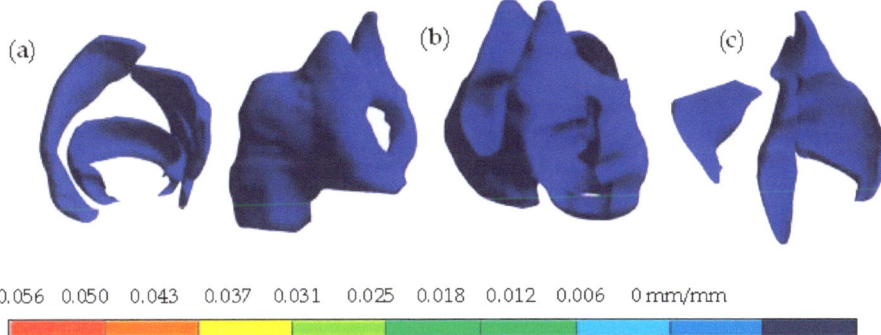

Figure 14. Total elastic strain results. (**a**) Collateral and annular ligaments of the radius. (**b**) Elbow joint capsule (front–rear view). (**c**) Collateral ligaments of the ulna.

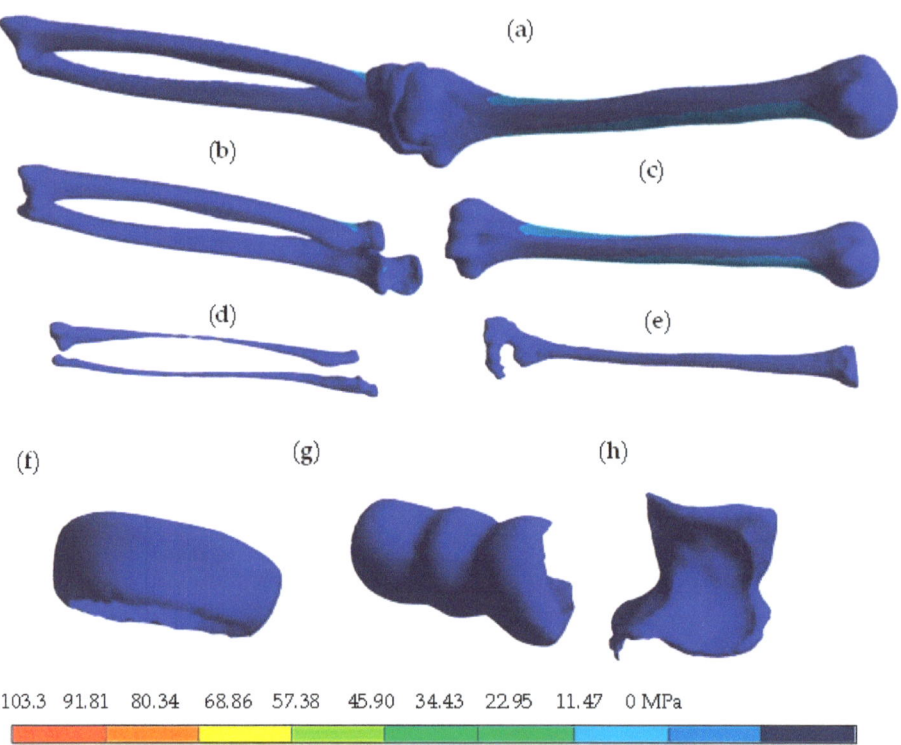

Figure 15. Von Mises's stress results. (**a**) Complete model of the elbow joint. (**b**) Radius–ulna (cortical bone). (**c**) Humerus cortical bone. (**d**) Radius–ulna (trabecular bone). (**e**) Humerus trabecular bone. (**f**) Radius cartilage. (**g**) Cartilage of the humerus. (**h**) Ulna cartilage.

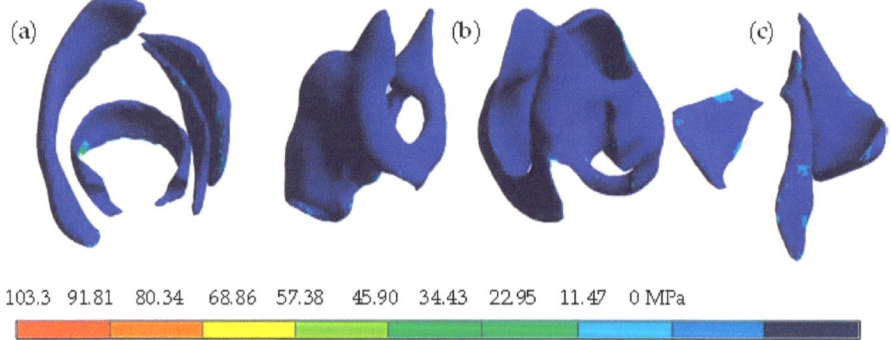

Figure 16. Von Mises's stress results. (**a**) Collateral and annular ligaments of the radius. (**b**) Elbow joint capsule (front–rear view). (**c**) Collateral ligaments of the ulna.

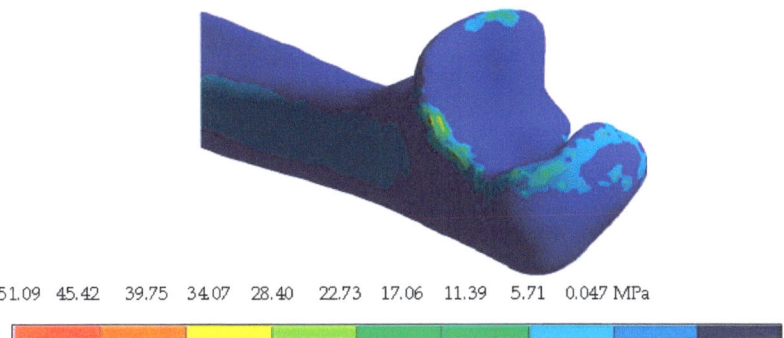

51.09 45.42 39.75 34.07 28.40 22.73 17.06 11.39 5.71 0.047 MPa

Figure 17. Von Mises's stress results for individual analysis of the ulna.

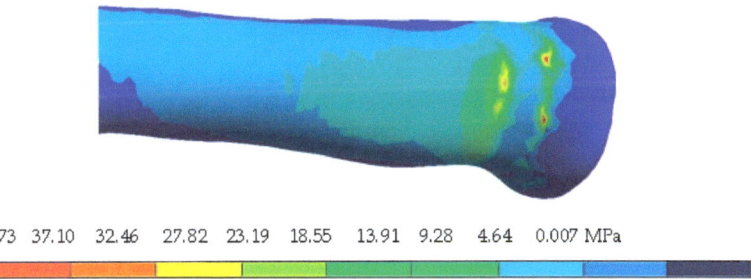

41.73 37.10 32.46 27.82 23.19 18.55 13.91 9.28 4.64 0.007 MPa

Figure 18. Von Mises's stress results for individual analysis of the radius.

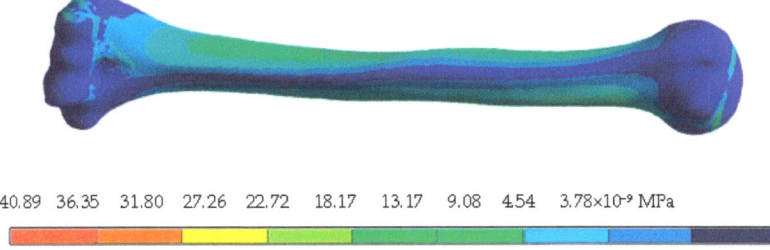

40.89 36.35 31.80 27.26 22.72 18.17 13.17 9.08 4.54 3.78×10⁻⁹ MPa

Figure 19. Von Mises's stress results for individual analysis of the humerus.

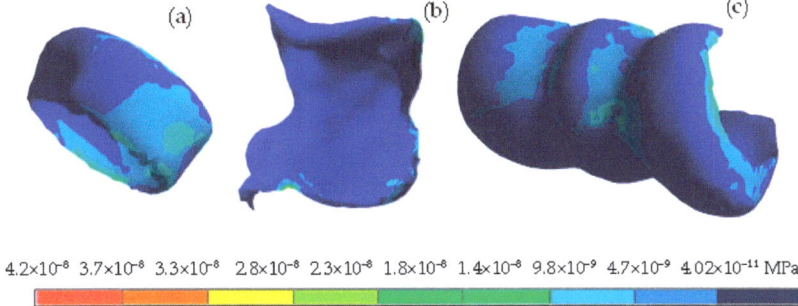

4.2×10⁻⁸ 3.7×10⁻⁸ 3.3×10⁻⁸ 2.8×10⁻⁸ 2.3×10⁻⁸ 1.8×10⁻⁸ 1.4×10⁻⁸ 9.8×10⁻⁹ 4.7×10⁻⁹ 4.02×10⁻¹¹ MPa

Figure 20. Von Mises's stress results for individual cartilage analysis: (**a**) radius, (**b**) ulna, (**c**) humerus.

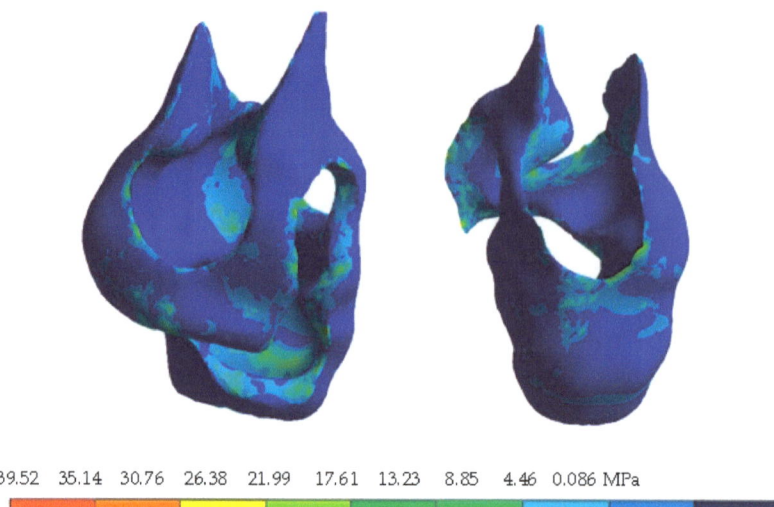

Figure 21. Von Mises's stress results for individual analysis of the capsule joint.

5. Discussion

Although there are currently different types of medical treatments for conditions that affect the human body, they have disadvantages because one cannot establish a diagnosis without compromising the integrity of the patient. Technology could be a supporting tool since the constant evolution in this area allows us to continue researching and providing solutions to different problems of the human body facing adversity. New technologies generate alternatives for surgical procedures, preventive methodologies, and corrective treatments. Numerical analyses are a reliable option for representing biological systems because they can simulate biological tissues in a three-dimensional manner, to which the conditions of its environment are applied. This study develops a methodology to produce a numerical biomodel for the simulation of the elbow joint and implementation of digital tools to perform a numerical evaluation (complemented with physics and structural mechanics knowledge). By developing a structural numerical evaluation of the healthy joint by the Finite Element Method, we obtained results showing how the structure behaves under the effect of compressive loading. The load distribution along the longitudinal axis and isochromatic changes can be distinguished where a maximum and minimum tensile stress is present, where the maximum represents the area prone to injury or even a fracture that could occur in this biological system. A biomodel is generated with characteristics that resemble the human body because it is developed from computerized axial tomography, which represents the bones, cartilage, and ligaments. Although the biofidelity of the biomodel can be questioned, it is clear that the characteristics of the biomodel represent 90% of the human morphology of the bone structure. It is worth mentioning that the internal structure that constitutes the biological tissue is too complex, so computerized tomography can be used to produce similar external dimensions. To quantify the error between the human component and the biomodel, it would be necessary to extract the human bone and obtain the mismatch percentage. The research objective was to produce biomodels and numerical evaluations so that diagnosis can be developed without affecting the integrity of the patient. Regarding the benefits of carrying out this type of research project where a biomodel is used, there is no doubt that it can cover several areas where medical diagnoses are implemented for the development of preventive and corrective treatments for a specific condition that affects the bone and joint structures of the human body. According to the results, the maximum total displacement occurs when the compressive load is applied, causing the bones (radius and ulna) to tend to separate at the interosseous membrane. Also, the strain describes the load tendency effect that affects the cartilage in the trochlea of the humerus zone. These results indicate the areas where the generation of cartilage wear begins. Finally, regarding the general stress distribution data, there is a change in isochromatic colors that is shown at the longitudinal part of the humerus and the section of the proximal part of the radius, initiating the volume reduction of these elements, and these changes tend to generate small lesions or even a crack in the bone. To better highlight the isochromatic changes that demonstrate how the stress is distributed in each component, an individual evaluation was performed. With this evaluation, the critical zones showing the maximum stresses are better appreciated, with smaller stress fields in the ulna, radius, and humerus. It can be stated that the affected area is located at the capsule joint. It can be concluded that at these points the load exceeds the structural resistance of the component. Also, there will be a separation between the capsule joint and the cortical bone, which can generate a joint effusion that causes pain. The authors have carried out projects where different methodologies were used for the development of biomodels applied to rehabilitation work and bone diseases, where it is considered an innovative process in medicine, biology, and dentistry [19–24].

6. Conclusions

The numerical evaluation presented has the advantage that the biomodel developed has a biofidelity that allows it to represent the morphological characteristics of the bones that constitute the elbow joint. The biological system is considered a continuous solid that has a defined volume suitable for developing the numerical analysis that applies the Finite Element Method. The results obtained showed the presence of stress concentrators and areas prone to injury or fractures. The von Misses stress results showed that, for the general analysis of the assembly, a slight isochromatic change is present in the proximal part of the humerus. The numerical analysis of individual components shows how the maximum stress is concentrated in the area where the ligaments are related to the bones. On the other hand, it was observed in the analysis that the elastic limit of the biological system was not exceeded. The results obtained and the behavior shown in this case (by the biomodel) can be validated by performing experimental tests. However, this is nearly impossible due to the cost, the risk to the patient, and established hygienic regulations. Numerical analysis can avoid experimental procedures, reduce costs, reduce time, and could be closer to reality. This shows that the application of these technological tools can influence different medical areas. All the results obtained are shown in Appendix A, Tables A1–A4. With this type of model, one can also add and simulate fractures in the bone or injuries that affect the joint, such as injuries to the ligaments or cartilage, because the human body degenerates as it completes its life cycle. Also, characterizing wear on the elbow joint is generated by developing repetitive or overextension movements that are commonly generated by the practice of sport, directly affecting the cartilage. Additionally, in the field of sports, the representation of bones with this method can be used to measure how the biological tissue is degenerating by carrying out a previous study when the joint is healthy or presents a previous injury and implementing a measurement period, so that at the end of this a new model is made to observe how much the biological tissue that is being studied has degenerated. It can also be used when a fracture occurs to determine how it is regenerated during the healing process, with the objective of determining whether there are malformations during this period. Finally, this biomodel can be used to generate a prosthesis design in a personalized manner. It can even develop bone prototypes using 3D printers with the purpose of developing bone models implementing biocompatible materials.

Author Contributions: Conceptualization, D.M.-A., G.U.-S. and B.R.-Á.; methodology, D.M.-A., G.U.-S., B.R.-Á. and G.M.U.-C.; validation, D.M.-A., G.U.-S., B.R.-Á., M.M.-M. and A.T.-E.; formal analysis, D.M.-A., G.U.-S., B.R.-Á. and M.I.C.-C.; investigation, D.M.-A., G.U.-S., B.R.-Á. and G.M.U.-C.; resources, D.M.-A., G.U.-S., B.R.-Á. and J.M.G.-C.; writing—original draft preparation, D.M.-A., G.U.-S., B.R.-Á. and A.S.-C.; writing—review and editing, D.M.-A., G.U.-S., B.R.-Á. and A.U.-L.; visualization, D.M.-A., G.U.-S., B.R.-Á. and M.I.C.-C.; supervision, D.M.-A., G.U.-S. and B.R.-Á.; project administration, D.M.-A., G.U.-S., B.R.-Á. and G.M.U.-C. All authors have read and agreed to the published version of the manuscript.

Funding: This research received no external funding.

Institutional Review Board Statement: Not applicable.

Informed Consent Statement: Not applicable.

Data Availability Statement: Not applicable.

Acknowledgments: The authors gratefully acknowledge the Instituto Politécnico Nacional, Consejo Nacional de Humanidades Ciencias y Tecnologías for supporting this research and Francisco Carrasco Hernández.

Conflicts of Interest: The authors declare no conflict of interest.

Appendix A

Table A1. Summary of general results of numerical evaluation of the humerus.

Concept	Cortical Bone		Trabecular Bone		Cartilage	
	Maximum	Minimum	Maximum	Minimum	Maximum	Minimum
Total displacement (mm)	3.80	0	3.70	0	3.87	3.32
Directional displacement, X axis (mm)	1.16	−0.21	1.02	−0.071	1.03	0.02
Directional displacement, Y axis (mm)	0.010	−1.57	0.008	−1.51	−1.42	−1.58
Directional displacement, Z axis (mm)	0.002	−3.46	0.007	−3.28	−2.97	−3.53
Elastic Strain	0.005	-1.85×10^{-8}	0.015	5.69×10^{-5}	0.056	0.0001
Elastic Strain, X axis	0.001	−0.002	0.007	−0.005	0.018	−0.023
Elastic Strain, Y axis	0.0008	−0.0006	0.008	−0.006	0.014	−0.005
Elastic Strain, Z axis	0.001	−0.002	0.005	−0.005	0.025	−0.019
Von Mises stress (MPa)	33.5	0	11.65	0	4.02×10^{-8}	3.68×10^{-11}
Nominal X-axis stress (MPa)	25.46	−36.62	11.28	−8.86	1.35×10^{-8}	1.69×10^{-8}
Nominal Y-axis stress (MPa)	10.99	−6.80	2.47	−2.35	1.14×10^{-8}	-4.67×10^{-9}
Nominal Z-axis stress (MPa)	15.68	−15.85	4.22	−4.24	1.95×10^{-8}	1.44×10^{-8}
Maximum principal stress (MPa)	27.29	−5.50	12.98	−1.27	2.50×10^{-8}	-8.46×10^{-10}
Middle principal stress (MPa)	10.78	−10.63	2.67	−2.25	6.04×10^{-9}	-2.47×10^{-9}
Minimum principal stress (MPa)	5.63	−37.19	1.15	−10.79	9.68×10^{-10}	-2.13×10^{-8}
XY shear stress (MPa)	7.89	−6.84	2.39	−2.09	7.73×10^{-9}	-8.98×10^{-9}
YZ shear stress (MPa)	6.57	−8.47	1.92	−2.45	5.06×10^{-9}	-7.18×10^{-9}
XZ shear stress (MPa)	13.45	−11.04	4.20	−5.52	9.51×10^{-9}	-1.34×10^{-8}

Table A2. Summary of general results of numerical evaluation of the ulna.

Concept	Cortical Bone		Trabecular Bone		Cartilage	
	Maximum	Minimum	Maximum	Minimum	Maximum	Minimum
Total displacement (mm)	10.26	3.26	10.07	3.68	4.11	3.31
Directional displacement, X axis (mm)	1.99	0.08	1.82	0.37	0.92	0.07
Directional displacement, Y axis (mm)	−1.41	−2.90	−1.52	−2.85	−1.43	−1.61

Table A2. *Cont.*

Concept	Cortical Bone		Trabecular Bone		Cartilage	
	Maximum	Minimum	Maximum	Minimum	Maximum	Minimum
Directional displacement, Z axis (mm)	−2.90	−9.69	−3.32	−9.50	−2.97	−3.68
Elastic Strain	0.006	5.92×10^{-6}	0.017	0.0001	0.04	2.87×10^{-5}
Elastic Strain, X axis	0.002	−0.002	0.009	−0.007	0.02	−0.015
Elastic Strain, Y axis	0.0007	−0.0006	0.001	−0.002	0.004	−0.003
Elastic Strain, Z axis	0.001	0.002	0.006	−0.004	0.017	−0.017
Von Mises stress (MPa)	48.72	0	14.41	0	3.43×10^{-8}	1.75×10^{-11}
Nominal X-axis stress (MPa)	35.08	−47.64	12.72	−9.83	1.73×10^{-8}	-1.15×10^{-8}
Nominal Y-axis stress (MPa)	7.83	−10.74	2.25	−2.42	3.84×10^{-9}	-2.84×10^{-9}
Nominal Z-axis stress (MPa)	11.63	−15.83	3.97	−3.55	1.37×10^{-8}	-1.35×10^{-8}
Maximum principal stress (MPa)	37.32	−5.19	13.79	−1.34	2.23×10^{-8}	-2.11×10^{-10}
Middle principal stress (MPa)	8.75	−11.18	3.55	−3.45	6.17×10^{-9}	-3.82×10^{-9}
Minimum principal stress (MPa)	4.85	−50.81	1.22	−10.07	6.83×10^{-10}	-1.81×10^{-8}
XY shear stress (MPa)	7.95	−7.14	3.18	−5.15	6.12×10^{-9}	-6.36×10^{-9}
YZ shear stress (MPa)	9.47	−8.48	2.08	−2.78	7.35×10^{-9}	-4.25×10^{-9}
XZ shear stress (MPa)	12.52	−14.16	7.12	−5.06	1.31×10^{-8}	9.61×10^{-9}

Table A3. Summary of overall results of numerical evaluation of radius.

Concept	Cortical Bone		Trabecular Bone		Cartilage	
	Maximum	Minimum	Maximum	Minimum	Maximum	Minimum
Total displacement (mm)	10.54	3.85	10.34	4.00	4.16	3.82
Directional displacement, X axis (mm)	2.30	0.66	2.18	0.80	1.18	0.64
Directional displacement, Y axis (mm)	−1.54	−3.01	−1.57	−2.96	−1.53	−1.61
Directional displacement, Z axis (mm)	−3.44	−9.88	−3.56	−9.69	−3.40	−3.67
Elastic Strain	0.005	5.34×10^{-6}	0.016	5.34×10^{-6}	0.03	0.0001
Elastic Strain, X axis	0.002	−0.002	2.07	−3.48	0.008	−0.010
Elastic Strain, Y axis	0.0005	−0.0007	5.83	−5.57	0.006	−0.0010
Elastic Strain, Z axis	0.002	−0.001	0.009	−0.007	0.011	−0.009
Von Mises stress (MPa)	37.32	0	14.22	0	2.16×10^{-8}	7.42×10^{-11}
Nominal X-axis stress (MPa)	38.11	36.65	9.70	−8.77	6.73×10^{-6}	-8.00×10^{-9}
Nominal Y-axis stress (MPa)	7.01	−7.96	2.07	−3.48	5.22×10^{-9}	-1.65×10^{-9}
Nominal Z-axis stress (MPa)	15.17	−13.84	5.83	−5.57	9.33×10^{-9}	-7.03×10^{-9}
Maximum principal stress (MPa)	41.53	−4.99	11.56	−1.21	1.56×10^{-8}	-4.33×10^{-10}
Middle principal stress (MPa)	8.40	−7.45	2.02	−2.37	4.52×10^{-9}	4.23×10^{-9}
Minimum principal stress (MPa)	5.16	−37.00	0.93	−11.2	9.94×10^{-10}	-1.13×10^{-8}
XY shear stress (MPa)	10.83	−5.84	3.87	−2.33	2.72×10^{-9}	-4.05×10^{-9}
YZ shear stress (MPa)	4.17	−11.38	2.77	−2.40	8.94×10^{-9}	-2.24×10^{-9}
XZ shear stress (MPa)	−11.09	−11.09	7.52	−4.36	3.15×10^{-9}	-1.77×10^{-8}

Table A4. Summary of general results of numerical assessment of the elbow joint.

Concept	Capsule Joint		Ligaments of the Radius		Ligaments of the Ulna	
	Maximum	Minimum	Maximum	Minimum	Maximum	Minimum
Total displacement (mm)	4.53	2.76	4.20	3.51	4.19	3.36
Directional displacement, X axis (mm)	1.25	−0.01	1.27	0.38	0.43	−0.08
Directional displacement, Y axis (mm)	−1.26	−1.66	−1.44	−1.61	−1.45	−1.65
Directional displacement, Z axis (mm)	−2.41	−3.87	−3.06	−3.71	3.03	−3.83
Elastic Strain	0.006	2.00×10^{-5}	0.017	2.09×10^{-6}	0.012	1.08×10^{-6}
Elastic Strain, X axis	0.004	−0.004	−0.008	−0.006	0.006	−0.004
Elastic Strain, Y axis	0.002	−0.001	0.008	−0.004	0.001	−0.001
Elastic Strain, Z axis	0.003	−0.004	0.005	−0.007	0.004	−0.005
Von Mises stress (MPa)	37.66	0	103.3	0	73.49	0
Nominal X-axis stress (MPa)	34.22	−40.48	102.6	−39.28	30.39	−38.10
Nominal Y-axis stress (MPa)	17.71	−22.10	52.39	−21.20	15.36	−20.77

Table A4. *Cont.*

Concept	Capsule Joint		Ligaments of the Radius		Ligaments of the Ulna	
	Maximum	Minimum	Maximum	Minimum	Maximum	Minimum
Nominal Z-axis stress (MPa)	18.15	−25.81	65.00	−62.19	34.97	−20.42
Maximum principal stress (MPa)	34.32	−12.02	115.19	−15.52	38.52	−7.87
Middle principal stress (MPa)	18.96	−21.66	63.34	−28.37	24.06	−18.40
Minimum principal stress (MPa)	11.27	−43.95	39.42	−94.40	12.73	−49.20
XY shear stress (MPa)	15.52	−12.91	25.26	−26.15	7.73	−17.11
YZ shear stress (MPa)	7.54	−9.14	42.17	−5.95	12.38	−28.54
XZ shear stress (MPa)	13.41	−19.75	28.34	−25.33	19.07	−14.26

References

1. Willing, R.T.; Lalone, E.A.; Shannon, H.; Johnson, J.A.; King, G.J.W. Validation of a finite element model of the human elbow for determining cartilage contact mechanics. *J. Biomech.* **2013**, *46*, 1767–1771. [CrossRef] [PubMed]
2. Garzón-Alvarado, D.A.; Duque-Daza, C.A.; Ramírez-Martínez, A.M. On the emergence of biomechanics and computational mechanobiology: Computational experiments and recent findings. *Rev. Cuba. Investig. Bioméd.* **2009**, *28*, 83–101.
3. Urbanowieza, E.M.; Ramíreza, E.I.; Ruiz, O.; Ortiza, A. Analysis by finite element parcel of a Thompson®hip prosthesis under four different load conditions. In Proceedings of the XXI Annual International Congress of the SOMIM, Pachuca, México, 22–24 September 2021; pp. 24–31.
4. López-Liévano, A.; López-Liévano, D.R.; Caicedo-Ortiz, H.E.; González-Rebattú, A. Biomodeling of the components of the human middle ear using magnetic resonance imaging. *Scientist* **2017**, *21*, 3–8.
5. Kumar, S.; Kumar, J. A review on application of finite element modelling in bone biomechanics. *Perspect. Sci.* **2016**, *8*, 696–698.
6. Goel, V.K.; Singh, D.; Bijlani, V. Contact areas in human elbow joints. *J. Biomech. Eng.* **1982**, *104*, 169–175. [CrossRef]
7. Lohfeld, S.; Barron, V.; McHugh, P.E. Biomodels of Bone: A Review. *Ann. Biomed. Eng.* **2005**, *33*, 1295–1311. [CrossRef]
8. Ruiz-Santiago, F.; Castellano-García, M.; Guzmán-Álvarez, L.; Tello-Moreno, M. Computed tomography and magnetic resonance imaging in painful diseases of the spine; Respective contributions and controversies. *Radiology* **2011**, *53*, 116–133.
9. Cristea, A.F. Mechanical stress and strain properties, regarding the elbow joint. *Acta Tech. Napoc.-Ser. Appl. Math. Mech. Eng.* **2014**, *57*, 179–188.
10. Jardini, A.L.; Larosa, M.A.; Filho, R.M.; Zavaglia, C.A.D.C.; Bernardes, L.F.; Lambert, C.S.; Kharmandayan, P. Cranial reconstruction: 3D biomodel and custom-built implant created using additive manufacturing. *J. Cranio-Maxillofac. Surg.* **2014**, *42*, 1877–1884. [CrossRef]
11. Oliveira, M.; Sooraj Hussain, N.; Dias, A.G.; Lopes, M.A.; Azevedo, L.; Zenha, H.; Santos, J.D. 3-D biomodelling technology for maxillofacial reconstruction. *Mater. Sci. Eng. C* **2008**, *28*, 1347–1351. [CrossRef]
12. Nareliya, R.; Kumar, V. Finite element application to a femur bone: A review. *J. Biomed. Bioeng.* **2012**, *3*, 57–62.
13. Cisneros-Hidalgo, Y.; González-Carbonell, R.; Ortiz-Prado, A.; Jacobo-Almendáriz, V.; Puente-Álvarez, A. Modelo mechanobiológical of a human tibia to determine its response to external mechanical stimuli. *Cuba. J. Biomed. Res.* **2015**, *34*, 54–63.
14. Mastache-Miranda, O.A.; Urriolagoitia-Sosa, G.; Marquet-Rivera, R.A. Three-dimensional reconstruction for use in medicine and biomechanics. *MOJ Appl. Bionics Biomech.* **2018**, *2*, 310–331.
15. Marquet-Rivera, R.A.; Urriolagoitia-Sosa, G.; Romero-Ángeles, B.; Vázquez-Feijoo, J.A.; Urriolagoitia-Calderón, G. Computational biomodelling and numerical analysis as means of diagnostic and odontological prognosis. *MOJ Appl. Bionics Biomech.* **2018**, *2*, 262–263.
16. Wu, D.; Isaksson, P.; Fergusson, S.J.; Persson, C. Young´s modulus of trabecular bone at the tissue level: A review. *Acta Biomater.* **2018**, *78*, 1–12. [CrossRef] [PubMed]
17. Flores-Renteria, M.A.; Ortíz-Domínguez, M.; Cruz-Avilés, A.; López-Sánchez, F. Bone mechanics: A review of bone remodeling, Ingenuity and Consciousness. *Sci. Bull. Super. Sch. Ciudad. Sahagún* **2018**, *9*, 1–15.
18. Mendoza, A. Study of the mechanical properties of the bone system. *J. Eng. Res.* **1991**, *23*, 14–19.
19. Martinez-Mondragon, M.; Urriolagoitia-Sosa, G.; Romero-Ángeles, B.; Maya-Anaya, D.; Martínez-Reyes, J.; Gallegos-Funes, F.J.; Urriolagoitia-Calderón, G.M. Numerical Analysis of Zirconium and Titanium Implants under the Effect of Critical Masticatory Load. *Materials* **2022**, *15*, 7843. [CrossRef]
20. Hernández-Vázquez, R.A.; Romero-Ángeles, B.; Urriolagoitia-Sosa, G.; Vázquez-Feijoo, J.A.; Vázquez-López, Á.J.; Urriolagoitia-Calderón, G. Numerical analysis of masticatory forces on a lower first molar considering the contact between dental tissues. *Appl. Bionics Biomech.* **2018**, *2018*, 4196343. [CrossRef]
21. Marquet-Rivera, R.A.; Urriolagoitia-Sosa, G.; Hernández-Vázquez, R.A.; Romero-Ángeles, B.; Mastache-Miranda, O.A.; Urriolagoitia-Calderón, G. High biofidelity 3D biomodel reconstruction from soft and hard tissues (knee), FEM, and 3D printing: A three-dimensional methodological proposal. *BioMed Res. Int.* **2021**, *2021*, 6688164.

22. Hernández-Vázquez, R.A.; Urriolagoitia-Sosa, G.; Marquet-Rivera, R.A.; Romero-Angeles, B.; Mastache-Miranda, O.A.; Vázquez-Feijoo, J.A.; Urriolagoitia-Calderon, G. High-biofidelity biomodel generated from three-dimensional imaging (cone-beam computed tomography): A methodological proposal. *Comput. Math. Methods Med.* **2020**, *2020*, 4292501. [CrossRef] [PubMed]
23. Marquet-Rivera, R.A.; Urriolagoitia-Sosa, G.; Romero-Ángeles, B.; Hernández-Vázquez, R.A.; Mastache-Miranda, O.A.; Cruz-López, S.; Urriolagoitia-Calderón, G. Numerical Analysis of the ACL, with Sprains of Different Degrees after Trauma. *Comput. Math. Methods Med.* **2021**, *2021*, 2109348. [CrossRef] [PubMed]
24. Hernández-Vázquez, R.A.; Romero-Ángeles, B.; Urriolagoitia-Sosa, G.; Vázquez-Feijoo, J.A.; Marquet-Rivera, R.A.; Urriolagoitia-Calderón, G. Mechanobiological analysis of molar teeth with carious lesions through the finite element method. *Appl. Bionics Biomech.* **2018**, *2018*, 1815830. [CrossRef] [PubMed]

Disclaimer/Publisher's Note: The statements, opinions and data contained in all publications are solely those of the individual author(s) and contributor(s) and not of MDPI and/or the editor(s). MDPI and/or the editor(s) disclaim responsibility for any injury to people or property resulting from any ideas, methods, instructions or products referred to in the content.

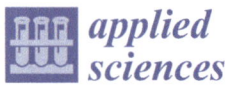

Article

The Spatial Characteristics of Intervertebral Foramina within the L4/L5 and L5/S1 Motor Segments of the Spine

Piotr Nowak [1], Mikołaj Dąbrowski [1,*], Adam Druszcz [2] and Łukasz Kubaszewski [1]

[1] Adult Spine Orthopaedics Department, Poznan University of Medical Sciences, 61-545 Poznan, Poland; pinowak@orsk.pl (P.N.); zaklad.sbk@ump.edu.pl (Ł.K.)
[2] Department of Neurosurgery, Provincial Specialist Hospital in Legnica, 59-220 Legnica, Poland
* Correspondence: mdabrowski@ump.edu.pl

Simple Summary: Lumbar foraminal stenosis (LFS) is a common pathology accompanying diseases of the spine, such as osteoarthritis, scoliosis, and spondylolisthesis. It affects patients of all ages and can cause lumbar radiculopathy. Lumbar radiculopathy symptoms, such as sharp pain in the back or legs, which may worsen with certain activities, weakness or loss of reflexes in the legs, numbness of the skin, "pins and needles", or other abnormal sensations (paresthesia) in the legs, are particularly troublesome for patients and hinder their daily activities. It is important to constantly improve the methods of LFS imaging diagnostics. In this article, we analyzed the three-dimensional shape of the root canals in the lower part of the lumbar spine, based on CT scans. The obtained results made it possible to assess how the shape of the intervertebral foramina is related to factors such as age, sex, and motor neuron level. The research conducted is an introduction to a better understanding of the pathology of LFS, which will improve the conservative and surgical treatment of spinal diseases.

Citation: Nowak, P.; Dąbrowski, M.; Druszcz, A.; Kubaszewski, Ł. The Spatial Characteristics of Intervertebral Foramina within the L4/L5 and L5/S1 Motor Segments of the Spine. *Appl. Sci.* **2024**, *14*, 2263. https://doi.org/10.3390/app14062263

Academic Editor: Claudio Belvedere

Received: 21 November 2023
Revised: 27 February 2024
Accepted: 27 February 2024
Published: 7 March 2024

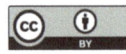

Copyright: © 2024 by the authors. Licensee MDPI, Basel, Switzerland. This article is an open access article distributed under the terms and conditions of the Creative Commons Attribution (CC BY) license (https://creativecommons.org/licenses/by/4.0/).

Abstract: The prevalence of lower back pain and radicular pain in the population requires more and more accurate diagnostic methods to more effectively prevent and treat patients with these ailments. In this paper, we focused on one of the causes of lower back pain and radicular pain—lumbar foraminal stenosis (LFS). The aim of the study is to assess the morphometry of the intervertebral canals in the lumbar spine at the levels of the L4/L5 and L5/S1 motor segments. The obtained results showed correlations between the circumference and the surface area on individual cross-sections of the intervertebral canals at the L4/L5 and L5/S1 levels and determined the approximate shape of the root canal and its variability. On this basis, we were able to determine the influences of the patient's age and sex on the morphometric parameters of the intervertebral canals at the L4/L5 and L5/S1 levels. Further research is needed in this area, taking into account additional factors influencing the shape of intervertebral canals.

Keywords: lumbar foraminal stenosis; spinal stenosis; 3D reconstruction; surface area; lumbar foraminal measurements

1. Introduction

Spinal stenosis is characterized by a reduction in the cross-sectional area of the spinal canal, leading to upper or lower motor neuron deficits and associated neurological symptoms depending on the site of compression [1].

Spinal stenosis is a relatively common medical problem. It concerns mainly geriatric patients. Spinal stenosis in younger patients is a consequence of congenital malformations. On the other hand, in people over 50 years old, it is the result of progressive degenerative changes. Epidemiological studies have shown that 5/100,000 people and 80% of people over 70 years of age may suffer from spinal stenosis [2]. Epidemiological trends suggest that, in the coming decades, the number of diagnosed cases of stenosis will increase. In adults over 65 years undergoing spinal surgery, the leading diagnosis is lumbar spinal stenosis (LSS) [3].

Lumbar foraminal stenosis (LFS) is a common cause of lower limb radiculopathy (8–11%), negatively affecting patients' quality of life and daily activities [4,5].

LFS is common in middle-aged populations, where degenerative changes in the bones and facet joints, hyperplasia of the flava ligament, and herniated discs may contribute to the narrowing of the spinal foramen.

Spinal canal stenosis can affect various anatomical structures within it. Stenosis is diagnosed in the central canal where the spinal cord is located. In such cases, stenosis in the anteroposterior dimension is observed, which leads to the compression of the nerve elements and reduced blood supply to the spinal cord in the cervical section and cauda equina in the lumbar section. The medical problem discussed in this part of the article may also concern the intervertebral canals, i.e., the channels through which the nerve roots exit the spinal cord. In the course of stenosis, compression is observed as a result of a herniated intervertebral disc, the overgrowth of facet joints and ligaments, or the unstable displacement of one vertebral body relative to the level below. The third anatomical structure that can be affected by spinal stenosis is the lateral recess, which occurs only in the lumbar spine. The lateral recess is the area along the epiphyse where the nerve root enters just before exiting through the intervertebral canal, and may be compressed due to hypertrophy of the facet joint [3].

Symptoms for LFS have been observed in patients with degenerative disc disease, scoliosis, spondylolysis, spondylolisthesis and spondylolytic spondylolisthesis. Hypertrophic ligamentum flavum (LF) and osteophytes are occasionally seen in patients with LFS. However, these types of symptoms do not always indicate the development of LFS. Therefore, it is necessary to improve the diagnostic procedures related to the described disease entity [6]. It is estimated that stenosis of the intervertebral foramina is a problem for about 8–11% of the population [7]. Pathologies occurring within the intervertebral disc may lead to changes in the parameters of the intervertebral foramina. With cranial subluxation of the upper articular process of the lower vertebra, the height and area of the intervertebral foramen decrease. Osteophytes of the facet joint and hypertrophic ligamentum flavum contribute to the reduction in the width and area of the foramen in the anterior–posterior dimension [8]. Changes occurring within the spinal canal may lead to compression of the lumbar nerve and dorsal root ganglion and result in the appearance of symptoms characteristic of spinal canal impingement [7].

Due to the fact that treatment in the case of LFS does not always mean a return to full fitness and pain relief, research continues, the aim of which is, among others, to learn the importance of the size of the intervertebral foramina in the appearance of spinal stenosis.

An accurate diagnosis of spinal stenosis is difficult to make. This is due to the lack of consensus on definitive diagnostic criteria and the requirement for consistency between physical symptoms and imaging features. In particular, Tominaga et al. [9] believe that clinicians should make a diagnosis based on a thorough physical examination and consistent imaging findings, including X-ray, computed tomography (CT), and magnetic resonance imaging (MRI) [9].

The utilization of intervertebral foramen evaluation as a diagnostic tool is relevant in conditions that involve the compression of neurovascular structures within the foramen [10]. A commonly employed technique for categorizing lesions within the spinal canal was introduced by Lee and colleagues [11]. This approach relies on magnetic resonance imaging (MRI) to examine the area surrounding the spinal nerve roots, assessing any reduction or absence of free space around these structures that may lead to contact with the elements defining the intervertebral foramen. A more recent classification system refined the accuracy of the previous one [12]. It should be noted that these categorizations do not denote absolute values but are instead unique analyses of MRI-obtained images.

Computed tomography-based LFS classification (CT Haleem–Botchu) is compatible with the MRI classification system [13].

The morphological characteristics of the intervertebral foramen of the lumbar spine are described as oval, round, and tear-like; however, variability in the narrowing of the foramen is observed [14].

The limited number of papers in the presented scope was the starting point for the search for quantitative assessments of the size of the intervertebral foramen. Due to the epidemiology of spinal degeneration, two lower motor segments within the lumbar spine were selected for analysis.

The aim of this study is to present the results of measurements of the intervertebral foramen in various cross-sections, forming the image of the intervertebral canal, and to compare their morphology between the L4/5 and L5/S1 segments.

2. Materials and Methods

2.1. Patients

This research was conducted on a population of 89 patients (44 women and 45 men) of W. Dega University Hospital in Poznan [15]. The oldest participant was 89 years old and the youngest was 22 years old (mean 53.4 ± 16.4). All patients that qualified for the study reported complaints in the L4/L5 and L5/S1 segment of the spine.

This study included individuals with lower back pain who had undergone lumbar spine CT.

The exclusion criteria were as follows: scoliosis, asymmetry of the position and shape of the pelvis, lumbar spondylolisthesis, lumbar spinal stenosis, spinal deformity, foraminal stenosis, spondylolysis, disc disease, isthmic lysis, herniated disc, root symptoms, history of lower limb pain and numbness, history of lumbar spine trauma, infection, and surgery.

Through verbal communication, individuals were informed that their scans would be anonymized, excluding personally identifiable information (except age and gender). Anonymized images were explicitly designated for research or educational purposes, and rigorous exclusion criteria were applied, excluding scans without explicit consent. No new protocol was used and the CT scans were derived from standard retrospective investigations based on images of patients with lumbar spine-related disorders. We informed local IRB committees.

2.2. Morphometric Measurement

Our CT imaging process involves utilizing a multi-detector CT scanner. The scan parameters include a slice thickness of 1–2 mm, covering the range from L3 to S1. During the procedure, patients were positioned in a supine position with a focus on maintaining a neutral alignment of the spine. The image acquisition followed a standard lumbar spine protocol, ensuring a systematic approach to data collection.

CT scans of the patients were transformed using InVesalius, Meshmixer, 3D Builder, and GOM programs to obtain a three-dimensional image. In the obtained spatial visualization, the space of the root canal and the measurement planes were defined.

The process of defining the root canal involved several steps. Since root canals can vary in their spatial arrangement depending on the evaluated motor segment, the primary factor used to define the root canal was the course of the long axis of the epiphysis that bordered the upper part of the canal. Subsequently, the cross-section of the root canal was determined to align with the axis of the pedicle, which formed the upper opening of the canal. The analysis specifically focused on the bony boundaries, disregarding any soft tissue contours like the intervertebral disc and joint capsule. To complete the outline of the root canal where the intervertebral disc outline was eliminated, a line was added, connecting the lower posterior edge of the upper vertebral body to the posterior upper edge of the lower vertebra.

The obtained root canal contour was used to measure its maximum vertical dimension (MaxY). The maximum vertical dimension represents the longest section within the contour, perpendicular to the end plate of the vertebral body below (Figure 1).

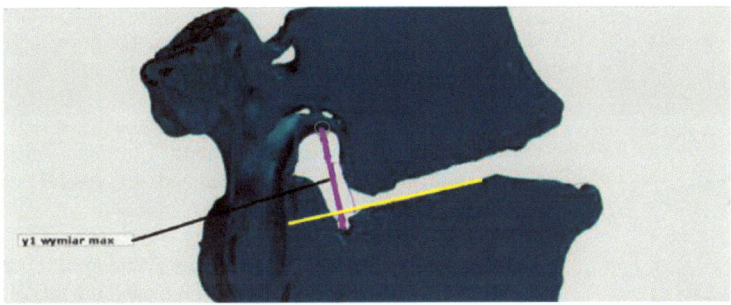

Figure 1. Measurement method. Purple line represents the maximum vertical dimension [y1 wymiar max]; the yellow line represents the endplate of the vertebral body.

The two senior orthopedic surgeons had an average of 10 years' experience with CT.

The surface area measurement method consisted of the following steps. In the first phase, the maximum vertical dimension of the L4/L5 root canal was determined. In the next stage of the measurement, the maximum vertical dimension of the root canal L4/L5 was applied to the visualization of the cross-section. Knowing the vertical dimension of the channel is expressed in mm, we calculated how many pixels fit in a square with a side equal to the vertical dimension. In this way, the scale was established as the number of pixels that fit in 1 mm^2 of the area in the cross-section visualization. In the last phase of the research, the cross-sectional area obtained was marked with a loop (Figure 2) and information on the number of pixels corresponding to the area of the selected area on the visualization was read. Then, using the proportion, the surface area of the intervertebral foramen cross section was calculated. We applied same procedure for L5/S1 root canal.

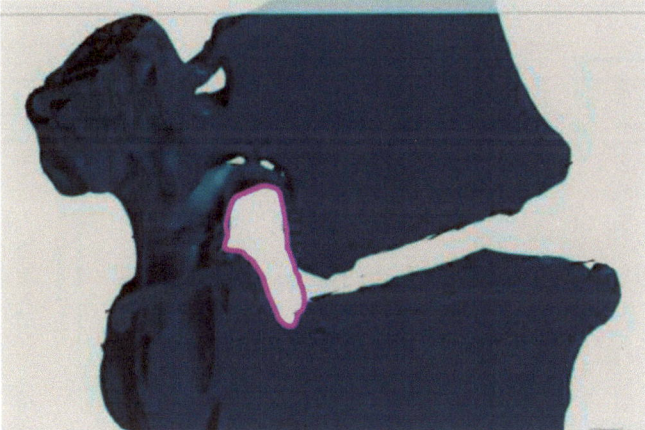

Figure 2. Surface area; close-up of the measured area from Figure 1. Purple line represents boundries of calculated surface area.

Sections I–III were defined as follows:
I. Halfway from the medial border of the root canal and the medial axis of the pedicle;
II. In the medial axis of the vertebral epiphysis;
III. Halfway from the lateral border of the root canal and the medial axis of the vertebral epiphysis

The dimensions of the cross-sections are given in mm, and the surface area in mm^2. The study population was divided into two age groups. The first was made up of people under 50, the second was made up of people over 50.

2.3. Segmentation

Segmentation was performed with a manual painter (sphere brush) (Slicer 3D). Once the segmentation mask was obtained, it was rendered into a 3D model.

2.4. Statistical Analysis

The analysis used Statistica software (Version 13.0, StatSoft Inc., Tulsa, OK, USA). To compare the impact of various factors on measurements of the intervertebral foramen, we used a Mann–Whitney U-test ($p < 0.05$). In addition, we determined the Spearman's rank correlation between measurements of the intervertebral foramen.

3. Results

The study population consisted of 89 people. Table 1 presents the general measurement values for motor segments L4/5 and L5/S1. This table includes data on the maximum horizontal value (MaxX), maximum vertical value (MaxY), minimum horizontal value (MinX), perimeter, and area. The left- and right-side results are shown for each segment. I–III indicate the numbers of the cross-sections used for the tests. In the L4/5 motion segment, the maximum value for MaxX was found in section III and was 11.7 mm for the right side and 11.1 mm for the left side. Similar patterns were found in the L5/S1 motion segment. MaxX had the highest value in section III and it was 12.2 mm (right side) and 10.8 mm (left side). The minimum value in the L4/5 movement segment is 10.3 mm, which was found in the second section (left side). For the L5/S1 segment, the minimum value was observed in the first section (left side) and this was 10.1 mm.

Table 1. Measurement results (mean ± SD in mm and area section in mm^2) for motion segment L4/5 and L5/S1 ($N = 89$). MaxX—Maximal Horizontal Dimension, MaxY—Maximal Vertical Dimension, MinX—Minimal Horizontal Dimension, NS—not statistically significant.

		L4/5			L5/S1		
		R	L	p	R	L	p
MaxX	I	10.2 ± 2.3	10.5 ± 2.5	NS	10.7 ± 3.5	10.1 ± 2.1	NS
	II	10.4 ± 2.1	10.3 ± 2	NS	11.2 ± 2.4	10.4 ± 2.5	NS
	III	11.7 ± 2.8	11.1 ± 2.5	NS	12.2 ± 2.5	10.8 ± 3.3	NS
	p	NS	NS		NS	NS	
MaxY	I	18.8 ± 3.6	19.3 ± 4	NS	17.2 ± 4.3	17.1 ± 4.4	NS
	II	17.6 ± 3.2	17.8 ± 3.4	NS	15.7 ± 3.8	16 ± 4	NS
	III	17.5 ± 3.7	17.3 ± 3.1	NS	15.1 ± 3.4	15 ± 4.3	NS
	p	NS	NS		NS	NS	
MinX	I	5.6 ± 2.9	5.7 ± 2.3	NS	6.2 ± 3.3	5.3 ± 2.4	NS
	II	5.4 ± 2.3	5.2 ± 2.2	NS	6.7 ± 7.5	5.4 ± 2.3	NS
	III	5.6 ± 2.4	5.8 ± 2.3	NS	6.2 ± 2.6	6.3 ± 2.6	NS
	p	NS	NS		NS	NS	
Circumference	I	53.5 ± 8.9	54.8 ± 9.2	NS	51 ± 11.6	49.3 ± 9.2	NS
	II	51 ± 8.1	51.1 ± 8	NS	49.1 ± 11.8	47.3 ± 9.9	NS
	III	52.5 ± 8.7	51.9 ± 7.7	NS	48.9 ± 8.6	47.5 ± 10.1	NS
	p	NS	NS		NS	NS	
Area	I	174.3 ± 52.2	173.9 ± 47.6	NS	152.2 ± 48.6	142.6 ± 44.1	
	II	158.7 ± 46.5	156.4 ± 48.7	NS	157 ± 73	140.3 ± 44	NS
	III	167.4 ± 53.1	166.8 ± 55.7	NS	158.9 ± 53.6	152.6 ± 65.2	NS
	p	NS	NS		NS	NS	NS

For Max Y, the maximum value was observed in I sections. For the L4/5 motion segment, it was 18.8 mm (right) and 19.3 mm (left sides), while in the L5/S1 motion segment, the maximum was 17.2 mm (right side) and 17.1 mm (left side). The smallest dimension was found in section III (left side). Its value was 17.3 mm. On the other hand, for the L5/S1 motion segment, the minimum value of Max Y was 15 mm (left side).

If the MinX parameter is taken into account, its highest L4/5 value was observed in the III section. This was 5.8 mm (right side). On the other hand, in the L5/S1 motion segment, it was 6.7 mm (right side, section II). The minimum MinX value for the L4/5 motion segment was 5.2 mm (left side, section II); in the L5/S1 motion segment, it was 5.3 mm.

The maximum value for the L4/5 circumference was found in segment I and this was 54.8 mm (section I). The minimum was observed in the case of section II and this was 51 mm. In the L5/S1 motor segment, the maximum value was 51× mm (right side, section I) and the minimum value was 47.3 mm (left side, section II).

In the case of surface area, the highest value of this indicator was found in section I and this amounted to 173.9 mm^2 (right side); the minimum value was observed on the right side and this was 156.4 mm^2 (section II). For the L5/S1 motor segment, the maximum value was 158.9 mm^2, which was found in section III (right side). In turn, the minimum value was 140.3 mm^2 (left side, II section).

Table S1 presents the results for the L4/5 motor segment, taking into account the gender criterion. Referring to the data related to the perimeter and surface area, differences in the average values of the mentioned parameters can be noticed. In women, in each analyzed cross-section, both the circumference and the surface area had a higher value. The site did not matter in this case. Table S2 presents the results for the L5/S1 motor segment, taking into account the gender criterion. In the male population, the mean circumference values were higher. For cross-sectional areas, higher values were noted in the female population.

Tables S3 and S4 present the results for the motor segments L4/5 and L5/S1, taking into account the age criterion. In the case of the L4/5 motor segment, age turned out to be a factor that influenced the value of the circumference. In the younger population, the circumference values for individual sections were higher. In the context of surface areas, such a relationship was observed for sections II and III. With regard to the motor segment L5/S1, it can be stated that the values of surface areas were higher in the younger population (excluding section I). The situation was similar in the context of circumference. In the older population, the mean circumference was only higher in section I (left side). Based on these results, it can be concluded that age and gender may be factors that affect the value of dimensions related to surface area and circumference.

In the subsequent part of this study, correlations between dimensions in individual sections will be shown. Tables S5–S7 present the Spearman's correlation coefficients for the measurement results (in mm) according to the L4/5 and L5/S1 motor section for sections I–III. In all cross-sections, significant positive correlations ($p > 0.5$) were found between the right and left sides between individual measurements in segment L4/5 and L5/S1, except for MaxX in cross-section II in L5/S1 (0.2).

The surface area correlated significantly and positively with the circumference in all cross-sections in the L4/5 and L5/S1 segments. This means that the larger the surface area, the higher the perimeter. Such a relationship is a prognostic indicator helpful in the process of diagnosing a patient with spinal canal stenosis. Based on this correlation, it can be concluded that the bony shape of the canals at individual levels was similar in the study population; greater irregularity would result in a lack of correlation between the surface area and the circumference. However, no such correlation with MinX was demonstrated. MaxX and MaxY positively correlated with the area in the L4/5 segment on the right and left. In the L5/S1 segment, MaxX and MaxY positively correlated with the surface area on the right side, while, on the left side, the values of the coefficient amounted to a maximum of 0.6, and there was no significant correlation between MaxX/Area in sections I and III.

In Tables S8–S13, the influence of gender on the correlation between individual measurements is analyzed. Table S8 presents the results of the correlation between the L4/5 and L5/S1 segments (Section 1) in the female population. The obtained data indicate the occurrence of correlations between measurements. It has been shown that the surface area (on the right side) correlates, among others, with the circumference. The same relationship is observed for the circumference and area on the left side. Positive correlations between individuals in the female population were also observed in Sections 2 and 3 (Tables S10 and S12). In the male population (Tables S9, S11 and S13), there were also correlations between measurements for individual segments.

Tables S14–S19 contain data that present the strength of the correlation between individual segments, taking into account the age criterion. In individual sections, the occurrence of positive correlations between individual measurements in the age groups created for the purpose of the analysis was demonstrated. Such data made it possible to determine that age is an element that can affect the correlations between individual dimensions.

Based on the obtained average measurement results, three-dimensional models of intervertebral canals at individual levels were created in order to better visualize their complicated spatial structure and the variability in dimensions in their course. Figure 3 visualizes the average dimensions of the canals at individual levels and cross-sections, while Figures 4–6 show exemplary 3D reconstructions of intervertebral canals at each level. According to the researchers, the obtained shape of the models correlates with the previous measurement results.

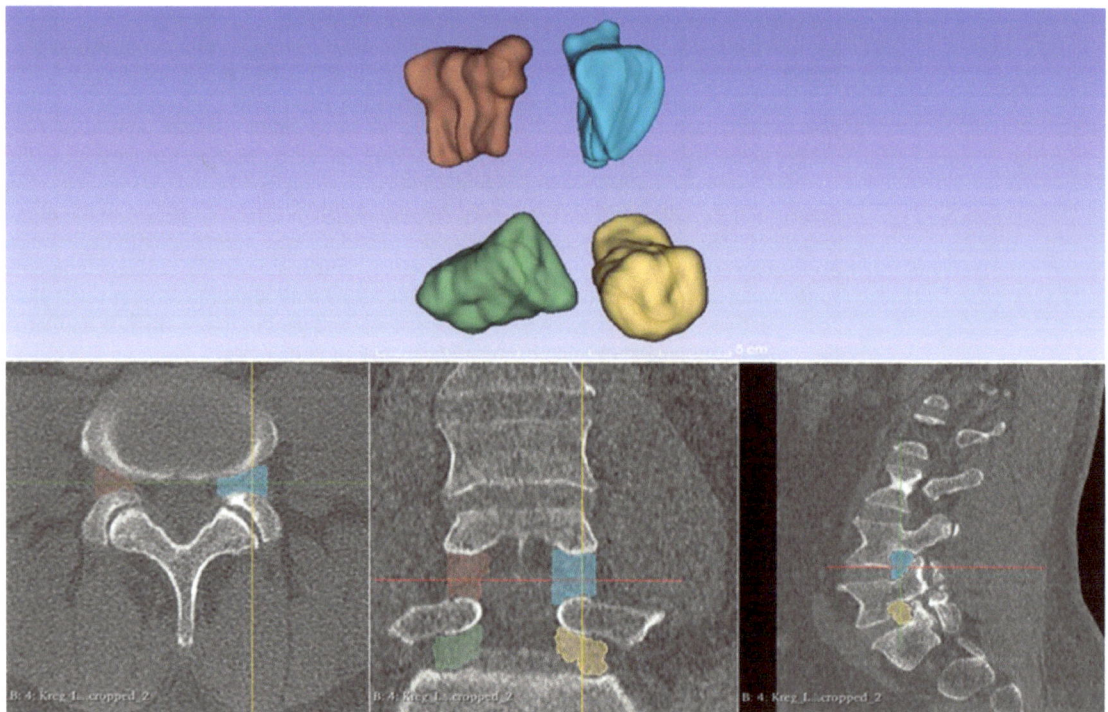

Figure 3. Screenshot from Slicer 3D showing the creation methodology for creating 3D models of the intervertebral foramina. The Supplementary Materials contain an animation presenting 3D models of intervertebral foramina [Video S1].

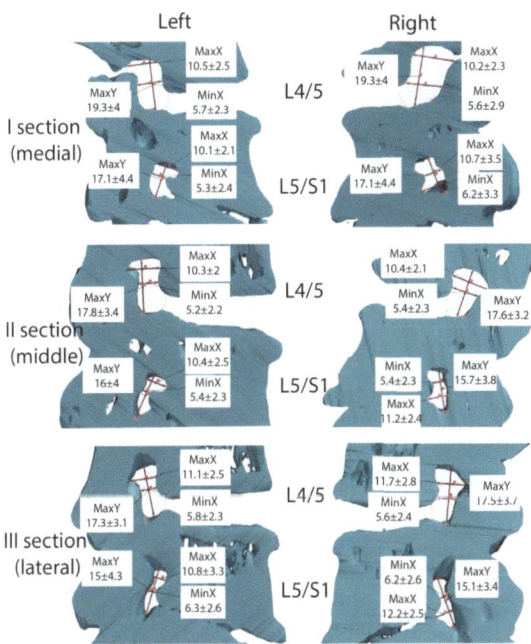

Figure 4. Average dimensions of the intervertebral foramina, L4/L5 and L5/S1, in individual sections. Left, right–side of the spine.

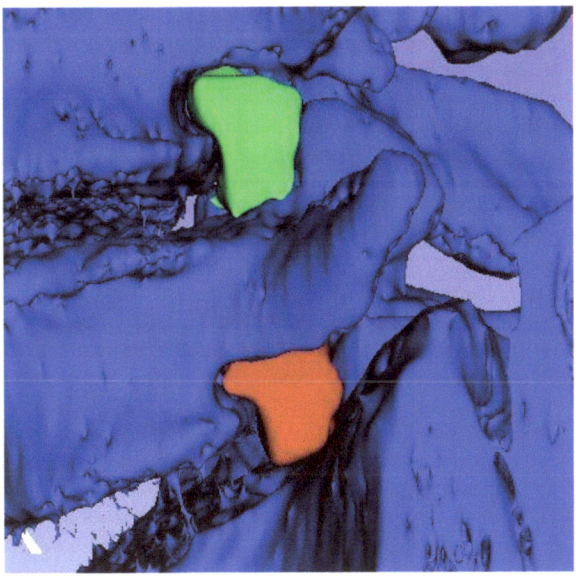

Figure 5. Sample 3D models of the intervertebral canals on the left side at L4/L5 (green) and L5/S1 (brown) before extracting them from the spine model.

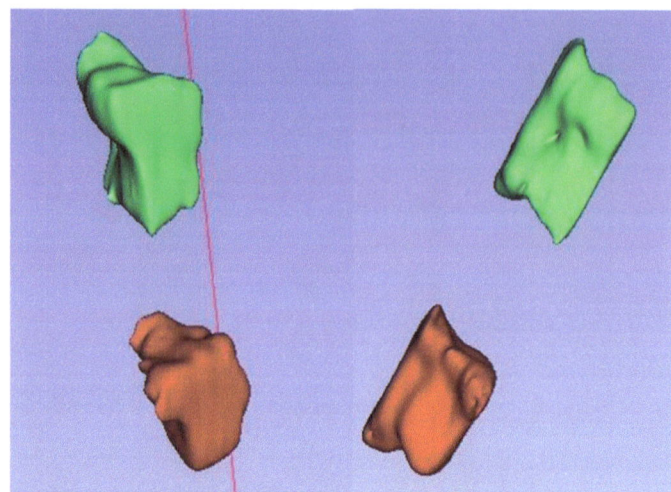

Figure 6. Sample 3D models of the intervertebral canals on the left side at L4/L5 (green) and L5/S1 (brown) lateral view (**left side**) and ventral view (**right side**).

4. Discussion

Osteoarthritis of the spine is currently a significant medical problem, especially in the context of the growing problem of an aging population. It is also important to strive to improve the quality of life of patients struggling with this disease. The main goal of the interventions undertaken is to relieve pain or significantly reduce it. However, surgical procedures do not always bring the expected results. This is due to inadequate qualifications for the procedure and the presence of individual risk factors in patients, such as comorbidities, factors related to mental state (depression), high BMI or smoking [16].

An important problem is also the correlation of anatomical abnormalities observed in radiological examinations with clinical symptoms [17].

In improving diagnostics, the possibility of using modern technologies in this process are important elements determining research activities in which attention is focused on the dimensions of the intervertebral foramens. It becomes important to establish the pathological factors that contribute to the compression of the nerve roots and thus the appearance of pain in the patient. Over the decades, the process of diagnosing back pain has developed significantly.

This was related to the greater availability of modern technologies in research practice. Morphometry has also benefited from the use of modern tools. The correlation between the results of radiological examinations and symptoms reported by patients is poorly recognized in the literature. There are no studies dealing with this topic in more detail. The ambition of the research conducted in this work was to establish such relationships. The authors were aware that identifying prognostic factors could influence the decision to perform surgery, as well as improve the clinical results of the procedures performed and thus have a positive impact on the quality of life of patients.

This article presents the results of research conducted on a group of 89 patients struggling with lower back pain. The main attention was focused on the surface area of individual cross-sections of the intervertebral foramen. Three cross-sections were developed with the help of 3D reconstruction tools and these were left- and right-sided cross-sections. The collected research material proved the correlation between the surface area and the circumference. The occurrence of such a relationship likely causes less pressure on the nerve root, which may prove useful in the process of diagnosing patients complaining of back pain. Attention was also paid to the age and gender of the patients participating in the study. In the studies in which the values of radiological parameters were analyzed, it was indicated that the individual characteristics of patients may be elements that interfere with diagnostic procedures [16]. In the course of our own research, we decided to analyze the influence of the sex and age of the respondents on the measurement values.

It has been shown in our study that there were positive correlations between individual measurements in the age groups created for the purpose of the analysis. Such data made it possible to determine that gender and age may affect the correlations between individual dimensions, which also have diagnostic value.

The prevalence of back pain is an important reason for conducting research aimed at even more accurately diagnosing the etiology of this type of disease. So far, the topic of the surface area of the intervertebral foramen, and its correlation with the other dimensions of this anatomical structure, have been poorly recognized. The research conducted shows that this is a direction that should be continued. Thanks to these, one can better understand the cause of pain, as well as the location of the pathology.

The issue of intervertebral foramen and their surface area has not been widely discussed in the literature. There is a lack of comprehensive research that addresses this issue in a holistic way. The topic of the dimensions of the intervertebral foramen appeared in the studies of Khalaf et al. [18]. The authors assessed the surface area, vertical, and horizontal dimensions of the intervertebral foramen. They tried to determine whether gender could be a factor differentiating these dimensions. The topic of intervertebral foramen was also reported by Giles [19], Fujiwara [20], and Lin [7]. The last of the studies cited showed that the anatomical parameters of the intervertebral foramen, assessed by preoperative MRI, were independently correlated with the results reported by patients with degenerative lumbar foramen stenosis. Reducing the width of the superior foramen was associated with better improvement in both functional status and quality of life after transforaminal lumbar interbody fusion (TLIF). The studies to date lack publications that would suggest significant associations between the anatomical parameters obtained from preoperative MRI and preoperative VAS results for leg pain, ODI, and EQ-5D. Sigmundsson et al. [21] showed a weak correlation between the area of the dural sac and walking distance, ODI, SF-36, EQ-5D, and the level of back and leg pain in patients with spinal canal impingement [21]. Kuittinen et al. (2014) also found no correlation between MRI results and symptoms or walking ability in patients with lumbar spinal stenosis [22].

Yan et al. reported a change in the geometry of the L4/5 foramen with age in men. They showed that the height of the hole decreased in each sagittal plane with age, while the width of the hole showed no significant difference [23].

Zhaoyang Qiu et al. analyzed the LS spine X-ray of healthy patients between 18 and 80 years of age. They found that the greatest changes in the shape of the intervertebral foramen occur in patients over 60 years of age compared to the population in the 40–60 bracket. The main changes were the parameters determined in relation to the upper articular process [24].

According to some authors, the measurements of the intervertebral canals made on cadavers are very similar to those obtained using imaging methods such as CT and MRI. However, cadaver studies are usually limited by small research samples and results are inconsistent across different authors. In contrast, imaging studies provide the ability to assess larger groups of patients relatively more easily and reproducibly, and thus allow more reliable results for further comparisons and analyses [24].

The measurement of intervertebral foramen (IVF) in the lumbar spine can be useful in clinical practice for several reasons, but its clinical significance may vary depending on the specific context and the patient's clinical presentation. Surgeons may measure the IVF to plan surgical procedures. Accurate measurements of the IVF can help determine the surgical approach and guide the removal of any obstructions causing nerve compression. Measuring the intervertebral foramen can also be valuable for tracking the progress of a patient's condition over time. It provides objective data to assess the effectiveness of treatments and whether the foramen has changed in size. In the field of spinal research, measurements of the intervertebral foramen can be valuable for studying spinal anatomy, pathophysiology, and treatment outcomes. Researchers can use these measurements to assess the impact of various interventions and contribute to the development of evidence-based clinical guidelines.

Research on the impact of surface area on the occurrence of pain should be continued. They should focus on issues related to the surface area of the intervertebral foramen and their impact on the nerve roots. Findings from such studies may help surgeons identify patients who will have a better prognosis after surgery.

The research carried out as part of this work had some limitations. The first was related to the relatively small research population. This fact was determined by the use of restrictive inclusion criteria in the study. The classification carried out at the inclusion stage in the studies made it possible to select patients who would fit their purpose. Another limitation of the study is the exclusive assessment of the bony morphology of the hole, which does not include the intervertebral disc and ligaments. Soft tissues should be included in future studies in order to gain more knowledge about the intervertebral foramen. Moreover, the primary CT data were only collected in the supine position, with no dynamic or axial positions. The morphology of the intervertebral foramen would change with position. A certain limitation is that the literature on the subject lacks data to which it would be possible to refer to for obtained results. Despite this, our research is of great value as it indicates a potential cause of pain and it should therefore be developed more widely.

5. Conclusions

This research aimed to investigate the relationships between the morphometric characteristics of intervertebral foramina at specific spinal levels and how factors such as age and sex affect these dimensions. The results demonstrated a significant correlation between the size and shape of the intervertebral foramina and these demographic variables, suggesting that understanding these variations is crucial for diagnosing and treating spinal conditions. Utilizing measurements and three-dimensional imaging techniques, the study mapped out the anatomical structure of the intervertebral foramina at the L4/L5 and L5/S1 motor segments, focusing on their bony configurations. Further exploration into how dynamic spinal movements and physiological loads influence these structures could provide deeper insights, potentially leading to more effective interventions for conditions affecting the intervertebral foramen.

Supplementary Materials: The following supporting information can be downloaded at https://www.mdpi.com/article/10.3390/app14062263/s1, Table S1: Measurement results (mean ± SD in mm, area section in mm^2) for motion segment L4/5 according to sex (N = 89). MaxX-Maximal Horizontal Dimension, MaxY-Maximal Vertical Dimension, MinX-Minimal Horizontal Dimension; Table S2: Measurement results (mean ± SD in mm. area section in mm2) for motion segment L5/S1 according to sex (N = 89). MaxX-Maximal Horizontal Dimension. MaxY-Maximal Vertical Dimension. MinX-Minimal Horizontal Dimension, Table S3: Measurement results (mean ± SD in mm) for motion segment L4/5 according to age groups (N = 89). MaxX-Maximal Horizontal Dimension. MaxY-Maximal Vertical Dimension. MinX-Minimal Horizontal Dimension, Table S4: Measurement results (mean ± SD in mm) for motion segment L5/S1 according to age (N = 89). MaxX-Maximal Horizontal Dimension. MaxY-Maximal Vertical Dimension. MinX-Minimal Horizontal Dimension, Table S5: Spearman correlation coefficients for measurement results (in mm) by motion segment L4/5 and L5/S1 for section I, Table S6: Spearman correlation coefficients for measurement results (in mm) by motion segment L4/5 and L5/S1 for section II, Table S7: Spearman correlation coefficients for measurement results (in mm) by motion segment L4/5 and L5/S1 for section III, Table S8: Spearman correlation coefficients for measurement results (in mm) by motion segment L4/5 and L5/S1 for women and section I, Table S9: Spearman correlation coefficients for measurement results (in mm) by motion segment L4/5 and L5/S1 for male and section I, Table S10: Spearman correlation coefficients for measurement results (in mm) by motion segment L4/5 and L5/S1 for women and section II, Table S11: Spearman correlation coefficients for measurement results (in mm) by motion segment L4/5 and L5/S1 for male and section II, Table S12: Spearman correlation coefficients for measurement results (in mm) by motion segment L4/5 and L5/S1 for women and section III, Table S13:

Spearman correlation coefficients for measurement results (in mm) by motion segment L4/5 and L5/S1 for male and section II, Table S14: Spearman correlation coefficients for measurement results (in mm) by motion segment L4/5 and L5/S1 age group < 50 and section I, Table S15: Spearman correlation coefficients for measurement results (in mm) by motion segment L4/5 and L5/S1 age group > 50 and section I, Table S16: Spearman correlation coefficients for measurement results (in mm) by motion segment L4/5 and L5/S1 for age group < 50 and section II, Table S17: Spearman correlation coefficients for measurement results (in mm) by motion segment L4/5 and L5/S1 age group > 50 and section II, Table S18: Spearman correlation coefficients for measurement results (in mm) by motion segment L4/5 and L5/S1 age group < 50 and section III, Table S19: Spearman correlation coefficients for measurement results (in mm) by motion segment L4/5 and L5/S1 age group > 50 and section II; Video S1: The animation presenting 3D models of intervertebral foramina L4/5 and L5/S1 [Video S1].

Author Contributions: Conceptualization, Ł.K.; methodology, Ł.K. and M.D; validation, Ł.K., A.D. and P.N.; formal analysis, P.N. and M.D.; investigation, P.N. and A.D.; data curation, Ł.K.; writing—original draft preparation, P.N.; writing—review and editing, Ł.K. and M.D.; supervision, Ł.K. All authors have read and agreed to the published version of the manuscript.

Funding: This research received no external funding.

Institutional Review Board Statement: Not applicable.

Informed Consent Statement: Not applicable.

Data Availability Statement: The data presented in this study are available on request from the corresponding author.

Conflicts of Interest: The authors declare no conflicts of interest.

References

1. Bai, Q.; Wang, Y.; Zhai, J.; Wu, J.; Zhang, Y.; Zhao, Y. Current understanding of tandem spinal stenosis: Epidemiology, diagnosis, and surgical strategy. *EFORT Open Rev.* **2022**, *7*, 587–598. [CrossRef]
2. Melancia, J.L.; Francisco, A.F.; Antunes, J.L. Spinal stenosis. *Handb. Clin. Neurol.* **2014**, *119*, 541–549. [CrossRef]
3. Raja, A.; Hoang, S.; Patel, P.; Mesfin, F.B. Spinal Stenosis. StatPearls; July 2022. Available online: https://www.ncbi.nlm.nih.gov/books/NBK441989/ (accessed on 18 May 2023).
4. Orita, S.; Inage, K.; Eguchi, Y.; Kubota, G.; Aoki, Y.; Nakamura, J.; Matsuura, Y.; Furuya, T.; Koda, M.; Ohtori, S. Lumbar foraminal stenosis, the hidden stenosis including at L5/S1. *Eur. J. Orthop. Surg. Traumatol.* **2016**, *26*, 685–693. [CrossRef] [PubMed]
5. Igari, T.; Otani, K.; Sekiguchi, M.; Konno, S.-I. Epidemiological Study of Lumbar Spinal Stenosis Symptoms: 10-Year Follow-Up in the Community. *J. Clin. Med.* **2022**, *11*, 5911. [CrossRef] [PubMed]
6. Fujita, M.; Inui, T.; Oshima, Y.; Iwai, H.; Inanami, H.; Koga, H. Comparison of Outcomes of Lumbar Interbody Fusion and Full-endoscopic Laminectomy for L5 Radiculopathy Caused by Lumbar Foraminal Stenosis. *Neurol. Med.-Chir.* **2022**, *62*, 270–277. [CrossRef] [PubMed]
7. Lin, Y.-T.; Wang, J.-S.; Hsu, W.-E.; Lin, Y.-H.; Wu, Y.-C.; Chen, K.-H.; Pan, C.-C.; Lee, C.-H. Correlation of Foraminal Parameters with Patient-Reported Outcomes in Patient with Degenerative Lumbar Foraminal Stenosis. *J. Clin. Med.* **2023**, *12*, 479. [CrossRef] [PubMed]
8. Choi, Y.K. Lumbar foraminal neuropathy: An update on non-surgical management. *Korean J. Pain* **2019**, *32*, 147–159. [CrossRef] [PubMed]
9. Tominaga, R.; Kurita, N.; Sekiguchi, M.; Yonemoto, K.; Kakuma, T.; Konno, S.-I. Diagnostic accuracy of the lumbar spinal stenosis-diagnosis support tool and the lumbar spinal stenosis-self-administered, self-reported history questionnaire. *PLoS ONE* **2022**, *17*, e0267892. [CrossRef]
10. Sievert, H.; Piedade, G.S.; McPhillips, P.; Vesper, J.; Slotty, P.J. The role of periradicular infiltration in dorsal root ganglion stimulation for chronic neuropathic pain. *Acta Neurochir.* **2021**, *163*, 2135–2140. [CrossRef] [PubMed]
11. Lee, S.; Lee, J.W.; Yeom, J.S.; Kim, K.-J.; Kim, H.-J.; Chung, S.K.; Kang, H.S. A practical MRI grading system for lumbar foraminal stenosis. *Am. J. Roentgenol.* **2010**, *194*, 1095–1098. [CrossRef]
12. Sartoretti, E.; Wyss, M.; Alfieri, A.; Binkert, C.A.; Erne, C.; Sartoretti-Schefer, S.; Sartoretti, T. Introduction and reproducibility of an updated practical grading system for lumbar foraminal stenosis based on high-resolution MR imaging. *Sci. Rep.* **2021**, *11*, 12000. [CrossRef] [PubMed]
13. Haleem, S.; Malik, M.; Guduri, V.; Azzopardi, C.; James, S.; Botchu, R. The Haleem–Botchu classification: A novel CT-based classification for lumbar foraminal stenosis. *Eur. Spine J.* **2020**, *30*, 865–869. [CrossRef]
14. Cinotti, G.; De Santis, P.; Nofroni, I.; Postacchini, F. Stenosis of lumbar intervertebral foramen: Anatomic study on predisposing factors. *Spine* **2002**, *27*, 223–229. [CrossRef]

15. Nowak, P.; Kubaszewski, Ł. Assessment of the Asymmetry of the Intervertebral Foramina within the Lower Motion Segments of the Lumbar Spine on the Computer Tomography Sections. *Symmetry* **2022**, *14*, 1967. [CrossRef]
16. Aaen, J.; Austevoll, I.M.; Hellum, C.; Storheim, K.; Myklebust, T.; Banitalebi, H.; Anvar, M.; Brox, J.I.; Weber, C.; Solberg, T.; et al. Clinical and MRI findings in lumbar spinal stenosis: Baseline data from the NORDSTEN study. *Eur. Spine J.* **2021**, *31*, 1391–1398. [CrossRef]
17. Splettstößer, A.; Khan, M.F.; Zimmermann, B.; Vogl, T.J.; Ackermann, H.; Middendorp, M.; Maataoui, A. Correlation of lumbar lateral recess stenosis in magnetic resonance imaging and clinical symptoms. *World J. Radiol.* **2017**, *9*, 223–229. [CrossRef] [PubMed]
18. Khalaf, A.M.; Yedavalli, V.; Massoud, T.F. Magnetic resonance imaging anatomy and morphometry of lumbar intervertebral foramina to guide safe transforaminal subarachnoid punctures. *Clin. Anat.* **2019**, *33*, 405–413. [CrossRef]
19. Giles, L.G. A histological investigation of human lower lumbar intervertebral canal (foramen) dimensions. *J. Manip. Physiol. Ther.* **1994**, *17*, 4–14.
20. Fujiwara, A.; An, H.S.; Lim, T.-H.; Haughton, V.M. Morphologic changes in the lumbar intervertebral foramen due to flexion-extension, lateral bending, and axial rotation: An in vitro anatomic and biomechanical study. *Spine* **2001**, *26*, 876–882. [CrossRef]
21. Sigmundsson, F.G.; Kang, X.P.; Jönsson, B.; Strömqvist, B. Correlation between disability and MRI findings in lumbar spinal stenosis: A prospective study of 109 patients operated on by decompression. *Acta Orthop.* **2011**, *82*, 204–210. [CrossRef]
22. Kuittinen, P.; Sipola, P.; Saari, T.; Aalto, T.J.; Sinikallio, S.; Savolainen, S.; Kröger, H.; Turunen, V.; Leinonen, V.; Airaksinen, O. Visually assessed severity of lumbar spinal canal stenosis is paradoxically associated with leg pain and objective walking ability. *BMC Musculoskelet. Disord.* **2014**, *15*, 348. [CrossRef] [PubMed]
23. Yan, S.; Wang, K.; Zhang, Y.; Guo, S.; Zhang, Y.; Tan, J. Changes in L4/5 Intervertebral Foramen Bony Morphology with Age. *Sci. Rep.* **2018**, *8*, 7722. [CrossRef] [PubMed]
24. Qiu, Z. X-ray measurement and analysis on parameters of intervertebral foramen in the lower lumbar spine associated with the superior articular process. *Clin. Surg. Res. Commun.* **2020**, *4*, 21–26. [CrossRef]

Disclaimer/Publisher's Note: The statements, opinions and data contained in all publications are solely those of the individual author(s) and contributor(s) and not of MDPI and/or the editor(s). MDPI and/or the editor(s) disclaim responsibility for any injury to people or property resulting from any ideas, methods, instructions or products referred to in the content.

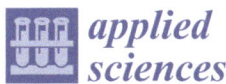

Article

Biomechanical Evaluation of Plantar Pressure Distribution towards a Customized 3D Orthotic Device: A Methodological Case Study through a Finite Element Analysis Approach

Jesus Alejandro Serrato-Pedrosa *, Guillermo Urriolagoitia-Sosa *, Beatriz Romero-Ángeles *, Guillermo Manuel Urriolagoitia-Calderón, Salvador Cruz-López , Alejandro Urriolagoitia-Luna, David Esaú Carbajal-López, Jonathan Rodolfo Guereca-Ibarra and Guadalupe Murillo-Aleman

Instituto Politécnico Nacional, Escuela Superior de Ingeniería Mecánica y Eléctrica, Sección de Estudios de Posgrado e Investigación, Unidad Profesional Adolfo López Mateos, Edificio 5, 2do, Piso, Biomechanics Group, Col. Lindavista, Del. Gustavo A. Madero, Ciudad de México 07320, Mexico; urrio332@hotmail.com (G.M.U.-C.); salvadorcruzlopezim@gmail.com (S.C.-L.); alex_ul56@hotmail.com (A.U.-L.); esaucarba99@hotmail.com (D.E.C.-L.); guerecatic@gmail.com (J.R.G.-I.); guadalupe.murillo.a95@gmail.com (G.M.-A.)
* Correspondence: alejandroserrato@live.com.mx (J.A.S.-P.); guiurri@hotmail.com (G.U.-S.); romerobeatriz97@hotmail.com (B.R.-Á.)

Abstract: Plantar pressure distribution is a thoroughly recognized parameter for evaluating foot structure and biomechanical behavior, as it is utilized to determine musculoskeletal conditions and diagnose foot abnormalities. Experimental testing is currently being utilized to investigate static foot conditions using invasive and noninvasive techniques. These methods are usually expensive and laborious, and they lack valuable data since they only evaluate compressive forces, missing the complex stress combinations the foot undergoes while standing. The present investigation applied medical and engineering methods to predict pressure points in a healthy foot soft tissue during normal standing conditions. Thus, a well-defined three-dimensional foot biomodel was constructed to be numerically analyzed through medical imaging. Two study cases were developed through a structural finite element analysis. The first study was developed to evaluate barefoot behavior deformation and stresses occurring in the plantar region. The results from this analysis were validated through baropodometric testing. Subsequently, a customized 3D model total-contact foot orthosis was designed to redistribute peak pressures appropriately, relieving the plantar region from excessive stress. The results in the first study case successfully demonstrated the prediction of the foot sole regions more prone to suffer a pressure concentration since the values are in good agreement with experimental testing. Employing a customized insole proved to be highly advantageous in fulfilling its primary function, reducing peak pressure points substantially. The main aim of this paper was to provide more precise insights into the biomechanical behavior of foot pressure points through engineering methods oriented towards innovative assessment for absolute customization for orthotic devices.

Keywords: plantar pressure; foot soft tissue; finite element analysis; medical imaging; 3D foot orthosis; orthotic devices; baropodometric testing

Citation: Serrato-Pedrosa, J.A.; Urriolagoitia-Sosa, G.; Romero-Ángeles, B.; Urriolagoitia-Calderón, G.M.; Cruz-López, S.; Urriolagoitia-Luna, A.; Carbajal-López, D.E.; Guereca-Ibarra, J.R.; Murillo-Aleman, G. Biomechanical Evaluation of Plantar Pressure Distribution towards a Customized 3D Orthotic Device: A Methodological Case Study through a Finite Element Analysis Approach. *Appl. Sci.* **2024**, *14*, 1650. https://doi.org/10.3390/app14041650

Academic Editors: Claudio Belvedere and Sorin Siegler

Received: 10 January 2024
Revised: 5 February 2024
Accepted: 6 February 2024
Published: 18 February 2024

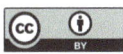

Copyright: © 2024 by the authors. Licensee MDPI, Basel, Switzerland. This article is an open access article distributed under the terms and conditions of the Creative Commons Attribution (CC BY) license (https://creativecommons.org/licenses/by/4.0/).

1. Introduction

Over recent years, there has been an increasing trend in the medical scientific community of studying and analyzing the print of plantar pressure distribution for an optimal understanding of the biomechanics of the foot relying on its load distribution. It is a reliable parameter for analyzing foot functions and provides further insights into the studies of the etiology of several lower limb musculoskeletal problems. Within the medical field, the measurement of these loads through footprints has been used from the oldest and most traditional methods, up until the development of computerized equipment specialized in this task, for accurately acquiring the pressure points on the foot externally [1–4]. The oldest tracing and sketching of footprint techniques, whether using any medical device or only paper and ink, has been established as a standard for the structural evaluation of the foot and body balance [5]. Innovative force platforms and pressure-sensing insoles are cutting-edge technologies for standing and dynamic pressure calculations [6–8].

Highly invasive and painful procedures are required to comprehend how these forces affect internal foot tissues. Thus, experimental tests (similar to compression tests) are usually performed on cadaveric feet, simulating their behavior under various amounts of load [9,10]. Obtaining the pressure points in the foot is considered one of the guidelines for understanding its normal and pathological function and determining stress behaviors, total displacements, total strains, and contact areas. These tests are remarkable approaches to understanding the complex foot mechanism of distributing loads within its unique capability of adapting to different ground geometries. Furthermore, pressure distribution varies from subject to subject since it is influenced by particular factors such as gender, age, race, and weight, to mention a few [11,12].

As it can be inferred from the above, a common problem for the multidisciplinary science of biomechanics is the professional equipment needed to perform studies and the fact that typically, to obtain better results, it is required to perform in vivo tests on the subject under investigation [13,14]. Employing a highly detailed segmented biomodel through medical imaging can provide an essential tool to assist the healthcare sector and biomechanics professionals and can partially replace and complement experimental testing.

Due to the increasing computational development, it has been possible to perform numerical analysis and obtain accurate and reliable estimates for various parts of the body, specifically through the finite element method (FEM) [15–17]. A 3D biological model is constructed by implementing the medical branch of imaging, which is considered a standard for obtaining complex geometries of human biological systems [18,19]. Numerical analyses are close estimations that solve complex problems utilizing partial differential equations. Such methods are forms of numerical–computational analysis, where these mathematical models are represented by a discretization of connected nodes, where a mesh-like layer covers the geometry analyzed, and the nodes are points joining the mesh. The discretization's complexity and finesse help obtain more accurate approximations of the problem's solution. Nonetheless, this requires high computational resources [20,21].

This research aims to deepen the knowledge and current perceptions of this lower extremity's biomechanical behavior to enhance the design of personalized plantar orthoses. Thus, the following research focuses on analyzing foot soft tissue behavior during normal standing conditions, obtaining the pressure points on the plantar surface, and designing a customized 3D model foot orthosis to re-evaluate pressure distributions. Likewise, this research also aims to provide relevant data on the intrinsic muscles of the foot and skin behavior under pressure and the direct effect of wearing a personalized 3D model total-contact foot orthosis.

2. Materials and Methods

2.1. Footprint Sketching

Before numerically analyzing foot soft tissue behavior to develop a 3D model insole, it is relevant to rely on sketching techniques to determine whether the foot of the participant can be considered a foot in normal conditions. Thus, it is possible to evaluate the state of the foot. Various static methods for obtaining such a footprint and analyzing foot structure exist. Indeed, these methods are advantageous due to their low cost, lack of specialized or sophisticated equipment, and ease of application. The method selected for its popularity and high reliability in foot classification criteria among biomechanical and medical researchers was the Hernández Corvo method [22]. Usually, this methodology uses sketching techniques using the photopodogram or the pedigraph. The photopodogram technique uses ink or paint to obtain the footprint when the subject steps on thermographic paper over a flat surface. Whereas the pedigraph method is very similar to the previous one, it differs in the subject stepping on a soft, foamy rubber surface filled with ink with a sheet placed underneath it. Subsequently, to analyze the results, perpendicular lines are drawn in different coincident sections along the length and width of the rearfoot and forefoot. The distance from the metatarsal area is X, and the site from the outer arch to the midfoot bearing surface is Y. When the measured lengths are obtained, an equation is applied that yields a result in the form of a percentage, which is further weighted in a broad and complete classification of foot types (Table 1) [23].

$$\text{H.C. (\%)} = \frac{(X - Y)}{X} * 100 \tag{1}$$

Table 1. Foot classification according to the Hernández Corvo method [22,23].

H. C. (%)	Foot Type
0–34	Flatfoot
35–39	Flatfoot–Normal
40–54	Normal
55–59	Normal–Cavus
60–74	Cavus Foot
75–84	Severe Cavus Foot
85–100	Extreme Cavus Foot

2.2. Biomodeling Methodology

The process by which 2D images are processed and converted to 3D matrices that generate models is known as segmentation, transforming the pixels of 2D visualizations into volumetric pixels, isovoxels, or simply voxels, in 3D [24].

Among the various programs, Simpleware ScanIP® 3.2 Build 1 and Materialise MIMICS® Research 21.0 stand out from the rest because of their advanced tools for generating 3D models. Specifically, to obtain the model of the foot, a computed tomography (CT) scan was used on a 30-year-old Mexican young adult in apparently healthy condition with a height of 1.80 m and a weight of 80 kg who usually exercises, having a regular complexion with a 24.7 kg/m^2 normal-range body mass index (BMI) and a foot in normal conditions (foot length of 256 mm and forefoot width of 137 mm). The described medical imaging study was conducted utilizing a high-resolution SIEMENS SOMATOM Emotion 16-slice configuration CT scan, which provided 16 images per second with a 0.6 mm distance between slices. Once the imaging study was performed, the visualization of the DICOM images and segmentation for constructing the 3D model were performed in Simpleware ScanIP® 3.2 Build 1. The reading of the tomographic study images in the program yielded a total number of slices in the transverse (axial) plane of 357, 260 in the sagittal plane, and 454 in the coronal (frontal) plane. A total of 1071 slices in all anatomical planes were obtained. Thus, it was possible to construct a well defined model of the foot of the participant.

The methodology employed to reconstruct the foot biomodel has been recognized as setting the guidelines in 3D biological tissue reconstruction [17,25]. The methods mentioned can be briefly described in the following points:

- Development of the medical imaging study (foot and ankle).
- Acquisition of images in DICOM format.
- Image importation into the Simpleware ScanIP® 3.2 Build 1 software.
- Determination of regions and tissues of interest (foot muscle and skin).
- Segmentation of soft tissue areas of interest through different masks.
- Implementation of smoothing tools to refine the 3D biomodel.
- Exportation of the biomodel to Materialise 3-Matic® Research 13.0 to fix any segmentation process error.
- In Materialise 3-Matic® Research 13.0, solidification of the model and application of a re-mesh to acquire uniform-size elements.

- Biological model exportation to a finite element method software to implement a numerical analysis.

With the particular research purpose of analyzing the pressure points on the sole, two soft tissue structures in the foot, skin, and muscle were modeled. There are 22 intrinsic muscles distributed in 4 different layers or volumes in a concentration of various tissues, mainly fatty tissue. Intrinsic muscles provide support and stability in the foot, in contrast to the extrinsic muscles responsible for movement and forces in the foot [26]. Therefore, it was decided to represent them as a solid encapsulated body of the total muscles. On the other hand, skin segmentation was defined as shown in the images of the imaging study.

As shown in Figure 1, the model is wholly segmented, avoiding empty pixels that could cause a subsequent failure due to a missing element. Likewise, the model is smoothed or rounded along its contour to prevent any peak or excess pixel from causing problems.

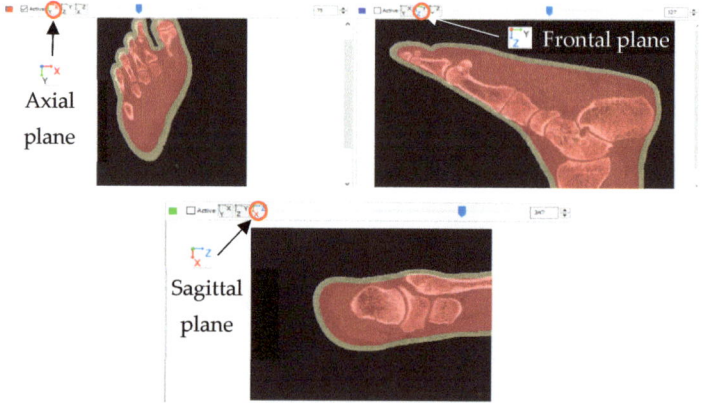

Figure 1. Plane views during the segmentation process. Axial plane section location corresponds to 21% of total slices. Frontal plane section location corresponds to 48.8% of total slices. Sagittal plane section location corresponds to 76.43% of total slices.

Once the model was wholly segmented and well defined, a rendering of the model was generated to smooth it and obtain more refined elements (Figure 2a). The product developed in the Simpleware ScanIP® 3.2 Build 1 software is considered a point cloud since it is hollow as a structure and not solid. Solidifying the obtained structure is mandatory to conduct a numerical analysis of the developed model. Therefore, the model generated from Simpleware ScanIP® 3.2 Build 1 was exported in an STL file extension to a computer-aided design (CAD) software capable of working with surfaces. A solidified realistic model can be achieved by refining the segmented model and closing gaps from the previous process. Notably, the design optimization software Materialise 3-Matic® Research 13.0 was used for this study to refine the surfaces to complete the model. Edges in the model were refined by using a smoothing tool. The assembly of the two solid elements (skin and muscles) and a re-meshing were added to the model to optimize its handling when numerically analyzing it (Figure 2b). Re-meshing provided uniform elements all over the complex foot geometry, allowing nodes to create a better connection among elements. This process increased the total number of nodes from 58,605 in elements with very different sizes to homogeneous elements with a total of 196,576 nodes.

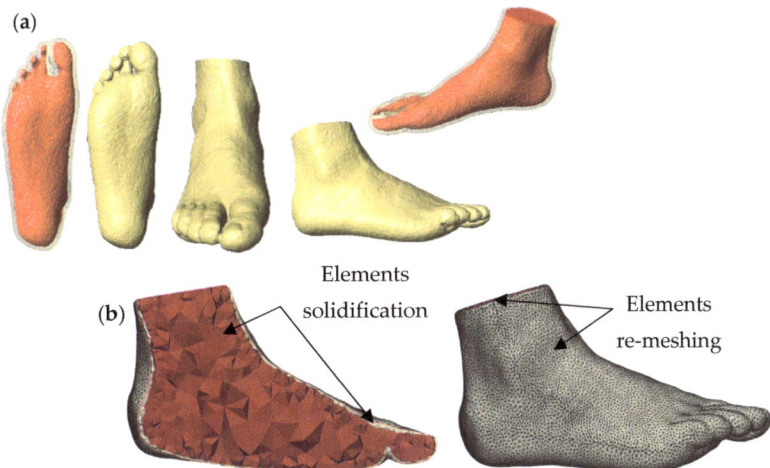

Figure 2. Generated biological models. (**a**) Implemented model from Simpleware ScanIP® 3.2 Build 1. (**b**) Solidification and re-meshing of the model from Materialise 3-Matic® Research 13.0.

2.3. Numerical Analysis of the Foot Biomodel

2.3.1. First Case Study

This first numerical analysis focused on studying the pressure points in the foot sole during standing, where the foot is considered in a neutral or medium support position since it is the most fundamental anatomical position of the foot to evaluate. Thus, in this position, the foot is structurally analyzed with an external agent in compression towards the plantar surface. The upper regions of the soft tissues were represented as fixed in all degrees of freedom, embedded, to simulate the effects of the supinator tissue constraints of the ankle. Likewise, all degrees of freedom were constrained at the top of the forefoot, instep, toes, and around the foot due to the softness of the tissues. In addition, a concrete plate with a vertical displacement was used as an external agent to simulate the impact produced on the sole by ground reaction forces. A 0.6 coefficient of friction between the foot and the ground was also set [27]. Figure 3 shows the representation of a free-body diagram for the loading and boundary conditions.

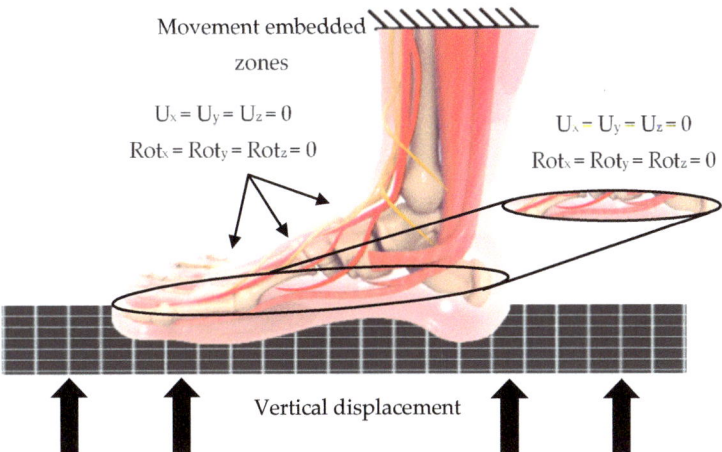

Figure 3. General biomodel free-body diagram. U refers to the displacement in the specified axis; Rot refers to rotation in the mentioned plane.

Soft tissues have extremely complex characteristics, being multilayer structures reinforced with collagen and with a nonlinear and anisotropic behavior, in addition to being considered hyperelastic and viscoelastic materials. For this study, the characteristics of the skin and muscle were simplified and considered with linear-elastic, continuous, homogeneous, and isotropic behavior, taking the values provided in the literature on foot biomechanical models by Luboz and Wu [28,29]. The assignment of two different mechanical properties for the muscle relied on developing an analysis with a partially conservative approach. In addition, the mechanical properties of the plate representing the ground were selected from the literature [30]. The mechanical property values can be seen in Table 2. Once the mechanical properties were assigned, the discretization process was developed using high-order 3D solid elements and generating 20 nodes per element. The analysis had three parts: skin, muscle encapsulation, and plate. A total of 371,120 elements and 196 576 nodes were obtained by fine and semi-controlled discretization (Figure 4). The discretization of the ground support was much less refined than that of the biomodel to save computational resources.

Table 2. Mechanical properties of the elements [28–30].

Material	Young's Modulus (MPa)	Poisson's Ratio
Foot skin	0.2	0.485
Foot muscles (Luboz)	0.06	0.495
Foot muscles (Wu)	1.08	0.49
Ground support	210,000	0.3

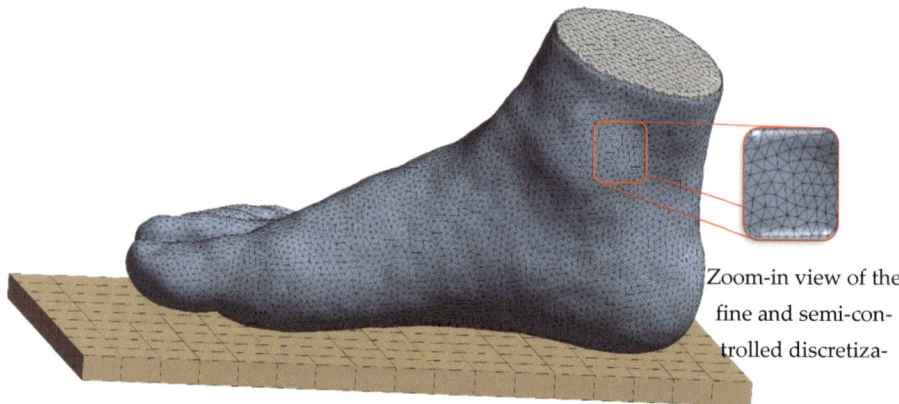

Zoom-in view of the fine and semi-controlled discretiza-

Figure 4. ANSYS Workbench® 2021 R2 model discretization.

Based on the established loading and boundary conditions, the upper area of the model, the forefoot, and the medial and lateral zones of the foot are also embedded. The constraint regions around the foot consist of a tape with a width of 2 mm relative to the dimensions of the modeled foot, avoiding an unreal lateral displacement when the load is applied. Likewise, the constraint in the instep and toe area has the same intention of controlling excessive vertical displacement. The external agent is assumed to be the plate, performing a vertical indentation to produce a displacement of 5 mm towards the plantar surface of the model to generate vertical loads. Since the weight of the person´s foot analyzed is 80 kg, an exerting force of 400 N is produced in each foot (Figure 5). According to experimental bases, there is a strong relationship when a force of 400 N produces a displacement magnitude of approximately 5 mm. Similarly, the foot has a constant displacement of between 4.8 and 5.6 mm while maintaining the anatomical position of balanced standing. In addition, evidence considers the application of an external agent within a displacement acting as a pressure rather than a load since it generates estimations closer to the natural behavior of the biomechanical characteristics of the plantar surface [29–33].

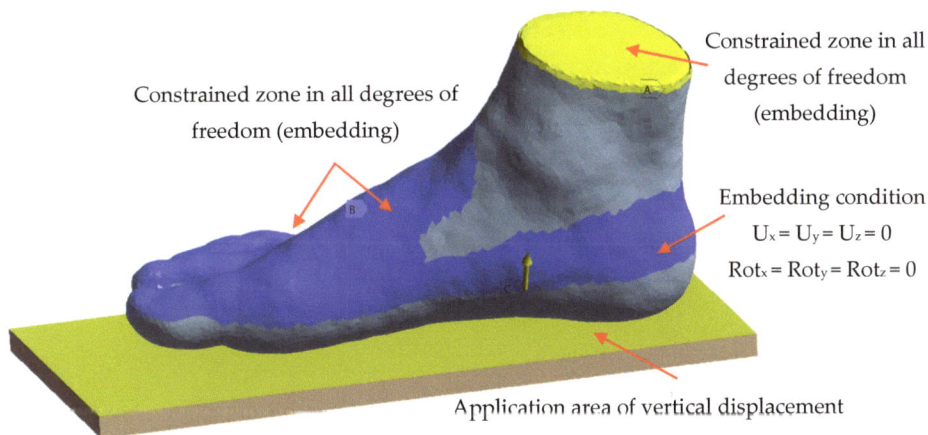

Figure 5. ANSYS Workbench® 2021 R2 loading and boundary condition assignment. U refers to the displacement in the specified axis; Rot refers to rotation in the mentioned plane.

2.3.2. Second Case Study

The second case study aimed to numerically evaluate the foot sole within the same anatomical position and mechanical principles, normal standing conditions. Nonetheless, a 3D personalized full-length total contact thermoplastic polyurethane (TPU) insole model was implemented between the foot sole contact points with the ground support to reduce pressure peaks. When an orthotic device is used, the insole cushioning effects absorb most ground reaction forces, and its performance is visualized in the biomechanical behavior results of the plantar region.

The employment of TPU as the insole material was due to several recent studies demonstrating its highly impressive characteristics; it has the qualities for use as an additively manufacturable material capable of being physically manufactured via fused filament fabrication (FFF), not requiring a high cost to produce and being suitable for 3D printing. Moreover, it has ideal mechanical properties for stress redistribution, compression strength support, and pain relief; in addition, it is biocompatible and sustainably advantageous for 3D printing manufacturing [34–41].

Many methodologies were reviewed to design an optimal biomodel closest to the specific right foot morphology of the participant. The refined 3D biological model developed for the numerical analysis was employed to obtain a positive foot impression from a box made in SpaceClaim® 2021 R2 CAD software, simulating a cast physically taken from an orthopedist (Figure 6a) [42,43]. The foot silhouette was sketched from the impression taken to generate the insole contour (Figure 6b). The 3D biomodel was placed right above the insole, using Boolean operations and working with surfaces to create a customized insole based on parametric designs set by specialized insole design software [44–47]. Working with surface modeling for the insole design allowed certain regions to be smoothed and the orthosis to be adjusted to foot morphology (Figure 6c). Factors such as total length, heel and toe thickness, width, and draft angle were considered. The insole has a 3 mm thickness, which is not a crucial factor for this case study evaluating the force distributions during regular standing since loads below 800 N are unimportant for 3D-printed devices made from TPU [48].

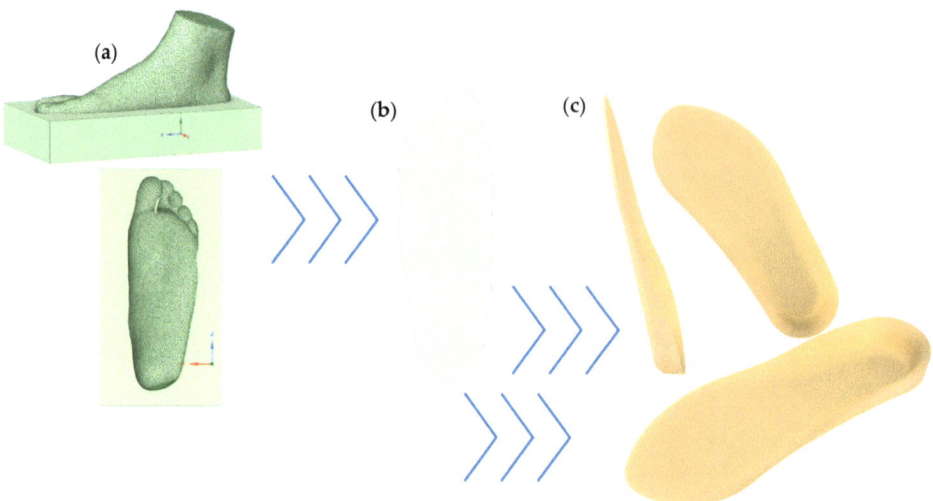

Figure 6. Process of design and development of the customized 3D model total-contact foot orthosis. (**a**) Foot impression from cast-taking simulation. (**b**) Foot contour sketching. (**c**) Final insole based on personal morphological characteristics.

To successfully import and numerically analyze the foot sole behavior within a customized full-contact insole under the same loading and boundary conditions, a new coefficient of friction of 0.5 was employed for foot–insole contact [34], and the same coefficient was used for plate–foot contact [27]. High-order 3D elements were established in the foot insole. From a high-order and semi-controlled discretization, 62,065 nodes and 34,816 elements were obtained (Figure 7). Furthermore, TPU mechanical properties were assigned to the designed orthotic device. These values were taken from previous research and literature (Table 3) [49,50].

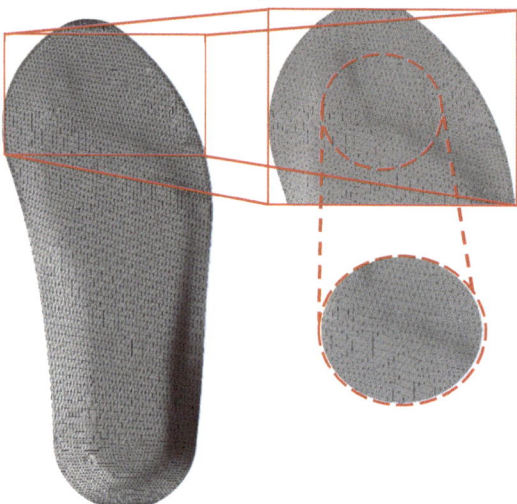

Figure 7. Foot orthosis discretization zoom-in views.

Table 3. Mechanical properties of TPU foot orthosis [49,50].

Material	Young's Modulus (MPa)	Poisson's Ratio
TPU	11	0.45

2.4. Experimental Baropodometric Testing

A baropodometric study was performed to validate the reliability of the assumptions and the biofidelity of the model. The medical software FreeSTEP® v.1.4.01 was employed along with the professional equipment from Sensor Medica®, and the foot was evaluated statically (Figure 8a). The contact surface, percentage, and geometric values of the load applied on the foot were measured. Likewise, the study obtained results from a stabilometric analysis and a 3D scan of the foot. Once the calibration and adjustment of the equipment were completed, the pressure between the ground and the plantar surface of the foot was measured when the participant was standing barefoot on the platform, the distribution of the plantar pressure, the maximum plantar pressure, and the center of pressure were recorded. To more precisely determine the distributed load along the sole, the foot was divided into six parts automatically by the software (Figure 8b). Figure 8c shows the anthropometric measurements of both feet. Using the values and sections provided by the software, the experimental results obtained were compared with the model's predictions solved by numerical analysis.

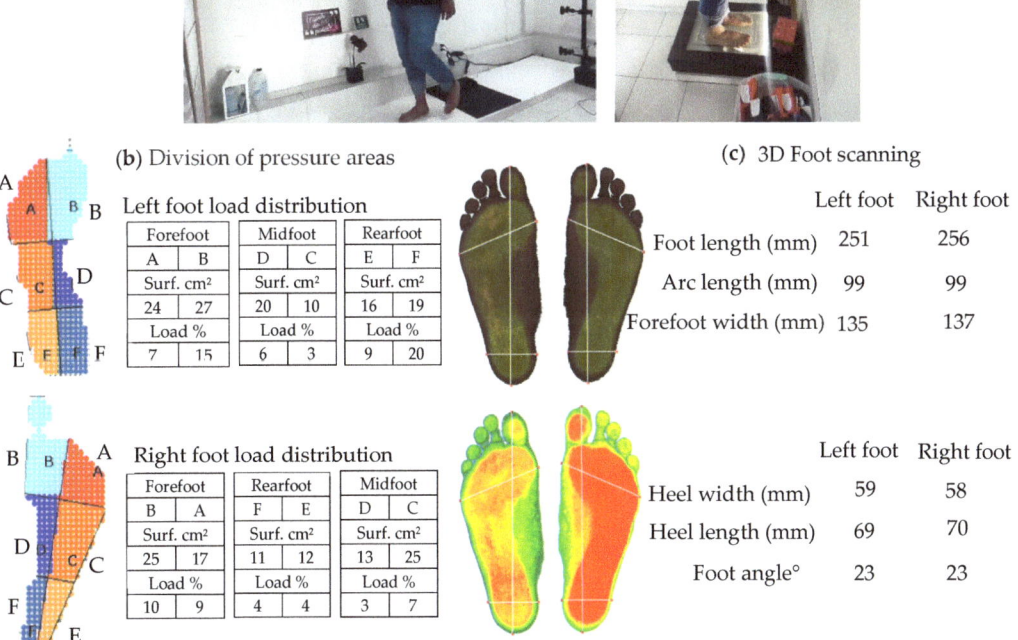

Figure 8. Baropodometric study. (**a**) Participant under experimental testing. (**b**) Sectioned regions of plantar pressure distribution. The abbreviation Surf in the tables refers to surface. (**c**) Three-dimensional anthropometric scanning.

3. Results
3.1. Footsketching Study Results

Several footprint sketches of the right foot of the participant were taken with different amounts of ink on the sole. These footprints were taken from a male young adult in his 30s. Using variations in the quantity of ink on the plantar surface allowed the observation of subtle changes in the plantar print that slightly changed the results. Despite slight variations in the percentages, they were very similar, resulting in the foot being classified as a normal foot type, as there was no tendency to fall into a Flatfoot–Normal or Normal–Cavus Foot classification. The results can be observed in Table 4 and Figure 9.

Table 4. Footprint results implementing the Hernández Corvo method.

Footprint	Percentage %	Foot Type
a	43.65	Normal
b	43.13	Normal
c	44.94	Normal
d	40.81	Normal

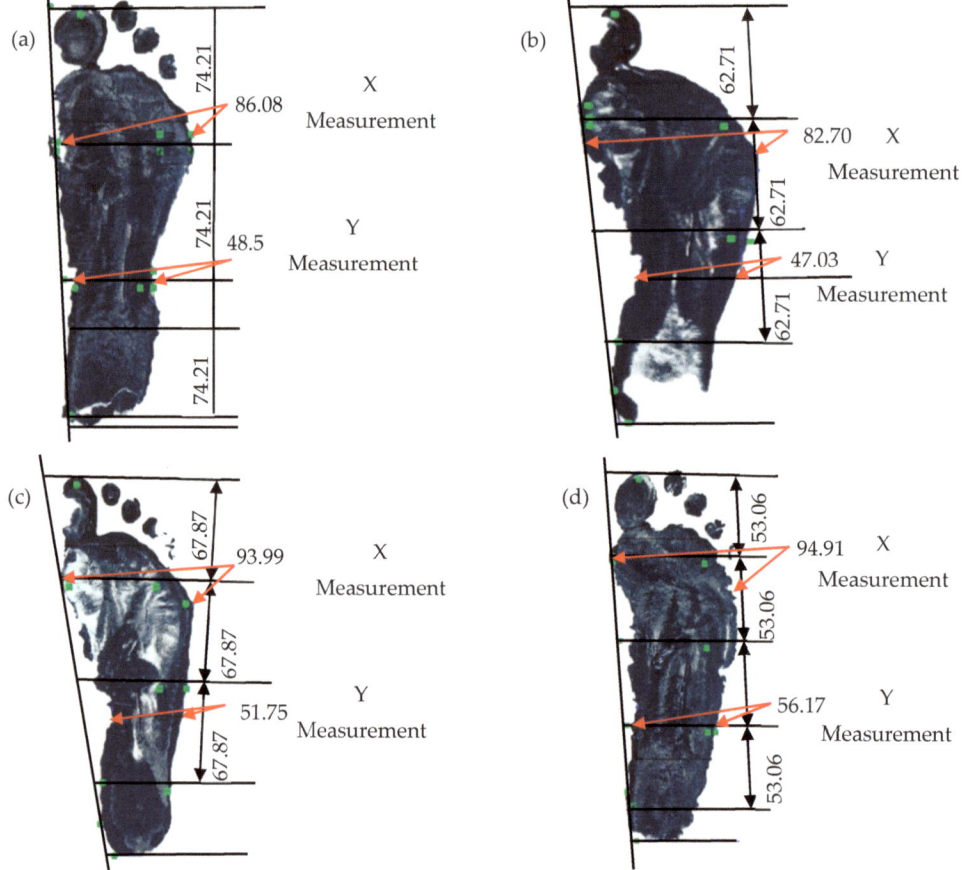

Figure 9. Footprint sketching results. (**a**) First trial. (**b**) Second trial. (**c**) Third trial. (**d**) Fourth trial.

3.2. First Case Study Results

Once the numerical analysis equations converged, results were obtained, mainly focusing on total deformation and von Mises stress due to representing a more precise behavior of the foot sole in both study cases. The visualization of the initial results corresponds to the less conservative model, corresponding to the mechanical properties proposed by Luboz (Figures 10 and 11), which has a lower Young's modulus value. The results obtained with the property defined by Wu are then shown (Figures 12 and 13).

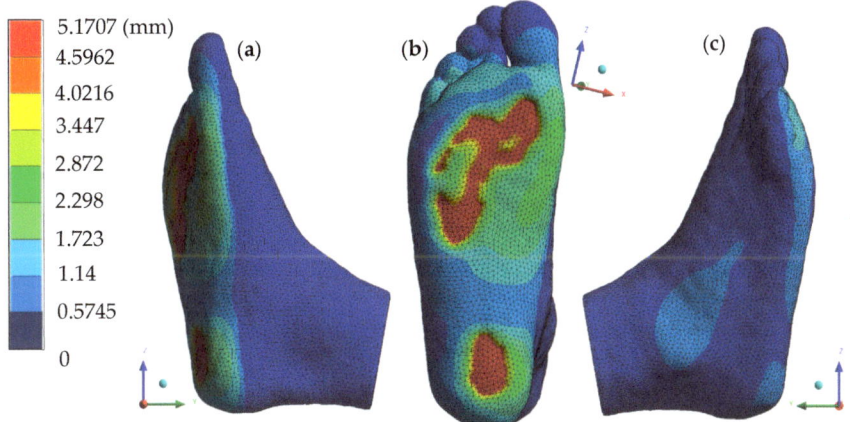

Figure 10. Total deformation (Luboz). (**a**) Left side view. (**b**) Plantar region. (**c**) Right side view.

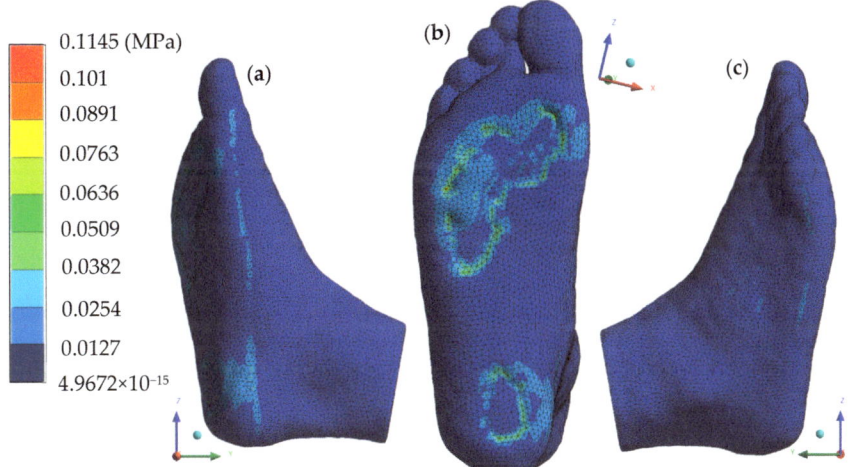

Figure 11. Von Mises stress (Luboz). (**a**) Left side view. (**b**) Plantar region. (**c**) Right side view.

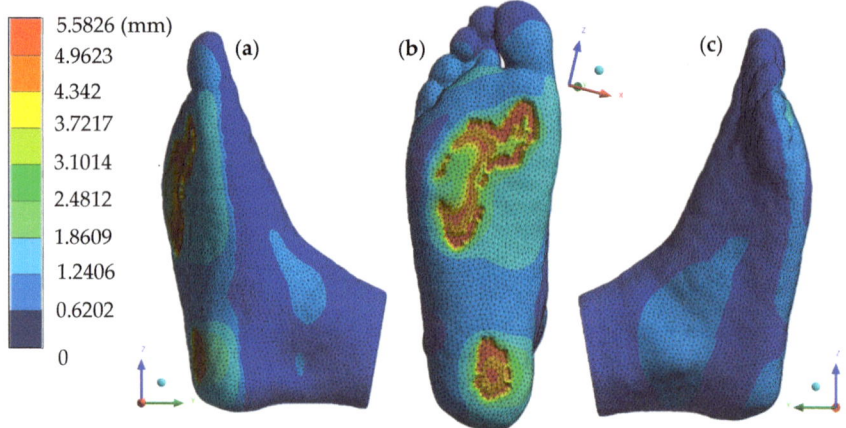

Figure 12. Total deformation (Wu). (**a**) Left side view. (**b**) Plantar region. (**c**) Right side view.

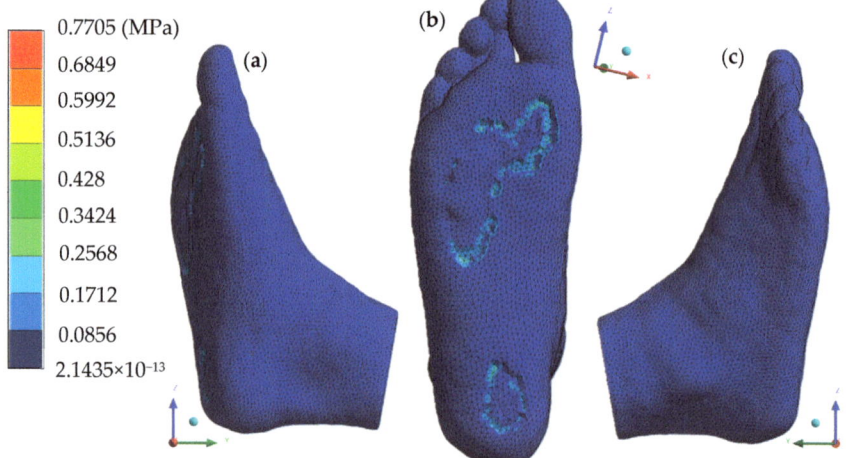

Figure 13. Von Mises stress (Wu). (**a**) Left side view. (**b**) Plantar region. (**c**) Right side view.

Results of Baropodometric Testing, Validation, and Comparison to First Case Study Results

A comparison of the plantar pressure points in the right foot sole between the experimental and numerical analysis proved the results to be extremely close for both mechanical properties for the encapsulating muscles, those proposed by Luboz and Wu. To compare and evaluate the stress concentration in these foot regions, von Mises stress theory values were considered; this theory is based on the difference in principal stresses. Therefore, this theory is optimal for the recreation of biological tissues since complex stress conditions and combinations of nominal and shear stresses are experienced in the plantar region under balanced standing. Furthermore, other researchers have widely used von Mises stress theory to measure and analyze the stress in the foot's plantar surface and soft tissues. The highest plantar pressure values obtained in the numerical analysis are around 0.050–0.063 MPa for the model with Luboz properties and 0.0856–0.1712 MPa for that with Wu properties. In comparison, the value registered in the baropodometric study yielded a 700 gr/cm^2 result, which is 0.0686 MPa (Figure 14). Thus, the numerical analysis predicted both highly trustworthy and precise results.

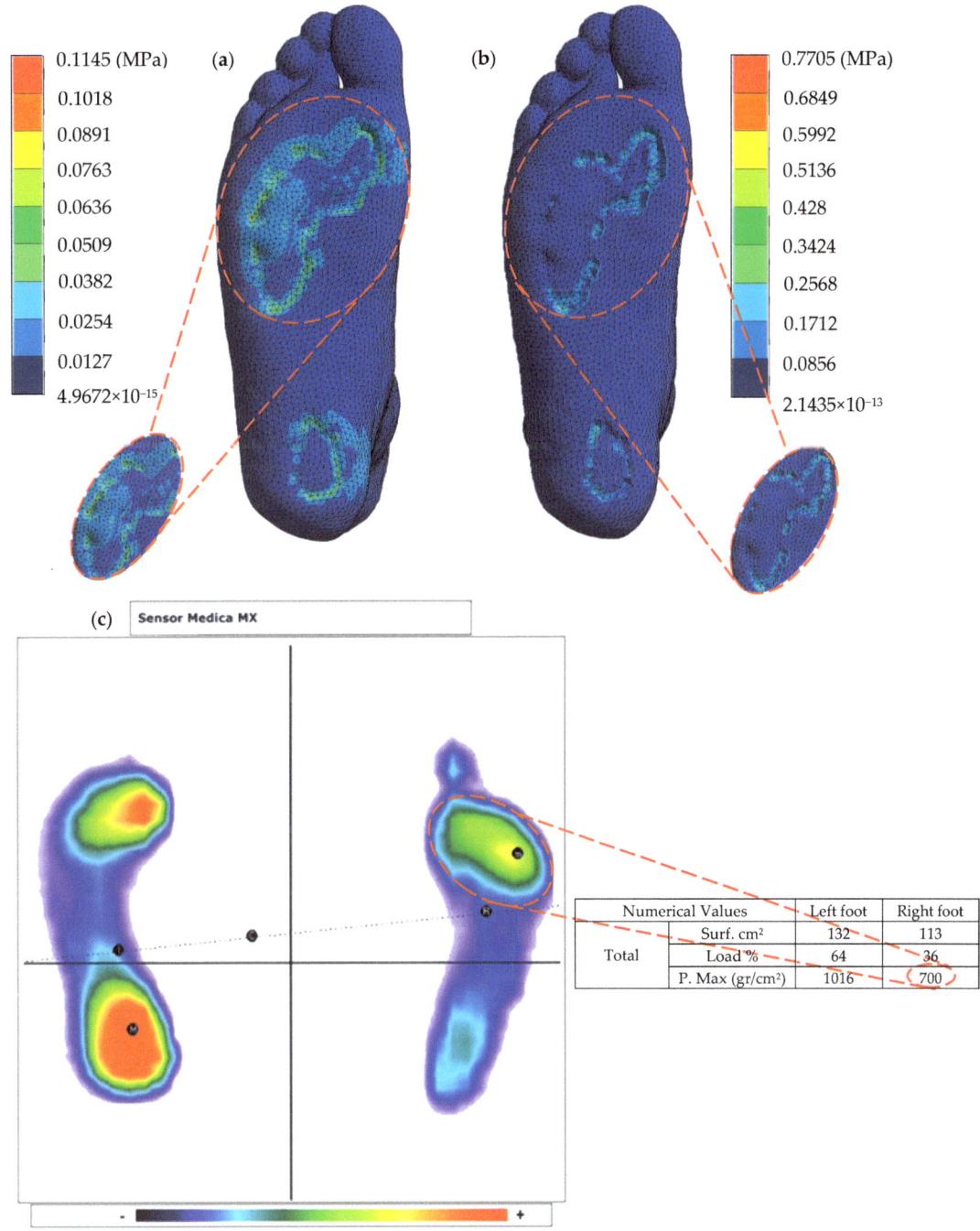

Figure 14. Comparison of numerical and experimental results. (**a**) Model with Luboz properties. (**b**) Model with Wu properties. (**c**) Baropodometric study. The abbreviation P. Max refers to maximum pressure.

3.3. Second Case Study Results

The results corresponding to the numerical evaluation employing the customized orthosis are presented for Luboz (Figures 15 and 16) and Wu (Figures 17 and 18), showing the cushioning effects redistributing pressure on the foot sole. All the maximum and minimum values obtained as results for both study cases can be found in Appendix A, Tables A1 and A2.

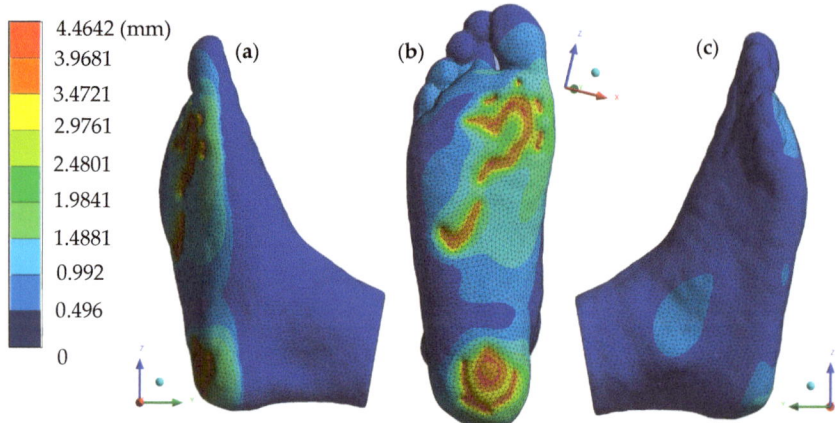

Figure 15. Total deformation with implementation of customized foot insole (Luboz). (**a**) Left side view. (**b**) Plantar region. (**c**) Right side view.

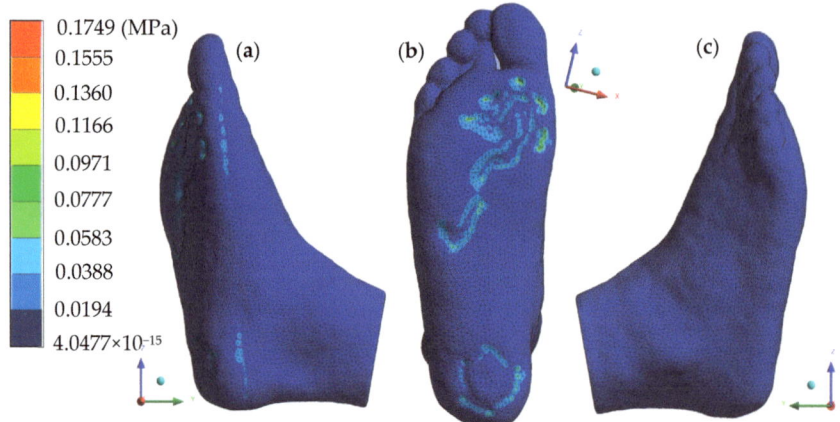

Figure 16. Von Mises stress with implementation of customized foot insole (Luboz). (**a**) Left side view. (**b**) Plantar region. (**c**) Right side view.

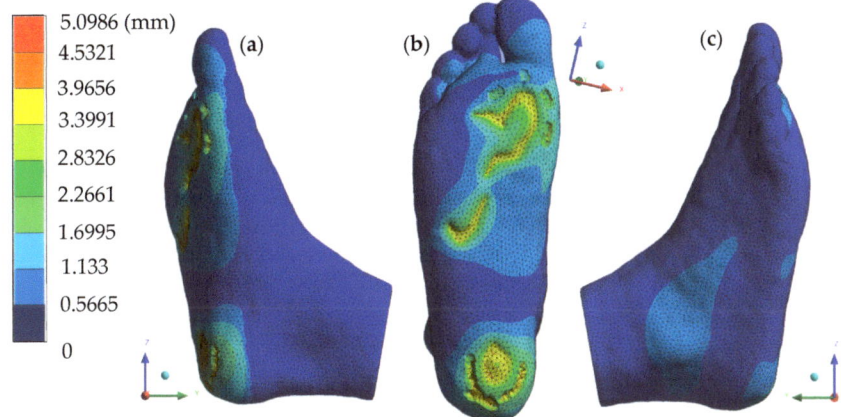

Figure 17. Total deformation with implementation of customized foot insole (Wu). (**a**) Left side view. (**b**) Plantar region. (**c**) Right side view.

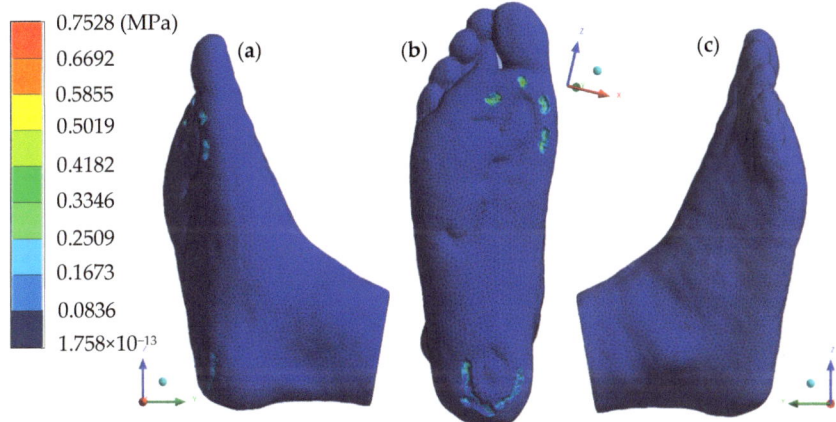

Figure 18. Von Mises stress with implementation of customized foot insole (Wu). (**a**) Left side view. (**b**) Plantar region. (**c**) Right side view.

4. Discussion

The human foot is among the most complex biological structures due to its remarkable functions, from locomotion to providing stability and support to the body, as it is the only human lower limb part having direct contact with the ground. Among these impressive functions, shock absorption is one of the most studied functionalities in medical and research fields, as it enables many functions, such as stabilization, body weight support, and surface adaptation.

A combination of experimental and numerical analyses allowed the acquisition of valuable data for analyzing the plantar foot region pressure points under normal standing conditions and providing a proper assessment in developing a personalized total-contact foot orthosis 3D model. This sophisticated methodology introduces segmentation procedures for reconstructing a three-dimensional foot model, representing an approach for feasibly reproducing different biological tissues. Despite representing foot muscles as an encapsulated element, the computational resource approach and intricateness set it apart as a highly elaborate three-dimensional biomodel construction.

In this research, mechanically recreating a static structural analysis in the standing condition predicted the appropriate behavior of the foot sole soft tissues, foot skin, and muscles. According to the medical literature, normal foot conditions present peak pressure points in the forefoot under the metatarsal heads, usually in the first or fifth, and the rearfoot in the heel while balanced standing is maintained. Numerical analysis showed a higher stress concentration in the forefoot region than in the rearfoot; mainly, the highest pressure was under the fifth metatarsal head. Thus, an equivalent representation in the plantar foot region for standard peak pressure values was obtained. In a validation of the finite element analysis, the pressure distributions were similar in the color scale depicted for both analyses. Thus, it was demonstrated that the participant tends to generate a higher pressure in the forefoot during balanced standing in normal conditions. Total elastic deformation results represent how the foot sole skin moves once it is in contact with the ground reaction force, having considerable values in regions with higher stress fields. Likewise, total elastic strain predicts the load tendency for the peak plantar pressure zones. The results for both models are in good agreement, adequately functioning when analyzed barefoot and within foot orthosis, employing the mechanical properties provided by Luboz and Wu. All the assumptions and considerations developed in the 3D modeling and finite element analysis for these foot soft tissues are considered precise. Since results are in good agreement and vary by very little, there is a standard error range between numerical and experimental testing.

The presented investigation stands out because it provides an innovative approach to analyzing the foot or any other biological tissue through finite element analysis since only soft tissues are considered. It is in contrast to most biological numerical analyses that require the reconstruction of bone tissue to analyze soft tissue shock absorption behavior. In addition, the detailed model developed and the fine discretization provide closer estimates as more differential partial equations converge into a solution.

Furthermore, both the material selection and geometry design of the customized 3D model insole were suitable because of the numerical prediction of lower peak pressure values and a uniform pressure redistribution along the foot sole, mainly reducing stress concentrations in most plantar regions where peak pressure points occurred when this anatomical position was maintained without the employment of any orthotic device. Foot sole regions presented a minor pressure increment, resulting in foot–insole contact. The initial numerical analysis utilizing the finite element method provides an appropriate assessment for the geometric design of a 3D model customized insole evaluation, firstly relying on analyzing the foot by itself (barefoot) and then considering both morphological and anthropometrical aspects to comprehend where there is a higher likelihood of peak pressure points occurring. The plantar orthosis material also has a significant role in the correct performance, commonly based on controlling foot functions or providing cushioning effects. TPU was ideal for relieving peak pressure points on tender spots, giving additional support, enhancing stability, and adding an extra layer to the plantar region.

Numerically analyzing pressure points in a foot, apparently under normal conditions, promotes a more thorough comprehension of real-life behavior under the simulated anatomical position. Deepening current knowledge about this subject could better implement numerical approaches for pathological foot analysis, giving proper medical evaluation towards rehabilitation. In addition to experimental validation, the present study closely aligns with extant investigations in foot finite element analysis modeling. Notably, whereas prior published studies predominantly focused on incorporating bony elements within their models, this work presents a unique aspect by exclusively considering the foot's soft tissues. This methodological distinction deviates from established approaches and thus represents a novel contribution to the existing body of literature. Numerical simulations' stress distribution results are in solid concordance with previous finite element analyses when evaluating barefoot balanced standing, reinforcing the observations reported regarding peak pressure values and the distribution of stress patterns in the plantar region [51–53], specifically when utilizing the muscles' mechanical properties provided by Luboz. At the same time, results obtained in the plantar surface, including the customized insole, correlate highly with other research papers that optimize insole design through numerical analyses [54–58]. Moreover, the plantar peak pressure values for the utilization of the personalized orthotic device are in substantial consensus with recent literature in insole construction combining additive manufacturing materials and traditional materials [49,59]. Nonetheless, the specific reconstructed model features differ from most foot finite element models in the literature; the results are in accordance due to two main reasons: utilizing a similar methodology to analyze balanced standing and the reconstruction of healthy foot models in similar patient populations in healthy conditions without foot pathology issues.

Despite this study demonstrating feasible results to be established as a solid methodology for numerical analyses in biological tissues, it is relevant to point out certain limitations of this research. While it is not a significant issue in employing this methodology, it is relevant to account for proper computational equipment to develop the numerical analyses quickly. Another issue that may compromise the reproducibility of this paper relies on the need for medical data to assign displacement magnitude, taking into account that defining the displacement value has a relationship with body weight but does not have a direct conversion. A fundamental limitation of this study is the use of data from a single, young, and healthy subject. This consideration restricts the generalizability of our findings to broader populations with diverse health conditions. While the proposed approach demonstrates promise in this specific case, further research is necessary to validate its efficacy and applicability in individuals with various health profiles. Future studies should include more extensive and diverse participant pools, incorporating individuals with various medical conditions and demographic characteristics.

5. Conclusions

Finite element analyses have been established as a powerful tool for evaluating biological tissues, providing valuable insights into understanding their complex behavior. This numerical engineering technique has the ambition to generate an even higher impact on the medical field. Notably, in the presented research, a proper assessment for creating a refined personalized 3D model orthotic device was employed through a numerical evaluation. Nonetheless, to use the described technique, it is mandatory to have strong mechanical knowledge and a high degree of expertise in segmentation and numerical analysis software in addition to having powerful computational equipment so that the methodology will not be time-consuming since biomodel refinement (biofidelity) and finite element analysis are directly related to computational features.

Numerical analysis can be applied to numerous approaches that, along with medical supervision, can trigger more sophisticated techniques when evaluating the outstanding but always complicated human body. It is relevant to mention that numerical analysis cannot replace experimental testing but results in an advantageous methodology complementing existing medical procedures predicting when the body may be susceptible to injuries and taking action when they occur. Furthermore, the interdisciplinary approaches from the union of medicine and engineering, biomechanics, and biomedicine, to mention a few, have facilitated the enhancement of current prostheses, orthoses, pre-surgical assistance and planning, and rehabilitation therapies. Moreover, the accelerated growth of additive manufacturing technologies has enabled new findings regarding new materials in assistive devices, with particular advantages such as easy access, affordability, and time efficiency.

Considering everything, the finite element analysis employed in this research can obtain estimations close to reality, validating engineering and mathematical methods as a reliable complementary tool regarding complex clinical assessment. Thus, the methods applied in the present work can change how traditional customization procedures in the medical field are currently carried out, with the concrete aim of creating personalized prosthetic and orthotic devices since the results obtained substantiate the utilization of numerical analysis in biological tissues, accurately predicting the behavior of these tissues under concrete circumstances. These methods provide an alternative to standard clinical procedures that are often time-consuming and expensive.

Author Contributions: Conceptualization, J.A.S.-P., G.U.-S. and B.R.-Á.; methodology, J.A.S.-P., G.U.-S., B.R.-Á. and G.M.U.-C.; validation, J.A.S.-P., G.U.-S., B.R.-Á., G.M.U.-C. and S.C.-L.; formal analysis, J.A.S.-P., G.U.-S., B.R.-Á. and D.E.C.-L.; investigation, J.A.S.-P., G.U.-S., B.R.-Á. and G.M.U.-C.; resources, J.A.S.-P., G.U.-S., B.R.-Á. and J.R.G.-I.; writing—original draft preparation, J.A.S.-P., G.U.-S., B.R.-Á. and G.M.-A.; writing—review and editing, J.A.S.-P., G.U.-S., B.R.-Á. and A.U.-L.; visualization, J.A.S.-P., G.U.-S., B.R.-Á. and A.U.-L.; supervision, J.A.S.-P., G.U.-S. and B.R.-Á.; project administration, J.A.S.-P., G.U.-S., B.R.-Á. and G.M.U.-C. All authors have read and agreed to the published version of the manuscript.

Funding: This research received no external funding.

Institutional Review Board Statement: The study was conducted in accordance with the Declaration of Helsinki and approved by the Ethics Committee of Biomechanics Group, Instituto Politécnico Nacional, Escuela Superior de Ingeniería Mecánica y Eléctrica, Sección de Estudios de Posgrado e Investigación, Unidad Profesional Adolfo López Mateos, 14 June 2023.

Informed Consent Statement: Informed consent was obtained from the participant involved in the study. Written informed consent has been obtained from the participant to publish this paper.

Data Availability Statement: All data generated or analyzed during this study are included within the article.

Acknowledgments: The authors gratefully acknowledge the Instituto Politécnico Nacional, Consejo Nacional de Humanidades Ciencias y Tecnologías, and Francisco Carrasco Hernández for supporting this research.

Conflicts of Interest: The authors declare no conflicts of interest.

Appendix A

Table A1. First case study summary of numerical evaluation results.

Type of Analysis	Luboz Properties		Wu Properties	
	Maximum	Minimum	Maximum	Minimum
Total deformation (mm)	5.1707	0	5.5826	0
Deformation X axis (mm)	2.4654	−1.403	1.7405	−1.2755
Deformation Y axis (mm)	5.1707	−0.7618	5.5737	−0.5247
Deformation Z axis (mm)	1.8151	−1.6289	1.5674	−1.5781
Total elastic strain (mm/mm)	0.6602	4.5741×10^{-16}	1.6765	4.4235×10^{-16}
Elastic strain X axis (mm/mm)	0.3623	−0.3095	0.9604	−0.6028
Elastic strain Y axis (mm/mm)	0.5329	−0.5899	0.7187	−1.4239
Elastic strain Z axis (mm/mm)	0.3541	−0.2437	0.6552	−0.5808
Nominal stress X axis (MPa)	0.1058	−0.1357	0.3503	−1.6429
Nominal stress Y axis (MPa)	0.1201	−0.179	0.3885	−1.8739
Nominal stress Z axis (MPa)	0.1014	−0.1526	0.2811	−1.6988
Shear stress XY plane (MPa)	0.0430	−0.038	0.2995	−0.2955
Shear stress YZ plane (MPa)	0.0357	−0.0373	0.1983	−0.2349
Shear stress XZ plane (MPa)	0.0217	−0.0203	0.1292	−0.1208
von Mises stress (MPa)	0.1145	4.9672×10^{-15}	0.7705	2.1435×10^{-13}
Maximum principal stress (MPa)	0.1222	−0.1313	0.4689	−1.5912
Minimum principal stress (MPa)	0.1010	−0.19	0.1887	−1.9227

Table A2. Second case study summary of numerical evaluation results.

Type of Analysis	Luboz Properties		Wu Properties	
	Maximum	Minimum	Maximum	Minimum
Total deformation (mm)	4.4642	0	5.0986	0
Deformation X axis (mm)	1.9254	−1.1515	1.9025	−1.2693
Deformation Y axis (mm)	4.4627	−0.5956	5.0832	−0.4367
Deformation Z axis (mm)	1.29	−1.3982	1.5646	−1.8064
Total elastic strain (mm/mm)	0.9865	7.3806×10^{-14}	2.6486	3.5677×10^{-16}
Elastic strain X axis (mm/mm)	0.5086	−0.2228	1.034	−0.6846
Elastic strain Y axis (mm/mm)	0.4684	−0.8719	0.8662	−2.0931
Elastic strain Z axis (mm/mm)	0.3331	−0.3519	1.1336	−0.6302
Nominal stress X axis (MPa)	0.0759	−0.2348	0.4053	−1.5162
Nominal stress Y axis (MPa)	0.0975	−0.4690	0.3665	−2.2535
Nominal stress Z axis (MPa)	0.0858	−0.3110	0.3382	−1.8223
Shear stress XY plane (MPa)	0.0585	−0.0548	0.4901	−0.3188
Shear stress YZ plane (MPa)	0.0529	−0.0417	0.3888	−0.3655
Shear stress XZ plane (MPa)	0.0240	−0.0173	0.1382	−0.1987
von Mises stress (MPa)	0.1749	4.0477×10^{-15}	0.7528	1.758×10^{-13}
Maximum principal stress (MPa)	0.1262	−0.2298	0.5284	−1.4975
Minimum principal stress (MPa)	0.0646	−0.4761	0.3214	−2.4995

References

1. Sun, Y.; Liang, S.; Yu, Y.; Yang, Y.; Lu, J.; Wu, J.; Cheng, Y.; Wang, Y.; Wu, J.; Han, J.; et al. Plantar pressure-based temporal analysis of gait disturbance in idiopathic normal pressure hydrocephalus: Indications from a pilot longitudinal study. *Comput. Methods Programs Biomed.* **2012**, *217*, 106691. [CrossRef]
2. Tang, X.; Wang, X.; Ji, X.; Wang, Y.; Chen, W.; Wei, Y.; Zhou, Y. Study on foot-type classification for young adults based on static and dynamic plantar pressure distribution. *Adv. Mech. Eng.* **2022**, *14*, 16878132221097904. [CrossRef]
3. Ang, C.K.; Solihin, M.I.; Chan, W.J.; Ong, Y.Y. Study of Plantar Pressure Distribution. *MATEC Web Conf.* **2018**, *237*, 01016. [CrossRef]
4. Zulkifli, S.S.; Wei, P.L. A state-of-the-art review of foot pressure. *Foot Ankle Surg.* **2020**, *26*, 25–32. [CrossRef] [PubMed]
5. Su, K.-H.; Kaewwichit, T.; Tseng, C.-H.; Chang, C.-C. Automatic footprint detection approach for the calculation of arch index and plantar pressure in a flat rubber pad. *Multimed. Tools Appl.* **2016**, *75*, 9757–9774. [CrossRef]
6. He, Y.-J.; Zheng, X.-L.; Wang, D.-F.; Mu, Z.-Z.; Li, G.-Y.; Fang, Z.-Z.; Fei, W.; Huan, K. Static and dynamic plantar pressure distribution in 94 patients with different stages of unilateral knee osteoarthritis using the footscan®platform system: An observational study. *J. Pharmacol. Exp. Ther.* **2023**, *29*, e938485. [CrossRef] [PubMed]
7. Mun, F.; Choi, A. Deep learning approach to estimate foot pressure distribution in walking with application for a cost-effective insole system. *J. Neuroeng. Rehabil.* **2022**, *19*, 4. [CrossRef]
8. Wafai, L.; Zayegh, A.; Woulfe, J.; Aziz, S.M.; Begg, R. Identification of Foot Pathologies Based on Plantar Pressure Asymmetry. *Sensors* **2015**, *15*, 20392–20408. [CrossRef]
9. Chen, D.-W.; Li, B.; Aubeeluck, A.; Yang, Y.-F.; Huang, Y.-G.; Zhou, J.-Q.; Yu, G.-R. Anatomy and biomechanical properties of the plantar aponeurosis: A cadaveric study. *PLoS ONE* **2014**, *9*, e84347. [CrossRef] [PubMed]
10. Zhu, G.; Wang, Z.; Yuan, C.; Geng, X.; Yu, J.; Zhang, C.; Huang, J.; Wang, X.; Ma, X. In vitro study of foot bone kinematics via a custom-made cadaveric gait simulator. *J. Orthop. Surg. Res.* **2020**, *15*, 346. [CrossRef]
11. Baxter, J.R.; Demetracopoulos, C.A.; Prado, M.P.; Gilbert, S.L.; Tharmviboonsri, T.; Deland, J.T. Graft shape affects midfoot correction and forefoot loading mechanics in lateral column lengthening osteotomies. *Foot Ankle Int.* **2014**, *35*, 1192–1199. [CrossRef]
12. Kohta, I.; Hosoda, K.; Masahiro, S.; Shuhei, I.; Takeo, N.; Hiroyuki, S.; Masateru, K.; Nobuaki, I.; Sadakazu, A.; Masahiro, J.; et al. Three-dimensional innate mobility of the human foot bones under axial loading using biplane x-ray fluoroscopy. *Foot Ankle Int.* **2017**, *4*, 171086.
13. Niu, W.; Yang, Y.; Fan, Y.; Ding, Z.; Yu, G. Experimental modeling and biomechanical measurement of flatfoot deformity. In Proceedings of the 7th Asian-Pacific Conference on Medical and Biological Engineering, Beijing, China, 22–25 April 2008.
14. Deepashini, H.; Omar, B.; Paungmali, A.; Amaramalar, N.; Ohnmar, H.; Leonard, J. An insight into the plantar pressure distribution of the foot in clinical practice: Narrative review. *Pol. Ann. Med.* **2014**, *21*, 51–56. [CrossRef]
15. Mastache-Miranda, O.A.; Urriolagoitia-Sosa, G.; Marquet-Rivera, R.A. Three-dimensional reconstruction for use in medicine and biomechanics. *MOJ Appl. Bionics Biomech.* **2018**, *2*, 310–331.
16. Martinez-Mondragon, M.; Urriolagoitia-Sosa, G.; Romero-Ángeles, B.; Maya-Anaya, D.; Martínez-Reyes, J.; Gallegos-Funes, F.J.; Urriolagoitia-Calderón, G.M. Numerical Analysis of Zirconium and Titanium Implants under the Effect of Critical Masticatory Load. *Materials* **2022**, *15*, 7843. [CrossRef]

17. Maya-Anaya, D.; Urriolagoitia-Sosa, G.; Romero-Ángeles, B.; Martinez-Mondragon, M.; German-Carcaño, J.M.; Correa-Corona, M.I.; Trejo-Enríquez, A.; Sánchez-Cervantes, A.; Urriolagoitia-Luna, A.; Urriolagoitia-Calderón, G.M. Numerical Analysis Applying the Finite Element Method by Developing a Complex Three-Dimensional Biomodel of the Biological Tissues of the Elbow Joint Using Computerized Axial Tomography. *Appl. Sci.* **2023**, *13*, 8903. [CrossRef]
18. García-Delgado, P.A.; Cabezas-Díaz, F.I.; Nieto-España, D.C.; Mogrovejo-Del Saltó, V.N. Imagenología médica y anatomía radiológica. *Recimu* **2022**, *6*, 557–565. [CrossRef]
19. Lozano-Zalce, H. Ética médica e imagenología. *Acta Méd. Grupo Ángeles* **2017**, *15*, 5–7. [CrossRef]
20. Tekkaya, A.E.; Soyarslan, C. *CIRP Encyclopedia of Production Engineering*, 2nd ed.; Springer: Berlin/Heidelberg, Germany, 2019; pp. 677–683.
21. Koutromanos, L. *Fundamentals of Finite Element Analysis: Linear Finite Element Analysis*, 1st ed.; John Wiley & Sons: Chichester, UK, 2018; pp. 6–12.
22. Lara-Diéguez, S.; Lara-Sánchez, A.J.; Zagalaz-Sánchez, M.L.; Martínez-López, E.J. Análisis de los diferentes métodos de evaluación de la huella plantar. *RETOS Nuevas Tend. Educ. Física Deporte Recreación* **2011**, *19*, 49–53.
23. Luengas, L.; Díaz, M.; González, J. Determinación de tipo de pie mediante el procesamiento de imágenes. *Ingenium Rev. Fac. Ing.* **2016**, *17*, 147–161.
24. Zabala-Travers, S. Biomodeling and 3D printing: A novel radiology subspecialty. *Ann. 3D Print. Med.* **2021**, *4*, 100038. [CrossRef]
25. Marquet-Rivera, R.A.; Urriolagoitia-Sosa, G.; Hernández-Vázquez, R.A.; Romero-Ángeles, B.; Mastache-Miranda, O.A.; Urriolagoitia-Calderón, G. High Biofidelity 3D Biomodel Reconstruction from Soft and Hard Tissues (Knee), FEM, and 3D Printing: A Three-Dimensional Methodological Proposal. *BioMed Res. Int.* **2021**, *2021*, 6688164. [CrossRef]
26. Jastifer, J.R. Intrinsic muscles of the foot: Anatomy, function, rehabilitation. *Phys. Ther. Sport* **2023**, *61*, 27–36. [CrossRef]
27. Zhang, M.; Mak, A.F.T. In vivo friction properties of human skin. *Prosthetics Orthot. Int.* **1999**, *23*, 135–141. [CrossRef]
28. Luboz, V.; Perrier, A.; Bucki, M.; Diot, B.; Cannard, F.; Vuillerme, N.; Payan, Y. Influence of the calcaneus shape on the risk of posterior heel ulcer using 3D patient-specific biomechanical modeling. *Ann. Biomed. Eng.* **2014**, *43*, 325–335. [CrossRef]
29. Wu, L. Nonlinear finite element analysis for musculoskeletal biomechanics of medial and lateral plantar longitudinal arch of Virtual Chinese Human after plantar ligamentous structure failures. *Clin. Biomech.* **2007**, *22*, 221–229. [CrossRef]
30. Su, S.; Mo, Z.; Guo, J.; Fan, Y. The effect of arch height and material hardness of personalized insole on correction and tissues of flatfoot. *J. Heath Eng.* **2017**, *2017*, 8614341. [CrossRef]
31. Tao, K.; Wang, D.; Wang, C.; Wang, X.; Liu, A.; Nester, C.J.; Howard, D. An in vivo experimental validation of a computational model of human foot. *J. Bionic Eng.* **2009**, *6*, 387–397. [CrossRef]
32. Parker, D.; Cooper, G.; Pearson, S.; Crofts, G.; Howard, D.; Busby, P.; Nester, C. A device for characterising the mechanical properties of the plantar soft tissue of the foot. *Med. Eng. Phys.* **2015**, *37*, 1098–1104. [CrossRef]
33. Smith, S.G.; Yokich, M.K.; Beaudette, S.M.; Brown, S.H.; Bent, L.R. Effects of foot position on skin structural deformation. *J. Mech. Behav. Biomed. Mater.* **2019**, *95*, 240–248. [CrossRef]
34. Tang, L.; Wang, L.; Bao, W.; Zhu, S.; Li, D.; Zhao, N.; Liu, C. Functional gradient structural design of customized diabetic insoles. *J. Mech. Behav. Biomed. Mater.* **2019**, *94*, 279–287. [CrossRef]
35. Rodríguez-Parada, L.; de la Rosa, S.; Mayuet, P.F. Influence of 3D-Printed TPU Properties for the Design of Elastic Products. *Polymers* **2021**, *13*, 2519. [CrossRef]
36. Rohm, K.; Manas-Zloczower, I. A micromechanical approach to TPU mechanical properties: Framework and experimental validation. *Mech. Mater.* **2023**, *180*, 104627. [CrossRef]
37. Choo, Y.J.; Boudier-Revéret, M.; Chang, M.C. 3D printing technology applied to orthosis manufacturing: Narrative review. *Ann. Palliat. Med.* **2020**, *9*, 4262–4270. [CrossRef]
38. Xu, T.; Shen, W.; Lin, X.; Xie, Y.M. Mechanical Properties of Additively Manufactured Thermoplastic Polyurethane (TPU) Material Affected by Various Processing Parameters. *Polymers* **2020**, *12*, 3010. [CrossRef]
39. Sreenivas-Reddy, B. 3D Printing for Foot. *MOJ Proteomic Bioinf.* **2017**, *5*, 165–169.
40. Davia-Aracil, M.; Hinojo-Pérez, J.J.; Jimeno-Morenilla, A.; Mora-Mora, H. 3D printing of functional anatomical insoles. *Comput. Ind.* **2018**, *95*, 38–53. [CrossRef]
41. Orsu, B.; Shaik, Y.P. Compression Strength Analysis of Customized Shoe Insole with Different Infill Patterns Using 3D Printing. *Open Access Libr. J.* **2022**, *9*, 1–13. [CrossRef]
42. Cheng, K.-W.; Peng, Y.; Chen, T.L.-W.; Zhang, G.; Cheung, J.C.-W.; Lam, W.-K.; Wong, D.W.-C.; Zhang, M. A Three-Dimensional Printed Foot Orthosis for Flexible Flatfoot: An Exploratory Biomechanical Study on Arch Support Reinforcement and Undercut. *Materials* **2021**, *14*, 5297. [CrossRef]
43. Hsu, C.-Y.; Wang, C.-S.; Lin, K.-W.; Chien, M.-J.; Wei, S.-H.; Chen, C.-S. Biomechanical Analysis of the FlatFoot with Different 3D-Printed Insoles on the Lower Extremities. *Bioengineering* **2022**, *9*, 563. [CrossRef]
44. Peng, Y.; Wang, Y.; Wong, D.W.-C.; Chen, T.L.-W.; Chen, S.F.; Zhang, G.; Tan, Q.; Zhang, M. Different Design Feature Combinations of Flatfoot Orthosis on Plantar Fascia Strain and Plantar Pressure: A Muscle-Driven Finite Element Analysis with Taguchi Method. *Front. Bioeng. Biotechnol.* **2022**, *10*, 853085. [CrossRef]
45. Jonnala, U.K.; Sankineni, R.; Kumar, Y.R. Design and development of fused deposition modeling (FDM) 3D-Printed Orthotic Insole by using gyroid structure. *J. Mech. Behav. Biomed. Mater.* **2023**, *145*, 106005. [CrossRef]

46. Hu, C.-W.; Dabnichki, P.; Baca, A.; Nguyen, C.T.; Pang, T.Y. Preventive strategy of flatfoot deformity using fully automated procedure. *Med. Eng. Phys.* **2021**, *95*, 15–24. [CrossRef]
47. Zuñiga, J.; Moscoso, M.; Padilla-Huamantinco, P.G.; Lazo-Porras, M.; Tenorio-Mucha, J.; Padilla-Huamantinco, W.; Tincopa, J.P. Development of 3D-Printed Orthopedic Insoles for Patients with Diabetes and Evaluation with Electronic Pressure Sensors. *Designs* **2022**, *6*, 95. [CrossRef]
48. Lee, H.; Eom, R.-I.; Lee, Y. Evaluation of the Mechanical Properties of Porous Thermoplastic Polyurethane Obtained by 3D Printing for Protective Gear. *Adv. Mater. Sci. Eng.* **2019**, *2019*, 5838361. [CrossRef]
49. Nouman, M.; Dissaneewate, T.; Chong, D.Y.R.; Chatpun, S. Effects of Custom-Made Insole Materials on Frictional Stress and Contact Pressure in Diabetic Foot with Neuropathy: Results from a Finite Element Analysis. *Appl. Sci.* **2021**, *11*, 3412. [CrossRef]
50. Yang, L.; Wang, X.; Deng, Q. Customized Design of Insoles for Pressure Relief via FEM. In *Design Studies and Intelligence Engineering*, 1st ed.; Jain, C.L.; Balas, V.E.; Wu, Q.; Shi, F., Eds.; IOS Press: Hangzhou, China, 2022; Volume 347, pp. 172–181.
51. Cheung, J.T.-M.; Zhang, M.; An, K.-N. Effects of plantar fascia stiffness on the biomechanical responses of the ankle–foot complex. *Clin. Biomech.* **2004**, *19*, 839–846. [CrossRef]
52. Wang, Y.; Li, Z.; Wong, D.W.-C.; Cheng, C.-K.; Zhang, M. Finite element analysis of biomechanical effects of total ankle arthroplasty on the foot. *J. Orthop. Transl.* **2017**, *30*, 55–65. [CrossRef]
53. Brilakis, E.; Kaselouris, E.; Xypnitos, F.; Provatidis, C.G.; Efstathopoulos, N. Effects of foot posture on fifth metatarsal fracture healing: A finite element study. *J. Foot Ankle Surg.* **2012**, *51*, 720–728. [CrossRef]
54. Cheung, J.T.-M.; Zhang, M. A 3-dimensional finite element model of the human foot and ankle for insole design. *Arch. Phys. Med. Rehabil.* **2005**, *86*, 353–358. [CrossRef]
55. Hsu, Y.-C.; Gung, Y.-W.; Shih, S.-L.; Feng, C.-K.; Wei, S.-H.; Yu, C.-H.; Chen, C.-S. Using an optimization approach to design an insole for lowering plantar fascia stress—A finite element study. *Ann. Biomed. Eng.* **2008**, *36*, 1345–1352. [CrossRef]
56. Natali, A.N.; Forestiero, A.; Carniel, E.L.; Pavan, P.G.; Dal Zovo, C. Investigation of foot plantar pressure: Experimental and numerical analysis. *Med. Biol. Eng. Comput.* **2010**, *48*, 1167–1174. [CrossRef]
57. Niu, J.; Liu, J.; Zheng, Y.; Ran, L.; Chang, Z. Are arch-conforming insoles a good fit for diabetic foot? Insole customized design by using finite element analysis. *Hum. Factors Ergon. Manuf.* **2020**, *30*, 303–310. [CrossRef]
58. Jafarzadeh, E.; Soheilifard, R.; Ehsani-Seresht, A. Design optimization procedure for an orthopedic insole having a continuously variable stiffness/shape to reduce the plantar pressure in the foot of a diabetic patient. *Med. Eng. Phys.* **2021**, *98*, 44–49. [CrossRef] [PubMed]
59. Ghazali, M.J.; Ren, X.; Rajabi, A.; Zamri, W.F.H.W.; Mustafah, N.M.; Ni, J. Finite Element Analysis of Cushioned Diabetic Footwear Using Ethylene Vinyl Acetate Polymer. *Polymers* **2021**, *13*, 2261. [CrossRef] [PubMed]

Disclaimer/Publisher's Note: The statements, opinions and data contained in all publications are solely those of the individual author(s) and contributor(s) and not of MDPI and/or the editor(s). MDPI and/or the editor(s) disclaim responsibility for any injury to people or property resulting from any ideas, methods, instructions or products referred to in the content.

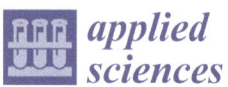

Article

Numerical Evaluation Using the Finite Element Method on Frontal Craniocervical Impact Directed at Intervertebral Disc Wear

Alfonso Trejo-Enriquez *, Guillermo Urriolagoitia-Sosa *, Beatriz Romero-Ángeles *, Miguel Ángel García-Laguna, Martín Guzmán-Baeza, Jacobo Martínez-Reyes, Yonatan Yael Rojas-Castrejon, Francisco Javier Gallegos-Funes, Julián Patiño-Ortiz and Guillermo Manuel Urriolagoitia-Calderón

Instituto Politécnico Nacional, Escuela Superior de Ingeniería Mecánica y Eléctrica, Sección de Estudios de Posgrado e Investigación, Unidad Profesional Adolfo López Mateos Zacatenco, Lindavista, Ciudad de México C.P. 07320, Mexico; mgarcial2100@alumno.ipn.mx (M.Á.G.-L.); maguzmanb@ipn.mx (M.G.-B.); jmartinezr0617@ipn.mx (J.M.-R.); yrojasc1300@alumno.ipn.mx (Y.Y.R.-C.); fgallegosf@ipn.mx (F.J.G.-F.); jpatinoo@ipn.mx (J.P.-O.); gurriolagoitiac@ipn.mx (G.M.U.-C.)
* Correspondence: atrejoe2100tmp@alumnoguinda.mx (A.T.-E.); guiurri@hotmail.com (G.U.-S.); romerobeatriz97@hotmail.com (B.R.-Á.)

Abstract: Traumatic cervical pathology is an injury that emerges due to trauma or being subjected to constant impact loading, affecting the ligaments, muscles, bones, and spinal cord. In contact sports (the practice of American football, karate, boxing, and motor sports, among others), the reporting of this type of injury is very common. Therefore, it is imperative to have preventive measures so players do not suffer from such injuries, since bad practices or accidents can put their lives at risk. This research evaluated cervical and skull biomechanical responses during a frontal impact, taking into consideration injury caused by wear on the intervertebral disc. Intervertebral disc wear is a degenerative condition that affects human mobility; it is common in people who practice contact sports and it can influence the response of the cervical system to an impact load. The main objective of this work is to evaluate the effects caused by impact loading and strains generated throughout the bone structure (composed of the skull and the cervical spine). The numerical evaluation was developed using the finite element method and the construction of the biomodel from computational axial tomography. In addition, the numerical simulation allowed us to observe how the intervertebral disc's wear affected the cervical region's biomechanical response. In addition, a comparison could be made between a healthy system and a disc that had suffered wear. Finally, the analysis provided information valuable to understanding how an impact, force-related injury can be affected and enabled us to propose better physiotherapeutic procedures.

Keywords: numerical simulation; finite element method; biomodel; impact load

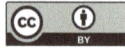

1. Introduction

Spinal cord injury is a problem that occurs in 80% of the entire general population (regardless of the job they perform). Principal activities causing these injuries are sports practice, working activities, and routine daily events [1,2]. However, people who practice a contact sport are at higher risk of developing cervical pathology. Among sports that stand out for producing this kind of injury is American football (where there is a 56% chance of developing a degenerative pathology) (Figure 1) [3]. Of all the injuries that can be caused, the one that stands out the most is cervical disc herniation in the lower area (C3–C7), which produces a fracture in the odontoid process [4,5]. The main reason for this is that the players constantly collide while practicing this sport. In addition, gym preparation for this sport includes weightlifting, which can overload participants' discs; with time, these discs can wear out, resulting in a disc rupture [6]. Disc rupture can be affected by spine anomalies, for example, the traumatic ones caused by head collisions [7]. In addition, degenerative injuries occur due to the misuse of anti-inflammatory drugs, being overweight, and weight loss [8]. To be able to observe critical effects generated by cervical pathology, a craniocervical biomodel (consisting of the skull, cervical vertebrae C1–C5, intervertebral discs, and spinal cord) was developed, and finite-element-method numerical analysis was performed to ensure it represented the reality of the injury effects as closely as possible [9]. These injuries, in some cases, generated a disability. Pathologies in the cervical spine are expected since players are exposed to constant physical contact (the most common impacts are frontal ones) [10]. The injury mechanisms generated by impacts cause traumatism to the skull, and the cervical spine is exposed to hyperextension movements with lateral flexion, which causes wear to develop due to the force of the hoof impact [11]. The craniocervical frontal effect depends on the impact force, which can result in serious neck injuries. The severity of these injuries depends on age and the time of exposure to this activity [12], which is a measurement factor due to the probability of wear on the intervertebral discs. This can occur more in a player at a professional level than a player at a nonprofessional level [13].

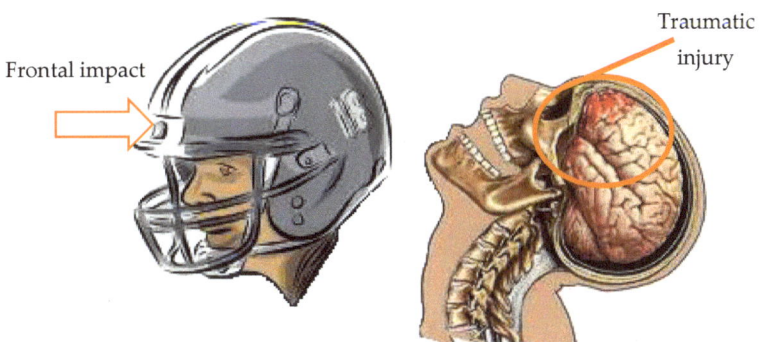

Figure 1. Frontal impact and possible effects.

Numerical analysis is a powerful tool for understanding the effects of frontal impact related to the biomechanical behavior of the neck and spine [14]. It is applied to simulate and predict the physical responses of these biological tissues under different loading conditions [15]. The implementation of this technology assists in evaluating the biomechanical behavior of biological systems through the use of computerized axial tomography. By performing a tomographical study, the biological tissue structure can be recreated in a 3D manner. This paper develops a complex biomodel by introducing the skull, cervical spine, intervertebral discs, and spinal cord [16]. Two cases of study are presented. The first study case considers a subject in a healthy condition, while the second study numerically simulates wear in the intervertebral disc [17,18]. This numerical analysis aimed to evaluate how intervertebral disc wear affects the biomechanical response of the neck and spine during a frontal impact. The described biomodels were analyzed by implementing the finite element method, which was used to simulate the behavior of tissues and bone structures [19]. The numerical analysis aimed to provide relevant data for the design of safety measures for players and for injury prevention in individuals with intervertebral disc wear. By better understanding the injury mechanisms and how they interact with disc wear, the development of effective strategies could be improved to minimize risks and progress safety for players playing this sport at a professional level [20]. Biomodels allow us to observe the behaviors of bone structures exposed to impact in a real situation since they are based on the use of tomography in medical diagnosis. However, biomodelling brings the scenario closer to reality by being three-dimensional because you can see the severity of the injury, which helps in proposing prevention or recovery treatment that can be performed in a personalized way. With the craniocervical biomodelling presented in this paper, you can see the behavior of a joint complex before an impact where one can see the damage's severity before a surgical operation, thereby allowing one to work with rehabilitation and physiotherapeutic treatment. Analyzing the entire joint complex is crucial since it allows us to visualize its behavior in the event of an impact. Other authors have only analyzed the skull or the cervical spine, distancing their studies from accuracy. This is why, with cervical degenerative pathology, the study using the biomodel allows us to analyze existing prostheses with different biocompatible materials in order to optimize them in the future [21,22].

2. Methods

To conduct numerical analysis of frontal impact on the skull, a craniocervical biomodel was developed. For this study, a male patient, an American football player who was 1.85 m tall and weighed 120 kg, was selected. The patient underwent computational axial tomography to produce images of the human skull, cervical region, discs, and spinal cord. The tomography was imported in DICOM format to the SCAN IP computer program and displayed in grayscale in order to visualize the cortical and trabecular bone of each part of the bone system in the different sections, which were displayed in three windows (representing views in the coronal, axial, and sagittal axes) [23,24]. These views allowed us to delimit the area of interest and develop the bones of the biomodel (Figure 2).

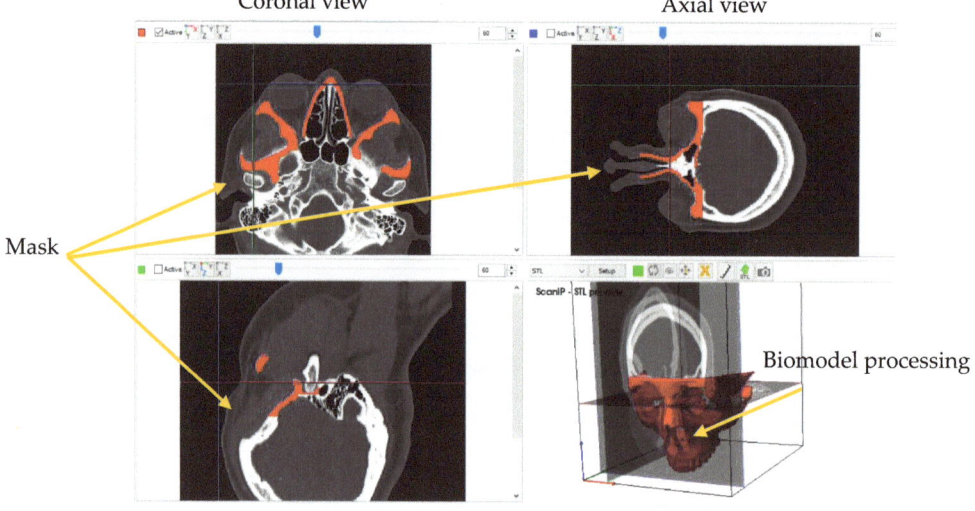

Figure 2. Patient's craniocervical computational tomography.

In Figure 3, the red mask represents the trabecular bone of the skull and the cervicals, yellow represents the cortical bone of the skull, blue represents the intervertebral discs, and pink represents the spinal cord. For the cervicals, C1 is represented by the green color, C2 the purple color, C3 the orange color, C4 the white color, and C5 the brown color. Once the masks were generated, they were exported in STL extension format and smoothing was applied to the surface of each of the components of the craniocervical system that made up the biomodel, which was developed through 3-Matic Medical software (a tool that allows the mesh to be corrected and simulates the wear on the intervertebral discs through material remotion) (Figure 4) [25].

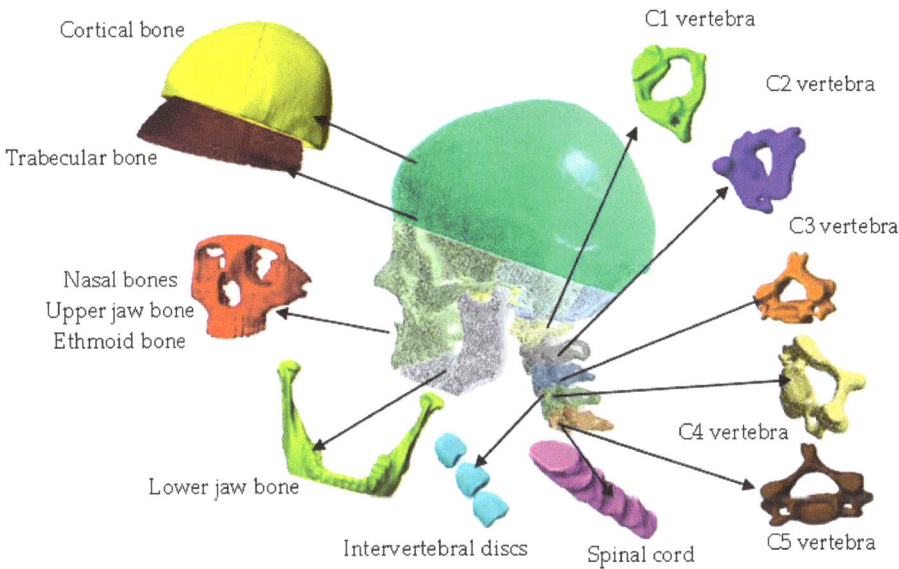

Figure 3. Biological system generated with masks.

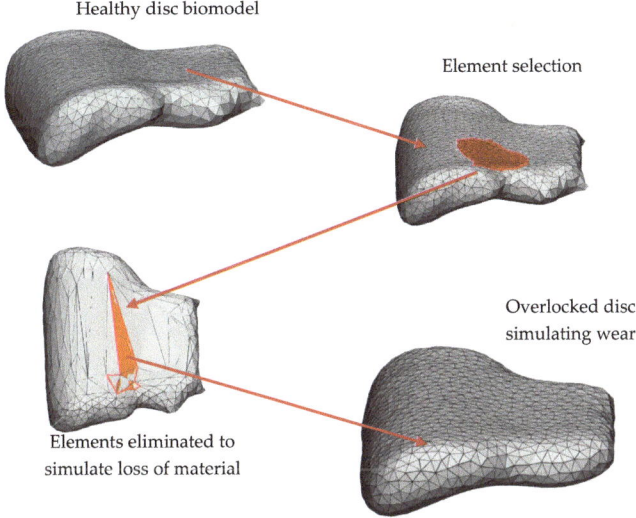

Figure 4. Wear process simulation on the intervertebral discs.

At the end of this process, biomodels of the cortical and trabecular bones (skull and cervical) were obtained along with ones for the bone marrow and intervertebral discs. Where a biomodel was considered to have high biofidelity and met the desired morphological characteristics, as the base with which it was performed was a tomography representing the craniocervical part of the bone system, the external dimensions of the contours of the bones (cortical and trabecular) were taken as references. Again, they were exported as STL files on which numerical evaluation was performed using the finite element method in the Ansys Workbench software [26].

Materials

Numerical analysis was performed by applying biomodeling, which was produced by computational tomography, and it was essential to assess the properties of the materials that describe the mechanical behavior of the biological tissues that were analyzed, which were as follows:

- Skull.
- Spinal cord.
- Cervical region: C1, C2, C3, C4, C5.
- Intervertebral disc.

The experimental analyses were the fundamental basis that supported the results obtained from the numerical studies. However, these results could be verified with significant technological development where economics are involved, saving time and material resources. For example, to understand the mechanical properties of the cervical and intervertebral disc, a numerical analysis of axial compression was carried out to support previous experimental research where the result was an approximation of 9.4%, which was acceptable [16]. Based on these results, the values considered for the cervical discs are presented in Tables 1 and 2 for the intervertebral discs. Table 3 shows the mechanical properties of the skull, which were obtained by numerical compression analysis [27].

Table 1. Mechanical properties assigned to the cervical bone [28].

Properties	Cortical Bone	Trabecular Bone
Young´s modulus	12,000 MPa	100 MPa
Density	1700 kg/m^3	0.14 g/cm^3
Poisson ratio	0.35	0.20

Table 2. Mechanical properties assigned to the intervertebral disc [29].

Properties	Nucleus Pulposus	Annulus Fibrosus
Young´s modulus	1 MPa	8.4 MPa
Density	997 kg/m^3	433 kg/m^3
Poisson ratio	0.40	0.35

Table 3. Mechanical properties are assigned to the skull bone [30].

Properties	Cortical Bone	Trabecular Bone
Young´s modulus	15,000 MPa	200 MPa
Density	1900 kg/m^3	430 g/cm^3
Poisson ratio	0.30	0.45

3. Numerical Analysis

For this work, two study cases were considered: a healthy case and a case where wear affected the intervertebral disc. The complex biomodel (the healthy and worn biomodel, respectively) was imported into the Ansys Workbench software, and the numerical simulation was carried out. The numerical analysis was a dynamic evaluation since the cervical spine was in motion, and the applied load was performed at high speed. Another aspect to consider was the properties of the previously explained materials, which based their studies on data in order to obtain the mechanical properties of each element that comprised the biological structure (the mechanical properties were declared). The biomodel considered 12 structural elements (bones and soft tissue) (Figure 3). Discretization was carried out in a semicontrolled manner by applying elements (producing 315,1321 nodes and 1,843,736 elements) (Figure 5). The material corresponding to each component of the biomodel was assigned.

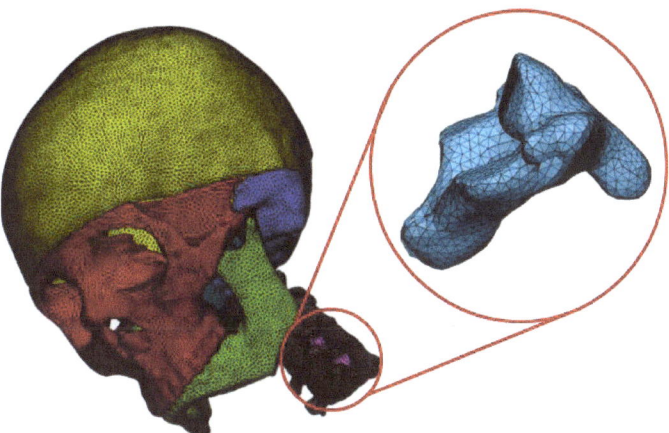

Figure 5. Discretized biomodel.

Then, the external agent conditions for the numerical simulation were introduced. First, the external agent applied for both study cases was considered as a pressure since the impact started in a specific area and the impact energy was distributed in a zone (Figure 6). Secondly, the boundary conditions (displacement and rotation restrictions) (Ux = Uy = Uz = 0, Rot XY = Rot YZ = Rot XZ = 0) were implemented in the lower zone of the C5 cervical region and spinal cord (Figure 7).

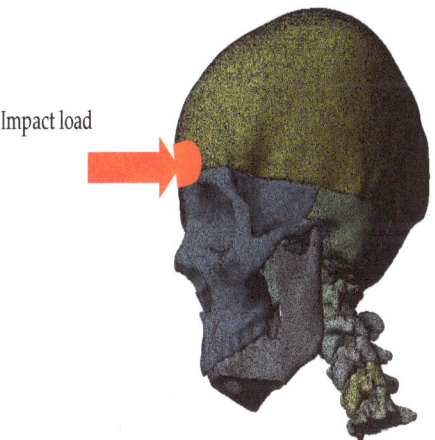

Figure 6. Loading application.

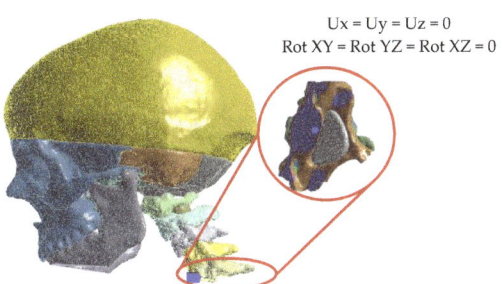

Figure 7. Application of the boundary conditions.

The National Standards Operations Committee for Athletic Equipment (NOCSAE) is a committee in the United States that certifies that the equipment used by players is the safest and takes care of the integrity of the person [30]. Every year, companies manufacturing American football helmets carry out evaluations with accelerometers inside the helmets to determine the impact force produced in a collision (around 30 g) [29]. Based on these results, for the numerical analysis, a force of 22 g was considered, which is the force exerted on a player in training camp, considering that they have experience collisions in practice than in a game. The conversion from g to m/s² is performed as follows:

$$22\ g \frac{9.81\ m/s^2}{1\ g} = 215.82\ m/s^2 \tag{1}$$

Knowing the acceleration and player's weight (120 kg), we calculate the impact load [31,32].

$$F = m\ a = (120\ kg)\ (215.82\ m/s^2) = 25{,}898.4\ N. \tag{2}$$

The impact begins punctually, and the way it develops covers a specific area, which is 10 cm in diameter at the front of the skull (Figure 8), onto which pressure is applied to observe the energy of the impact dispersed throughout the skeletal system. A circle was chosen in order to see the behavior of the entire joint complex. If a sphere was considered, it had a penetration effect in the contact area where the forces were distributed in different ways. The pressure calculation was performed with the data obtained from the force and the implemented area [31].

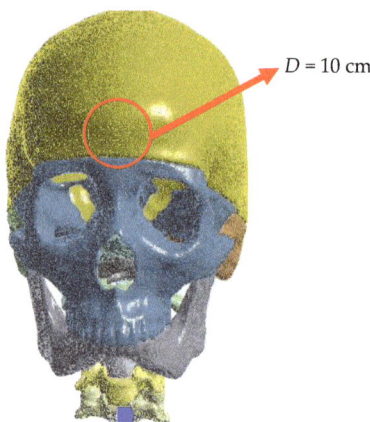

Figure 8. Impact area.

4. Results

It has been documented that American football players with disc wear develop severe headaches and suffer from reduced mobility [5, 6 y 17]. The main reason for this is that the disc no longer cushions the impact or helps movement. In addition, the disc, as it wears out, begins to move into the area of the spinal cord, exercising pressure on the nerve areas and the vertebrae, producing friction. This research work is based on two numerical analyses of a frontal impact. The first analysis considers the healthy intervertebral disc, and the second analyzes the intervertebral disc with wear. The most significant structural results in stress and displacement for both study cases are presented as follows (Figures 9–14) (Appendix A, Table A1).

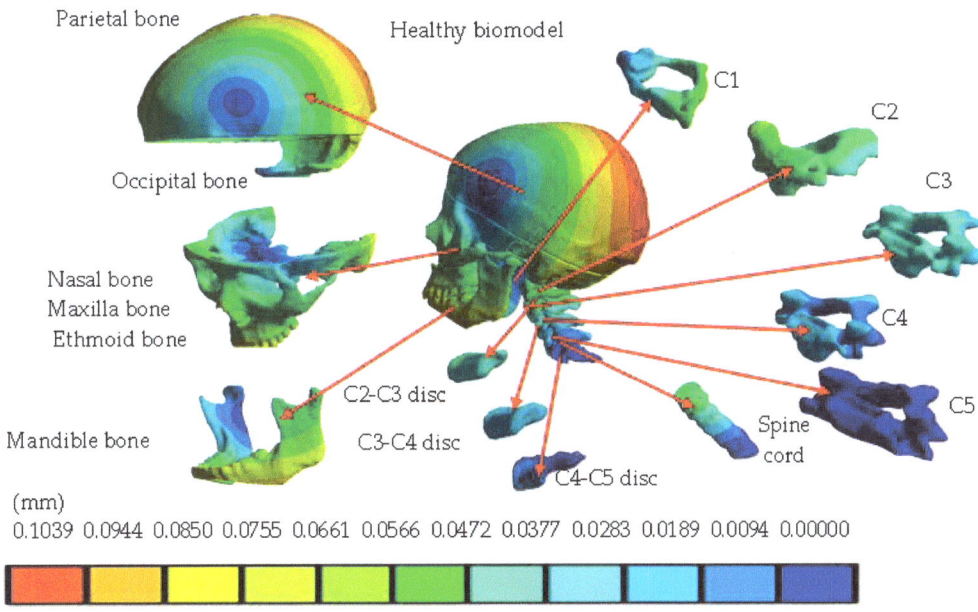

Figure 9. Total displacement for healthy biomodel by components.

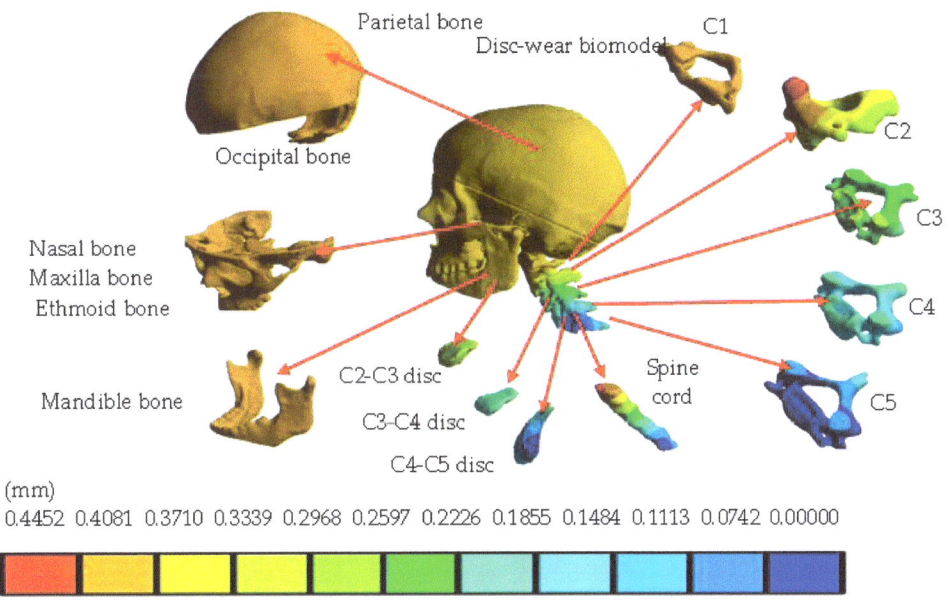

Figure 10. Total displacement for disc-wear biomodel by components.

Appl. Sci. **2023**, *13*, 11989

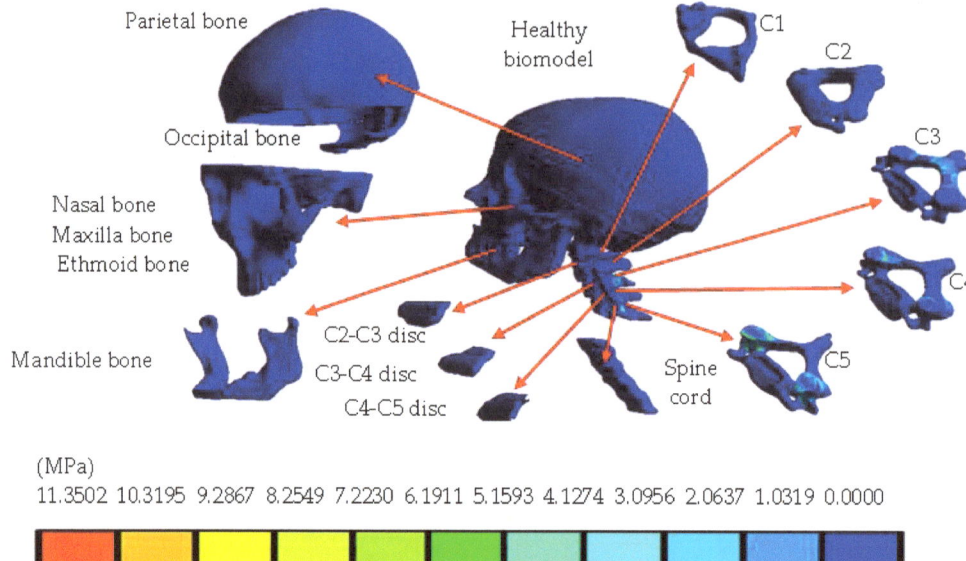

Figure 11. Von Mises stress for healthy biomodel by components.

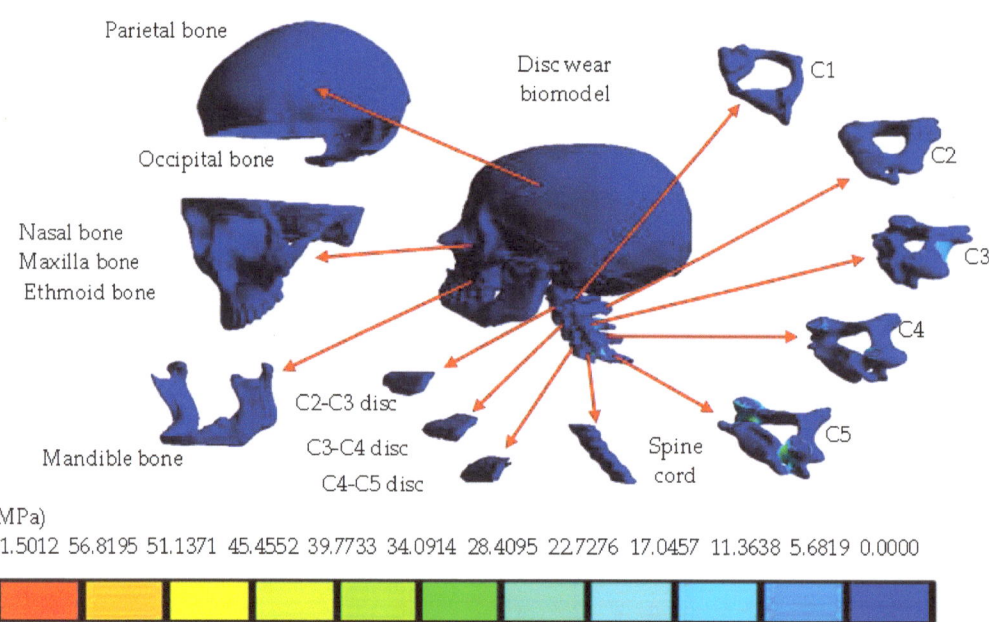

Figure 12. Von Mises stress for disc-wear biomodel by components.

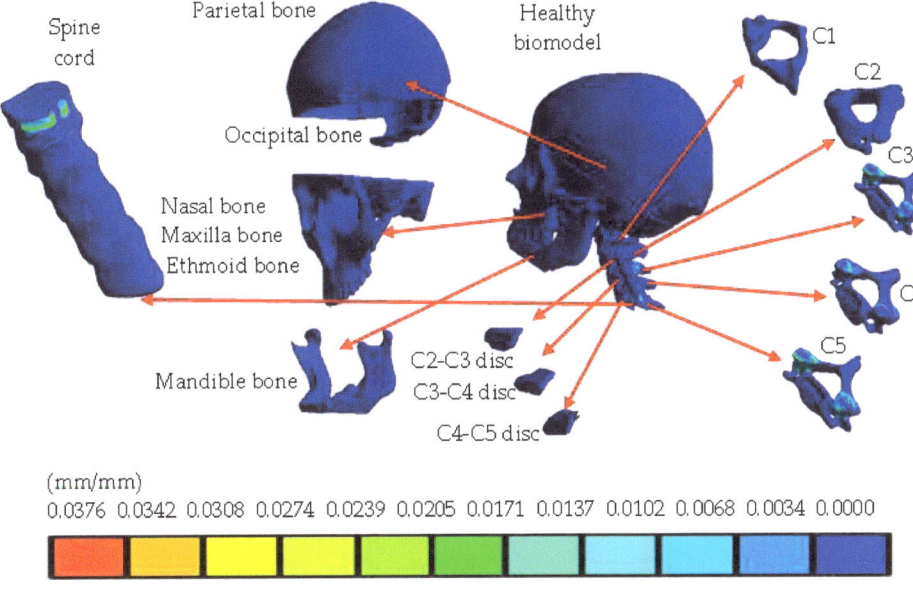

Figure 13. General equivalent strain for healthy biomodel by components.

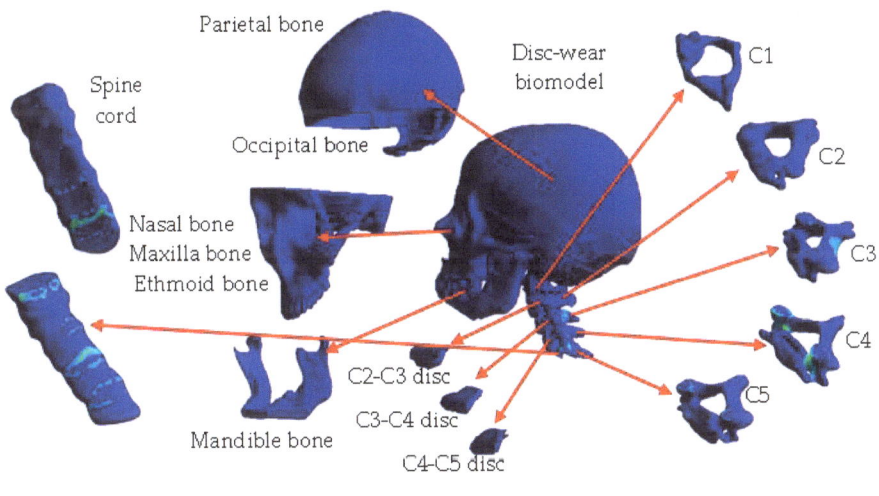

Figure 14. General equivalent strain for disc-wear biomodel by components.

Additionally, numerical analysis permitted the observation of substantial effects and estimated the damage produced by the disc's wear (Figures 15 and 16). In addition, a comparison between numerical cases being evaluated could be made. The numerical analyses were based on a free-body diagram to consider in a structural, mechanical manner the effects of the application of external agents and take into account the loading angles due to the displacement of the skull together with the cervical bones (Figures 17 and 18).

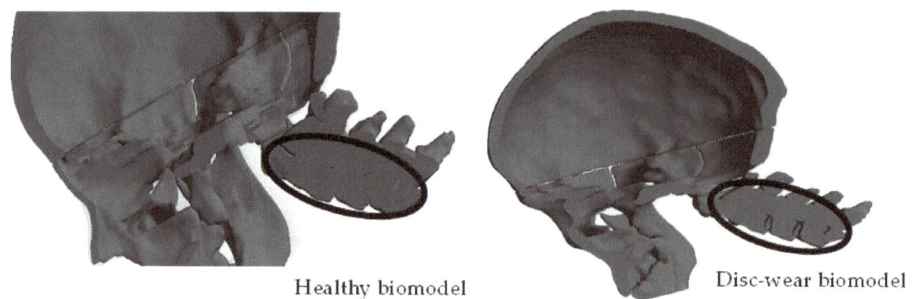

Figure 15. Comparison between cervical spine with healthy disc and cervical spine with disc wear.

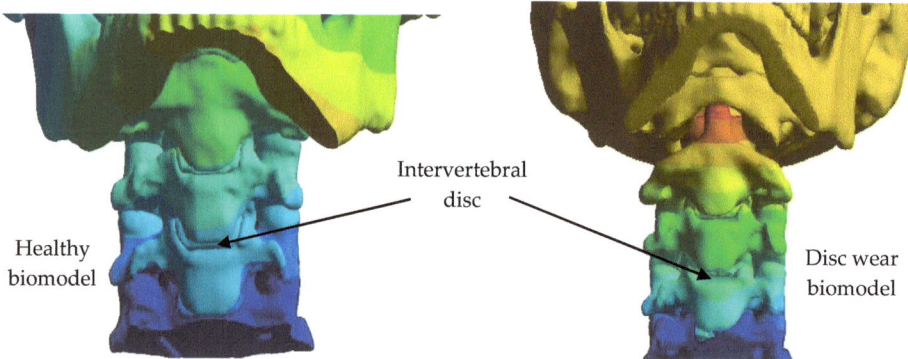

Figure 16. Zones implemented to visualize disc-wear nearness produced by impact loading.

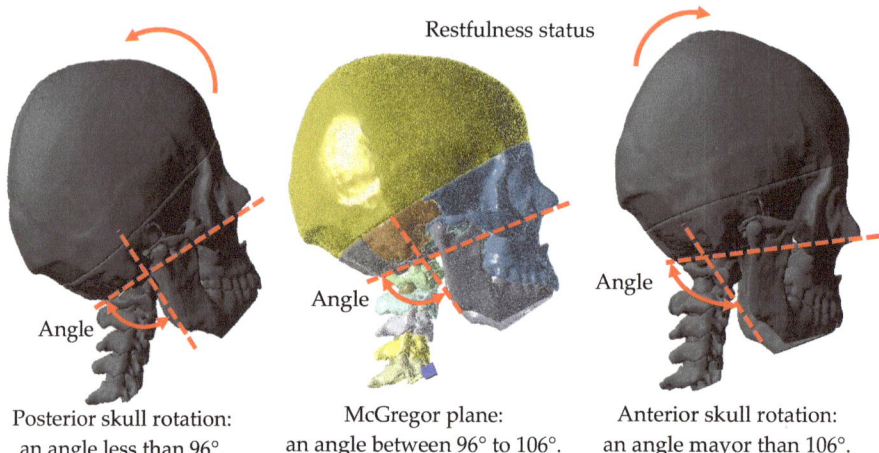

Figure 17. Comparison between free-body diagrams related to skull rotation angles that produce commotion.

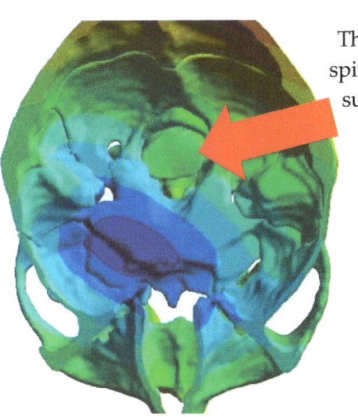 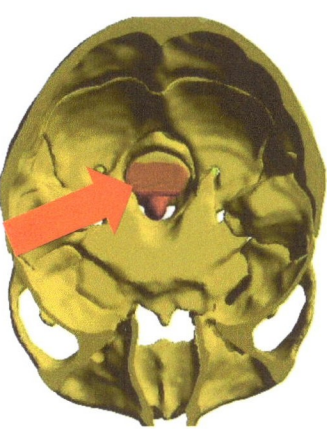

Figure 18. Graphical representation of discomfort effect when there is intervertebral disc wear.

5. Discussion

Even though computational technological development has opened the door for the development and representation of biological tissues in a three-dimensional way, it has not yet been possible to design a 100% faithful representation that meets the real morphological characteristics of a bone structure. The methodology applied for the development of the biomodel presented in this research work is considered to be of high biofidelity since the design is based on tomography to represent the biological tissue of the area of interest, which adapts to the contour of the structure, producing a biomodel that complies with the real morphology of the patient without compromising his physical integrity. This type of methodology is an auxiliary tool for designing complex biomodels with different biological tissues acting together. Having a more realistic image helps with the complexity of the implemented craniocervical biomodel since the research contemplates the development of a criterion that demonstrates, according to the displacements, how the impact energy is distributed throughout the entire joint complex. Comparisons can be made between the following scenarios: when the intervertebral disc has healthy conditions and when there is degenerative disc pathology. In addition, observations using unit deformations and stresses in the area most susceptible to injury can be performed. The remarkable thing about this research is that the results obtained could be beneficial for developing or improving preventive treatments or surgical procedures from a medical point of view. In addition, with this type of numerical analysis, intervertebral disc prostheses could be developed and optimized, considering different biocompatible materials and making comparisons in order to select the one that best suits the patient's conditions. It is essential to consider the entire joint complex because the impact begins at a point with a specific area and, from there, that impact energy is transmitted so that the work is carried out together, for this case study, in the skull. Hence, the cervical discs cushion the impact and one can observe their behavior with the spinal cord and, when you have the degenerative disc pathology, where that herniation occurs. On the other hand, other authors have only analyzed the skull, where the impact effect cannot be appreciated because the cervical and intervertebral discs with the spinal cord are missing. Finally, other authors have also only analyzed the cervical spine without all the elements that comprise it, and the skull, to show this effect [21,22].

6. Conclusions

With the results obtained in the numerical study, you can see the affected areas; you can deduce the reasons why players have symptoms of back and neck pain and, in very critical cases, severe headaches that limit their activities. Since the maximum efforts occur in susceptible areas of the vertebrae, more specifically in C3 to C5, where an isochromatic change can be seen in each structure, in addition to the displacement, it is observed how the part of the bone marrow is compressed, which causes the symptoms that directly affect the head, such as headaches. For analysis of the wear of the disc, it is observed how a space is generated that makes the cervical ones closer together, causing friction between both biological structures. With the effect of the external agent, the worn disc causes the cervical region to compact along its longitudinal axis without allowing movement or cushioning, so the most significant energy is transmitted directly to the skull as the process generates pressure on C1, limiting the patient's activities. It is essential to verify how the affected areas change with disc wear to better understand what causes damage to the bone structure. Research could also focus on supporting the search for feasible solutions to treat diseases or injuries caused by this type of physical activity, emphasizing this discipline and all those that involve high-impact physical contact. Even simple activities performed in daily activities, such as driving, are at risk of causing frontal impact when a road accident occurs. Obtaining a biomodel that represents the components of the skull and neck (which make up the craniocervical structure) that contains a high biofidelity of each element of the system will produce an analysis close to reality, which allows the evaluation of possible symptoms presented by a healthy biological group when having intervertebral disc wear, thereby assisting the health sector in providing a better structural mechanobiological understanding from the point of view of classical mechanics. This promotes the design of new surgical treatments and allows scholars to propose new rehabilitation methods for patients with this pathology.

Author Contributions: Conceptualization, A.T.-E., G.U.-S., and B.R.-Á.; methodology, A.T.-E., G.U.-S., B.R.-Á., and G.M.U.-C.; validation, G.U.-S., A.T.-E., B.R.-Á., M.Á.G.-L., and M.G.-B.; formal analysis, A.T.-E., G.U.-S., B.R.-Á., and F.J.G.-F.; investigation, A.T.-E., G.U.-S., B.R.-Á., and G.M.U.-C.; resources, A.T.-E., G.U.-S., and B.R.-Á.; writing—original draft preparation, A.T.-E., G.U.-S., and B.R.-Á.; writing—review and editing A.T.-E., G.U.-S., B.R.-Á., and J.M.-R.; visualization, A.T.-E., G.U.-S., B.R.-Á., and Y.Y.R.-C.; supervision, A.T.-E., G.U.-S., and B.R.-Á.; project administration, A.T.-E., G.U.-S., B.R.-Á., and J.P.-O. All authors have read and agreed to the published version of the manuscript.

Funding: This research received no external funding.

Institutional Review Board Statement: Not applicable.

Informed Consent Statement: Not applicable.

Data Availability Statement: Not applicable.

Acknowledgments: The authors gratefully acknowledge the Instituto Politécnico Nacional and the Consejo Nacional de Humanidades, Ciencias y Tecnologías, for the support of this research.

Conflicts of Interest: The authors declare no conflict of interest.

Appendix A

Table A1. Summary of general results of numerical evaluation.

Concept	Healthy Condition		Disc-Wear Condition	
	Minimal	Maximum	Minimal	Maximum
Total displacement (mm)	0	0.1039	0	0.4452
Displacement X axis (mm)	−0.0444	0.0653	−0.02043	0.00941
Displacement Y axis (mm)	−0.0724	0.0882	−0.3297	0.0911
Displacement Z axis (mm)	−0.0727	0.0531	−0.3163	0.1465
Total strain (mm/mm)	0	0.0376	0	0.0212
Strain X axis (mm/mm)	−0.0174	0.0082	−0.0042	0.0031
Strain Y axis (mm/mm)	−0.0204	0.0133	−0.0123	0.0044
Strain Z axis (mm/mm)	−0.0215	0.0108	−0.0117	0.0070
Von Mises stress (MPa)	0	11.3502	0	62.501

Table A1. *Cont.*

Concept	Healthy Condition		Disc-Wear Condition	
	Minimal	Maximum	Minimal	Maximum
Maximum principal stress (MPa)	−4.7549	12.6048	−14.507	59.984
Minimum principal stress (MPa)	−15.5285	3.4748	−68.268	6.4836
Maximum shear stress (MPa)	0	5.8328	0	34.632
Nominal stress X axis (MPa)	−8.0763	5.8252	−24.959	22.713
Nominal stress Y axis (MPa)	−11.9718	7.1022	−31.995	24.682
Nominal stress Z axis (MPa)	−14.9241	11.2437	−65.264	55.777
Shear stress XY plane (MPa)	−2.0796	2.3934	−11.901	12.005
Shear stress YZ plane (MPa)	−4.1420	5.1737	−25.828	25.919
Shear plane XZ plane (MPa)	−3.8517	3.3848	−11.612	21.842

References

1. Frank, R.M.; Beaulieu-Jones, B.; Sánchez, G.; Vopat, B.; Logan, C.; Price, M.D.; Provencher, M.T. Epidemiology of Injuries Identified at the NFL Scouting Combine and Their Impact on Performance in the National Football League: Evaluation of 2203 Athletes From 2009 to 2015. *Arthroscopy* **2017**, *33*, e101–e102. [CrossRef]
2. Craig, A.; Tran, Y.; Wijesuriya, N.; Middleton, J. Fatigue and tiredness in people with spinal cord injury. *J. Psychosom. Res.* **2012**, *73*, 205–210. [CrossRef] [PubMed]
3. Mez, J.; Daneshvar, D.H.; Kiernan, P.T.; Abdolmohammadi, B.; Alvarez, V.E.; Huber, B.R.; McKee, A.C. Clinico–pathological evaluation of chronic traumatic encephalopathy in players of American football. *JAMA* **2017**, *318*, 360–370. [CrossRef]
4. Gause, P.R.; Godinsky, R.J.; Burns, K.S.; Dohring, E.J. Lumbar disk herniations and radiculopathy in athletes. *Clin. Sports Med.* **2021**, *40*, 501–511. [CrossRef] [PubMed]
5. Mead, L.B.; Millhouse, P.W.; Krystal, J.; Vaccaro, A.R. C1 fractures: A review of diagnoses, management options, and outcomes. *Curr. Rev. Musculoskelet. Med.* **2016**, *9*, 255–262. [CrossRef]
6. Kumar, V.; Gaurav, A.; Dhatt, S.S.; Neradi, D.; Kumar, S.; Shetty, A. Traumatic cervical disc protruding postero-laterally mimicking lateral flexion type injury of cervical spine: A case report. *SN Compr. Clin. Med.* **2021**, *3*, 2060–2063. [CrossRef]
7. Benzakour, T.; Igoumenou, V.; Mavrogenis, A.F.; Benzakour, A. Current concepts for lumbar disc herniation. *Int. Orthop.* **2019**, *43*, 841–851. [CrossRef]
8. Khalid, M.; Tufail, S.; Aslam, Z.; Butt, A. Osteoarthritis: From complications to cure. *Int. J. Clin. Rheumatol.* **2017**, *12*, 160–167. [CrossRef]
9. Patel, P.D.; Canseco, J.A.; Houlihan, N.; Gabay, A.; Grasso, G.; Vaccaro, A.R. Overview of minimally invasive spine surgery. *World Neurosurg.* **2020**, *142*, 43–56. [CrossRef] [PubMed]
10. Wu, L.C.; Kuo, C.; Loza, J.; Kurt, M.; Laksari, K.; Yanez, L.Z.; Camarillo, D.B. Detection of American football head impacts using biomechanical features and support vector machine classification. *Sci. Rep.* **2017**, *8*, 855. [CrossRef] [PubMed]
11. Jakanani, G.; Kenningham, R.; Bolia, A. Active retropharyngeal hemorrhage from an acute thyrocervical artery injury: A rare complication of hyperextension cervical spine injury. *J. Emerg. Med.* **2012**, *43*, e39–e41. [CrossRef]
12. Mendoza-Puente, M.; Oliva-Pascual-Vaca, Á.; Rodriguez-Blanco, C.; Heredia-Rizo, A.M.; Torres-Lagares, D.; Ordoñez, F.J. Risk of headache, temporomandibular dysfunction, and local sensitization in male professional boxers: A case-control study. *Arch. Phys. Med. Rehabil.* **2014**, *95*, 1977–1983. [CrossRef] [PubMed]
13. Cejudo, A.; Centenera-Centenera, J.M.; Santonja-Medina, F. The Potential Role of Hamstring Extensibility on Sagittal Pelvic Tilt, Sagittal Spinal Curves and Recurrent Low Back Pain in Team Sports Players: A Gender Perspective Analysis. *Int. J. Environ. Res. Public Health* **2021**, *18*, 8654. [CrossRef]
14. Alizadeh, M.; Knapik, G.G.; Mageswaran, P.; Mendel, E.; Bourekas, E.; Marras, W.S. Biomechanical musculoskeletal models of the cervical spine: A systematic literature review. *Clin. Biomech.* **2020**, *71*, 115–124. [CrossRef]
15. Benítez, J.M.; Montáns, F.J. The mechanical behavior of skin: Structures and models for the finite element analysis. *Comput. Struct.* **2017**, *190*, 75–107. [CrossRef]
16. Zhu, J.B.; Zhou, T.; Liao, Z.Y.; Sun, L.; Li, X.B.; Chen, R. Replication of internal defects and investigation of mechanical and fracture behavior of rock using 3D printing and 3D numerical methods in combination with X-ray computerized tomography. *Int. J. Rock Mech. Min. Sci.* **2018**, *106*, 198–212. [CrossRef]
17. Urits, I.; Burshtein, A.; Sharma, M.; Testa, L.; Gold, P.A.; Orhurhu, V.; Kaye, A.D. Low back pain, a comprehensive review: Pathophysiology, diagnosis, and treatment. *Curr. Pain Headache Rep.* **2019**, *23*, 23. [CrossRef] [PubMed]
18. Li, F.; Liu, N.S.; Li, H.G.; Zhang, B.; Tian, S.W.; Tan, M.G.; Sandoz, B. A review of neck injury and protection in vehicle accidents. *Transp. Saf. Environ.* **2019**, *1*, 89–105. [CrossRef]
19. Chi, Q.; Liu, P.; Liang, H. Biomechanics Assist Measurement, Modeling, Engineering Applications, and Clinical Decision Making in Medicine. *Bioengineering* **2022**, *10*, 20. [CrossRef]

20. Zhang, J.K.; Alimadadi, A.; ReVeal, M.; Del Valle, A.J.; Patel, M.; O'Malley, D.S.; Mattei, T.A. Litigation involving sport-related spinal injuries: A comprehensive review of reported legal claims in the United States. *Spine J.* **2022**, *23*, 72–84. [CrossRef] [PubMed]
21. Rebatú, A.G.; Cárdenas, A.A.; Falfan, R.R.; Fernández, J.A.B. Análisis mecánico-estructural del injerto óseo en el segmento C3-C5 de la columna cervical como tratamiento de las fracturas con método de elementos finitos. *Rev. Espec. Médico-Quirúrgicas* **2013**, *18*, 195–199.
22. Carrasco Hernandez, F. Análisis Numérico de Cargas de Impacto Sobre Cráneo Humano. Ph.D. Thesis, Instituto Politécnico Nacional, Mexico City, Mexico, 2020; pp. 57–59.
23. Hernández-Vázquez, R.A.; Urriolagoitia-Sosa, G.; Marquet-Rivera, R.A.; Romero-Ángeles, B.; Mastache-Miranda, O.A.; Vázquez-Feijoo, J.A.; Urriolagoitia-Calderón, G.M. High-biofidelity biomodel generated from three-dimensional im-aging (cone-beam computed tomography): A methodological proposal. *Comput. Math. Methods Med.* **2020**, *2020*, 4292501. [CrossRef]
24. Hernández-Vázquez, R.A.; Romero-Ángeles, B.; Urriolagoitia-Sosa, G.; Vázquez-Feijoo, J.A.; Vázquez-López, Á.; Urriolagoitia-Calderón, G. Numerical analysis of masticatory forces on a lower first molar, considering the contact between dental tissues. *Appl. Bionics Biomech.* **2018**, *2018*, 4196363. [CrossRef] [PubMed]
25. Kumar, K.; Prasad, R.B. Stress analysis of cortical bone of the human femur. *Mater. Today Proc.* **2021**, *44*, 2054–2060. [CrossRef]
26. Correa-Corona, M.I.; Urriolagoitia-Sosa, G.; Romero-Ángeles, B.; Urriolagoitia-Luna, A.; Maya-Anaya, D.; Suarez-Hernández, M.d.l.L.; Trejo-Enríquez, A.; Urriolagoitia-Calderón, G.M. Application of the finite element model using 3D modeling of a human bone system with osteoporosis for biomedical and mechanical analysis. *MedCrave Online J. Appl. Bionics Biomech.* **2023**, *7*, 14–15.
27. Wang, J.L.; Parnianpour, M.; Shirazi-Adl, A.; Engin, A.E.; Li, S.; Patwardhan, A. Development and validation of a viscoelastic finite element model of an L2/L3 motion segment. *Theor. Appl. Fract. Mech.* **1997**, *28*, 81–93. [CrossRef]
28. Zambrano, L.; Lammardo, A.; Mller-Karger, C. Modelo numérico del anillo fibroso: Revisión del estado del arte. *Rev. Fac. Ing. Univ. Cent. Venez.* **2013**, *28*, 117–130.
29. Nieto, J.; Minor, A.; Alvarez, J. Determinación de esfuerzos en el cráneo humano por medio del método del elemento finito. In *Simposio de Ingeniería de Sistemas y Automática en Bioingeniería, Primer Congreso Español de Informática*; Thomson: Washington, DC, USA, 2005.
30. Breedlove, E.L.; Breedlove, K.M.; Bowman, T.G.; Lininger, M.R.; Nauman, E.A. Impact attenuation capabilities of new and used football helmets. *Smart Mater. Struct.* **2023**, *32*, 064004. [CrossRef]
31. Trejo Enriquez, A. Design of a Helmet to Dissipate Energy by Means of Finite Element Failure. Master's Thesis, Instituto Politécnico Nacional, Mexico City, Mexico, 2020; pp. 57–59.
32. Jacobson, B.H.; Conchola, E.G.; Glass, R.G.; Thompson, B.J. Longitudinal morphological and performance profiles for American, NCAA Division I football players. *J. Strength Cond. Res.* **2013**, *27*, 2347–2354. [CrossRef]

Disclaimer/Publisher's Note: The statements, opinions and data contained in all publications are solely those of the individual author(s) and contributor(s) and not of MDPI and/or the editor(s). MDPI and/or the editor(s) disclaim responsibility for any injury to people or property resulting from any ideas, methods, instructions or products referred to in the content.

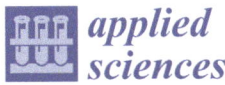

Review

Spine Deformity Assessment for Scoliosis Diagnostics Utilizing Image Processing Techniques: A Systematic Review

Nurhusna Najeha Amran [1], Khairul Salleh Basaruddin [2,3], Muhammad Farzik Ijaz [4,5,*], Haniza Yazid [1,3], Shafriza Nisha Basah [6], Nor Amalina Muhayudin [2] and Abdul Razak Sulaiman [7]

1. Faculty of Electronic Engineering & Technology, Universiti Malaysia Perlis, Arau 02600, Malaysia; hanizayazid@unimap.edu.my (H.Y.)
2. Faculty of Mechanical Engineering & Technology, Universiti Malaysia Perlis, Arau 02600, Malaysia; khsalleh@unimap.edu.my (K.S.B.); noramalina@unimap.edu.my (N.A.M.)
3. Medical Devices and Health Sciences, Sports Engineering Research Center (SERC), Universiti Malaysia Perlis, Arau 02600, Malaysia
4. Mechanical Engineering Department, College of Engineering, King Saud University, Riyadh 11421, Saudi Arabia
5. King Salman Center for Disability Research, Riyadh 11614, Saudi Arabia
6. Faculty of Electrical Engineering & Technology, Universiti Malaysia Perlis, Arau 02600, Malaysia; shafriza@unimap.edu.my
7. Department of Orthopaedics, School of Medical Science, Universiti Sains Malaysia, Kota Bharu 16150, Malaysia; abdrazak@usm.my
* Correspondence: mijaz@ksu.edu.sa

Citation: Amran, N.N.; Basaruddin, K.S.; Ijaz, M.F.; Yazid, H.; Basah, S.N.; Muhayudin, N.A.; Sulaiman, A.R. Spine Deformity Assessment for Scoliosis Diagnostics Utilizing Image Processing Techniques: A Systematic Review. *Appl. Sci.* 2023, 13, 11555. https://doi.org/10.3390/app132011555

Academic Editors: Jan Egger, Claudio Belvedere and Sorin Siegler

Received: 11 August 2023
Revised: 18 October 2023
Accepted: 19 October 2023
Published: 22 October 2023

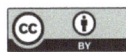

Copyright: © 2023 by the authors. Licensee MDPI, Basel, Switzerland. This article is an open access article distributed under the terms and conditions of the Creative Commons Attribution (CC BY) license (https://creativecommons.org/licenses/by/4.0/).

Abstract: Spinal deformity refers to a range of disorders that are defined by anomalous curvature of the spine and may be classified as scoliosis, hypo/hyperlordosis, or hypo/hyperkyphosis. Among these, scoliosis stands out as the most common type of spinal deformity in human beings, and it can be distinguished by abnormal lateral spine curvature accompanied by axial rotation. Accurate identification of spinal deformity is crucial for a person's diagnosis, and numerous assessment methods have been developed by researchers. Therefore, the present study aims to systematically review the recent works on spinal deformity assessment for scoliosis diagnosis utilizing image processing techniques. To gather relevant studies, a search strategy was conducted on three electronic databases (Scopus, ScienceDirect, and PubMed) between 2012 and 2022 using specific keywords and focusing on scoliosis cases. A total of 17 papers fully satisfied the established criteria and were extensively evaluated. Despite variations in methodological designs across the studies, all reviewed articles obtained quality ratings higher than satisfactory. Various diagnostic approaches have been employed, including artificial intelligence mechanisms, image processing, and scoliosis diagnosis systems. These approaches have the potential to save time and, more significantly, can reduce the incidence of human error. While all assessment methods have potential in scoliosis diagnosis, they possess several limitations that can be ameliorated in forthcoming studies. Therefore, the findings of this study may serve as guidelines for the development of a more accurate spinal deformity assessment method that can aid medical personnel in the real diagnosis of scoliosis.

Keywords: spine deformity; scoliosis diagnostic; image processing; medical images

1. Introduction

Three types of spinal deformities—scoliosis, lordosis, and kyphosis—are a set of disorders that are characterized by anomalous spinal curvature. A spine is deemed to be in good health when it is perfectly straight in the frontal plane, whereas it has lordosis in the lumbar and cervical region and kyphosis in the thoracic in the sagittal plane.

The most prevalent kind of deformity is scoliosis, which is a complicated three-dimensional curvature that is unable to be viewed from a single angle [1]. Scoliosis can be categorized into many types; hence, the most common scoliosis is adolescent idiopathic scoliosis, which can occur in and affects approximately 2% to 4% of adolescents [2]. Spinal deformity evaluation is a vital stage in deciding treatment since a good diagnosis of scoliosis can result in a better plan of care for scoliotic patients. Treatment is developed for scoliosis followed by diagnosis, which depends on the severity of the disease in the person [2–4], such as bracing, surgery, and changes in daily lifestyle.

Scoliosis can be confirmed through clinical examination and specific radiological exams with a key metric that is currently used by clinicians, which is the Cobb angle. Clinicians used a protractor to draw two lines that are perpendicular to each other where each line must lie at the most tilted vertebrae [3]. This process was undertaken to calculate the Cobb angle between the superior endplate of the upper extremity curvature and the inferior endplate of the lower extremity of the vertebrae [5]. Even though this measurement is the golden principle for identifying scoliosis, however, the measurement's accuracy can be questionable, as it is manually measured by the clinicians, which might lead to human error. The measurement also can vary from one clinician to another clinician due to their eye observation of the most curved vertebrae [6,7]. The Ferguson angle is an alternative measurement that identifies the three markers of a scoliotic curve: the geometric centers of the upper, apical, and lower vertebrae [1]. Both metrics require medical professionals to manually choose the vertebrae, which might result in bias based on the medical professionals that leads to inaccurate diagnosis. Typically, medical professionals need to know the patient's background, such as the patient's age, the size of the curve, the location of the curve, and the condition, in identifying scoliosis, so they know what they are dealing with when treating patients. The patient's age is an unreliable indicator of potential progression, while the degree of spinal curvature can be estimated by measuring the angle of the curve, thereby giving insight into its severity. According to the studies conducted by Shrestha et al. [7] and Horng [8], an individual can be considered to have no scoliosis if the Cobb angle measures less than 10 degrees. In cases when the Cobb angle ranges from 10 to 20 degrees, this indicates mild scoliosis, and scoliosis is classified as severe when the Cobb angle exceeds 40 degrees. Moreover, the Lenke Classification system [9] enables surgeons to obtain a comprehensive understanding of a patient's condition by assessing the location and type of curvature from a two-dimensional perspective.

Modern three-dimensional medical imaging offers emerging opportunities and potential in assessing spinal deformities. These opportunities offered by emerging imaging diagnostic equipment, such as computers and software applications, can avoid or lessen the shortcomings highlighted in the past and meet the demands of the medical community. The current diagnosis of scoliosis can be established via radiographic examination [10], and four imaging modalities that are relevant to the diagnosis are plane radiography (X-rays), computed tomography (CT), magnetic resonance imaging (MRI), and back surface topography (ST) [1]. While CT and MRI could provide detailed images of the spine in three dimensions, radiography can only provide a basic view of the spine in two potential projections—anterior–posterior and lateral. ST is a photogrammetric technique that involves reconstructing an object's forms, sizes, and relative placements. Hence, each modality has its pros and cons, which can affect the performance of the diagnosis.

Much research has investigated the assessment method in identifying scoliosis in every aspect to acquire a good diagnosis. The current body of research on the assessment methodology for diagnosing scoliosis through the utilization of image-processing techniques that can be applied in practical scenarios is restricted. What remains unknown is the optimal diagnostic mechanism that employs these approaches and that can be effectively executed in real-world scenarios.

In this regard, several researchers have attempted to create novel methods that might enhance the way spinal deformity is currently assessed, such as raster stereography, the artificial intelligence (AI) scoliosis detection method, and many more. There are studies on the golden parameter which is the Cobb Angle measurement, using AI methods performed by Vyas [11] and Sun [12] for detecting deformities. Research [13] on a new angle, a polar angle using non-invasive methods to assess scoliosis, also has been explored. Due to the recent development of these methods, there exists a scarcity of comprehensive reviews that concentrate on summarizing the assessment methods employed in diagnosing scoliosis deformities. In addition, certain reviews have a limited range that is not particularly relevant to our field of interest in image-processing approaches for scoliosis diagnosis. Previous reviews [14] focus on summarizing assessment methods and imaging modalities with chest and trunk deformation as the parameters. Considering the vast range of potential variables that can be employed in the assessment methods, including the parameters evaluated, imaging modality, plane, and software tool utilized, it is plausible that certain articles may have been inadvertently disregarded in previous reviews. Hence, the aim of this systematic review paper is to provide a summary and to gain an understanding systematically of the current and latest scoliosis diagnostic method that utilizes image processing techniques. It aims to find gaps and possible best variables that can be utilized in scoliosis deformity assessment methods that can be helpful for future works when developing accurate diagnostic methods. Therefore, the advantages and disadvantages of the diagnostic methods presented in this review paper can help to find appropriate methods to assess scoliosis severity.

2. Materials and Methods

The 2020 Preferred Reporting Items for Systematic Reviews and Meta-Analyses (PRISMA) standard [15] was followed for this systematic review.

2.1. Search Strategy

Article search was performed through the electronic databases and was restricted to ten years of publication. Three databases were used to obtain the articles, which were Scopus (2012–2022), ScienceDirect (2012–2022), and PubMed (2012–2022). The following search keywords were used to identify research addressing the assessment and diagnosis of spine deformities using imaging techniques: "spinal deformity", "assessment", "diagnostic," "treatment", and "image". The Boolean operator "AND" was used in searching the papers. The search was limited to only complete English textual articles and included research articles and studies only.

This study started with the PICO (Population, Intervention, Comparison, Outcome) strategy as follows: The population interested in this study was humans who encounter spinal deformity diseases, especially scoliosis, and the intervention of the interest was the assessment method to diagnose the scoliosis utilizing image processing techniques. The outcome of the interest was the effectiveness and how successful the method was in diagnosing scoliosis.

2.2. Eligibility Criteria

The articles were evaluated using following inclusion criteria: (1) studies regarding assessment methods to diagnose scoliosis using images, (2) Cobb and Ferguson angles or any parameters used as parameters to measure scoliosis, (3) full-text English research articles only, (4) reliability and/or validity of the scoliosis assessment measurement was evaluated, (5) included the selected search keywords in abstract and/or title and/or keywords of the study.

Exclusion criteria for articles were (1) studies with other spinal deformities (such as lordosis and kyphosis), (2) books, letters, survey or literature reviews, case reports, (3) not able to be accessed, (4) unavailable full-text articles, (5) studies that were not able to provide details of their methodology and protocol design study or experiment.

2.3. Selection and Screening of the Studies

The results of the search were assessed and retrieved according to the keywords by the two reviewers (N.N.A. and K.S.B.). Articles authored by the same individual were eliminated to prevent duplication. Titles and abstracts of the articles were read thoroughly, and a selection was made in accordance with the inclusion and exclusion criteria. A comprehensive analysis of the full-text articles was conducted in instances during the screening process if the articles disclosed inadequate information in the titles and abstract. The articles that were rejected were rescreened to prevent any unnoticed information. The final papers were subject to individual scrutiny by two reviewers in accordance with the established criteria for eligibility to reduce bias. In instances where there was contradiction, the two reviewers engaged in discussion to resolve the matter, ultimately reaching a consensus. This study did not impose any limitations on the subjects' ages, genders, body mass indices (BMIs), or medical histories.

2.4. Data Extraction

The relevant data extracted from each study were author and publication year, data characteristics, variables of scoliosis deformity assessment (imaging modality; parameters evaluated for scoliosis measurement; assessment method; software/tools used for scoliosis analysis), protocol or design study, and outcome measure.

2.5. Assessment of Research Quality

There is no standardized or validated method to evaluate the credibility of the identified articles. In this paper, the articles were assessed using a systematic quality method to analyze and review them by the two reviewers. This method can be instrumental in obtaining the most pertinent and significant information from the articles. Questions were adapted from previously published articles by Kavita et al. [16] and Wen et al. [17] as a reference to evaluate the credibility of the articles, and several questions were excluded, as they failed to justify spine deformity assessment and diagnosis. Some of the questions underwent modifications based on our aim in this study, which is imaging method. Each of the questions was valued with a score of "2" if it fulfilled the questions, whereas a score of "1" was valued if it had lack of detailed information. A score of "0" or "no" was given if there was no information provided and "NA" for questions that were not applicable. The questions are as follows below:

1. Has the objective of the study been articulated with clarity?
2. Does the study design have a clear and detailed outline?
3. Are the subject/data characteristics and details presented distinctly?
4. Is method used to assess the spinal deformity clearly defined and described?
5. Does the study involve imaging method to diagnose spine deformity?
6. Is parameter measured used in the method clearly described?
7. Does it use the appropriate numerical methods in data analysis, and is the analysis clearly verified or validated?
8. Does study have clear outcome?
9. Did the study state the limitations?
10. Does the study have a clear conclusion?

3. Results

3.1. Primary Search Results

Seventeen articles were selected after a meticulous screening procedure, and Figure 1 provides the selection procedure of the systematic review of the articles. A total of 1384 articles were identified based on the search keyword and research article criteria, with inclusion restricted to those written in the English language throughout the entire process. Following the process, 97 of these articles were identified as duplicates and eliminated. The titles and abstracts of the articles were reviewed to evaluate the relevancy of the article studies, and 983 articles were then eliminated. An additional screening was performed by reading the full text of the articles to ascertain the goals of the studies based on the eligibility criteria that were assessed, and 304 articles were eliminated. A total of 283 articles were rejected because the studies did not provide clear details on the methodology or the protocol or design of their study, while 49 articles were discarded because they were unable to satisfy the inclusion and exclusion criteria established. Some of the articles merely presented their methodological studies in a generic and ambiguous manner, lacking information pertaining to the whole diagnostic process and unable to provide clear objectives or results of their studies. There were 17 articles retrieved for further review that related to and met the criteria. The final articles were scientific research articles pertaining to the evaluation of scoliosis deformity that were deemed suitable for inclusion in this investigation. In this study, the researchers conducted empirical inquiries for their scholarly exploration, wherein they formulated and designed their inquiries that encompassed regulated variables and deliberate data. Certain researchers utilized randomized controlled studies in their studies, wherein they compared their approach with the existing method. Conversely, others adopted a single-case design, focusing solely on the development of their novel approach, providing their own control for comparison, and demonstrating the efficacy of their method instead of evaluating disparities with the current approach.

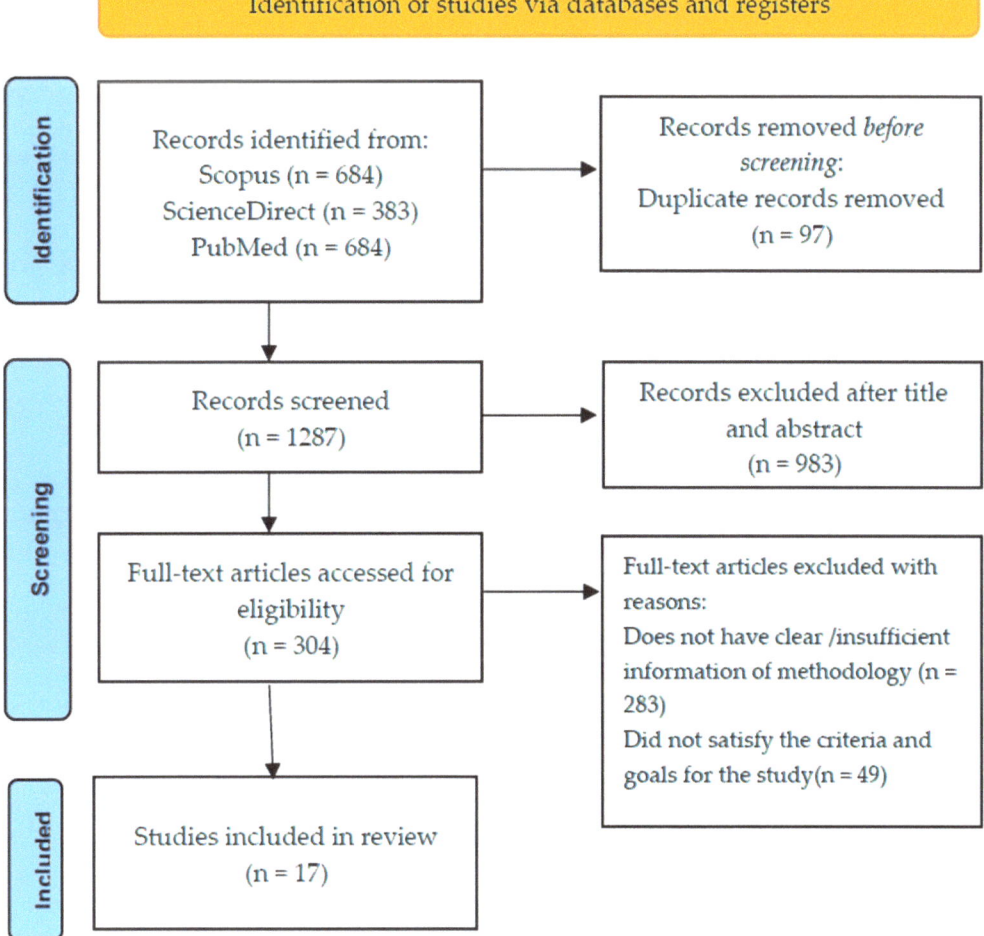

Figure 1. PRISMA flowchart of study selection procedure from reviewed articles.

3.2. Analyzed Data Quality of Assessment Articles

The quality scores of the 17 reviewed articles are presented in Table 1. The reviewed articles exhibit quality scores in the range of 70% to 95%. The articles with scores above 85% are considered good, as they satisfactorily answered all the questions and provided in-depth information regarding their objectives, design study, outcomes, and conclusions. Only 2 out of the 17 papers achieved a score of less than 80%, and most of them achieved more than 80%. These findings indicate the reviewed papers are of high quality.

3.3. Data Characteristics and Details

Table 2 presents a list of the data used from the 17 reviewed articles. The sources of the data can be categorized into two, which are the patients and images. Most of the articles used subjects that were patients to obtain images, and only four articles [18–21] used solely readily images as their dataset. Three studies used private datasets, and one paper did not state the source of the dataset. The number of subjects or data that participated in the studies varied with the highest being 3240 images and the lowest being 10 patients. Three studies involved a wide age range of individuals (aged between 11 and 86) [20,22,23], and ten studies focused on adolescents and middle-aged individuals (aged between 10 and 30 years old) [18,24–32], while four studies did not provide the age information of the dataset. Fourteen studies provided the required details of the data included in the investigations, such as the inclusion and exclusion criteria. The other three studies did not provide extensive and clear details on the dataset, which led to bias.

Table 1. Overall Rating Score of the Reviewed Articles.

Authors and Year	Questions										Overall Score	Overall (%)
	1	2	3	4	5	6	7	8	9	10		
Dubousset et al. (2014) [24]	1	2	2	1	1	2	2	2	2	1	16/20	80.0
Colombo et al. (2021) [25]	2	2	2	2	2	2	2	2	1	2	19/20	95.0
Yang et al. (2019) [18]	2	1	2	2	2	NA	1	2	1	1	14/18	77.8
Yildirim et al. (2021) [26]	2	2	2	2	2	1	2	2	1	0	16/20	80.0
Grunwald et al. (2023) [22]	1	2	2	2	1	2	1	2	1	2	16/20	80.0
Rothstock et al. [27]	2	2	1	2	2	2	1	2	1	2	17/20	85.0
Liu et al. (2022) [19]	2	2	2	2	2	1	2	2	1	1	17/20	85.0
Wang et al. (2015) [28]	2	2	2	2	2	2	2	2	1	1	18/20	90.0
Zheng et al. (2016) [29]	2	2	2	2	2	1	1	1	2	2	17/20	85.0
Lukovic et al. (2019) [30]	2	2	2	2	2	1	1	2	1	2	17/20	85.0
Navarro et al. (2019) [31]	2	2	2	2	1	1	2	2	2	2	18/20	90.0
Celan et al. (2015) [23]	2	1	2	2	0	2	2	2	0	1	14/20	70.0
Yang et al. (2022) [33]	2	2	1	2	2	2	2	2	1	2	18/20	90.0
Sikidar et al. (2022) [32]	2	2	2	2	0	1	2	2	1	2	16/20	80.0
Roy et al. (2020) [20]	2	2	1	2	2	2	2	1	1	2	17/20	85.0
Hurtado-Aviles et al. (2022) [21]	2	2	1	1	2	2	2	2	1	2	17/20	85.0
Glowka et al. (2020) [34]	2	2	1	2	2	2	2	2	0	1	16/20	80.0

Table 2. Data Characteristics and Details of the reviewed studies.

Authors	Data Sample	Number Subject/Data	Gender	Details of Subject/Data
Dubousset et al. [24]	Patients	49	Male: 4 Female: 45	Age: 13–17 years old
Colombo et al. [25]	Healthy and scoliotic patients	298	Male: 135 Female: 163	Inclusion criteria: - Age: 14–30 years old Male or female Exclusion criteria: - Clinical background of vertebrae pathological condition of vertebrae whether congenital or acquired. Medical history of vertebral fractures and/or vertebral surgery. Disc protrusion/hernia in any level of the spine diagnosis. Diagnosis of scoliosis is secondary to neurological, rheumatological, and/or congenital conditions. AIS diagnosis through X-rays with Cobb angle greater than 45°. Any neurological and/or rheumatological condition diagnosis.
Yang et al. [18]	Labeled images of unclothed backs and standing posterior–anterior X-ray images of spine or ultrasound images from normal and scoliosis patients	3240	Male: 1029 Female: 2211	Age: 10–20 years old Exclusion criteria: - Subjects exhibit nontrue scoliosis (attributed to pain or leg discrepancy, amongst other factors). Other spine disorders or abnormalities in the back region (such as soft tissue mass, thoracic cage diseases, etc.).
Yildirim et al. [26]	Patients	42	Male: 10 Female: 32	Age: 10–20 years old Caucasian ethnic group Exhibits a double spinal curve with convexity towards the right in thoracic region and convexity towards left in lumbar region. Exclusion criteria: - Gap between the umbilicus-medial malleolus and SIAS-medial malleolus on both right and left side must exceeds one centimeter.
Grunwald et al. [22]	Patients	10	Male: 5 Female: 5	Age: 11–50 years old Show signs of spinal deformation. Able to stand upright without support.
Rothstock et al. [27]	Patients	50	NM *	Age: 12–15 years old Adolescent idiopathic scoliosis patients and are scheduled to have initial bracing to eliminate any potential artifacts from prior treatments or operations.
Liu et al. [19]	X-ray images in anterior–posterior (AP) and lateral (LAT) position	400 images of 200 patients	NM *	Height–width ratios of the image ratio from 1.85 to 2.16. Average image resolution was 3560 × 1740 × 3 pixels and resized into 1024 × 512 × 3 pixels.

Table 2. *Cont.*

Authors	Data Sample	Number Subject/ Data	Gender	Details of Subject/Data
Wang et al. [28]	Patients	16	Female: 16	Inclusion criteria: Adolescent female Age: 10–18 years Cobb angle: 10°–80° No previous surgical treatments. MRI examination of the entire spine on the study day without the use of a brace.
Zheng et al. [29]	Patients	49	Male: 15 Female: 34	Age: 11–23 years Exclusion criteria: Have metallic implants. BMI higher than 25 kg/m^2. Cobb angle larger than 50°.
Lukovic et al. [30]	Patients	35	Male: 15 Female: 20	Age: 11 to 18 years
Navarro et al. [31]	Patients	61	NM *	Age: 7–18 years Eligibility criteria: Doctors requested to conduct a full-spine radiography. Have ability to maintain an upright position independently. Did not undergo surgical procedure in the spinal region. Absence of spina bifida, sixth lumbar vertebra, or fewer than 12 thoracic vertebrae.
Celan et al. [23]	Patients	275	Male: 129 Female: 146	Age: 16–82 years Distributed into 2 groups, which were scoliosis group that was clinically confirmed scoliosis (28 patients) and control group that was clinically confirmed physiological spinal curvatures (247 patients).
Yang et al. [33]	Patients	30	Male: 9 Female: 21	-
Sikidar et al. [32]	Patients	16	All female	Inclusion criteria: Age: 12–22 years Cobb angle: (healthy controls (HC) < 20°, 20° < mild scoliosis (MS) < 40°, severe scoliosis (SS) > 40°) Height range: 130–170 cm Weight range: 25–65 kg Exclusion criteria: Neurodegenerative disorders, such as ataxia, dystonia, Parkinson's, etc.
Roy et al. [20]	Computed tomography (CT) images	26	Male: 14 Female: 12	Age: 18 to 86 years
Hurtado-Aviles et al. [21]	X-ray images	21	NM *	Image resolution was 283.46 pixels/mm and printed in dimensions of 350 by 430 mm.

Table 2. Cont.

Authors	Data Sample	Number Subject/Data	Gender	Details of Subject/Data
Glowka et al. [34]	Patients	41	NM *	Inclusion criteria: Presence of a main curve either in thoracic or lumbar region. Imaging modalities conducted throughout duration of the hospitalization: high-quality plain-standing X-rays (PA and lateral) and thoracic and lumbar spine CT scans conducted as part of the preoperative protocol. Exclusion criteria: Scoliosis type other than the idiopathic, a lack of CT or PA and lateral standing X-ray data, and poor-quality X-rays.

* NM—Not mentioned.

3.4. Assessment Methods for Scoliosis Diagnosis

The goal of conducting a systematic review is to reduce the likelihood of potential biases by thoroughly searching and examining all published papers. All the characteristics and design studies in diagnosing scoliosis, such as the imaging modality/instrumentation, the parameter/landmark evaluated, the software or tools used, the assessment mechanism, and the plane/view used, have an influence on the accuracy and precision of the study. These variables have an impact on the method that must be considered in the evaluation of both the outcomes and inferences. Table 3 presents the variables utilized by the reviewed articles of the assessment method for scoliosis diagnosis. These data can help to provide supplementary information by comparing methods in scoliosis diagnosis studies.

The instrumentation or imaging modality is crucial in capturing the structure of the spine to obtain good image quality because it affects the accuracy of scoliosis diagnosis. Six out of eighteen studies used common and conventional imaging modalities, such as X-rays, computed tomography (CT), and ultrasounds [18–20,28,33,34], while other researchers [21–27,29–31,35] used uncommon instrumentation, like rasterstereography, cameras, EOS imaging, scanners, and 3D laser profilemeters. Special mention goes to Sikidar et al. [32], as the study did not collect data as images that used electromyogram (EMG) and ground reaction force (GRF) data.

The critical aspect of the diagnosis of scoliosis deformities is the parameters or landmarks evaluated during the assessment, as they are utilized as a metric that determines the existence of scoliosis in a person. The gold-standard parameter that current clinicians use is the Cobb angle, which [21,27] utilized in their studies. Study [18] provided no evaluated parameter, as the study used image processing for the assessment, whereas the authors constructed new parameters or improvised from the current parameter to evaluate scoliosis. The new parameters used for scoliosis evaluation are the vertebrae as a landmark [22,24], rasterstereographic measurements [25], the center of laminae (COL) [28], the Scolioscan angle [29], a digital image-based postural assessment (DIPA) [31], the bending asymmetry index (BAI) [33], EMG and GRF [32] data, and a 3D scoliosis angle [34].

Three possible approaches have been employed for the assessment method of scoliosis diagnosis where five scholarly articles devoted to the study of artificial intelligence [18,19, 25,27,32], nine articles studied image processing [20,22,24,26,28,31,33,34], and four articles studied building a system to diagnose scoliosis [21,23,29,30]. Digital image processing has become the most common form in the medical field, as it is the most efficient and cheapest method. Previous studies have tested scoliosis assessment by using various image processing techniques, including 3D reconstructions of the spine and rib cage [24], segmentation and superimposition [26], the COL [28], photogrammetry [31], the BAI method [33], automatic analysis and measurement of 3D spine images [20,34]. Studies on artificial intelligence implemented deep learning, machine learning, and supervised learning in the assessment of scoliosis, while computer-aided systems including graphic user interface (GUI) analysis tools, the Scolioscan system, the *ScolioMedIS* system, and 3D laser triangulation systems were built to identify and recognize scoliosis.

Four out of eighteen studies used MATLAB software for scoliosis diagnosis and analysis studies [18,20,30,31], and two studies [23,33] do not mention, while others used a variety of custom software.

Table 3. Variables of Scoliosis Deformity Assessment studies.

Authors	Instrumentation/ Imaging Modality	Parameters Evaluated for Scoliosis Measurement	Assessment Method of Scoliosis Diagnosis	Software/ Tools Used for Scoliosis Analysis
Dubousset et al. [24]	EOS imaging system	Thoracic: Thoracic volume, mean spinal penetration (SPIm), apical spinal penetration (SPIa) Spinal and pelvic: T4/T12 kyphosis, L1/S1 lordosis, Cobb angles of different curves; (lumbar, main thoracic, proximal thoracic), apical vertebral rotation (AVR), torsion index of main thoracic curve	Three-dimensional reconstructions of spine and rib cage from EOS low-dose biplanar stereoradiography	IdefX (version 4.8.4, Arts et Metiers ParisTech, Paris, France)
Colombo et al. [25]	Rasterstereography	Rasterstereographic Measurements: 40 VRS features including thoracic kyphosis angle, lumbar lordosis angle, lumbar fle'che, cervical fle'che, kyphotic apex	Supervised and unsupervised machine learning (ML)	Video–Raster– Stereography (VRS), Formetric 4D system
Yang et al. [18]	Camera X-ray Ultrasound	NA *	Deep learning algorithms (DLAs): Faster-RCNN and Resnet	MATLAB
Yildirim et al. [26]	Hand-held 3D scanner device	Distance, angle, and geometric measurements	Image processing after 3D scanning (segmentation and superimposition) and 3D analysis (point-to-point distance calculation and colored deviation map)	Artec studio software 2013, Netfabb Basic software (version 6.0.0146, Netfabb GmbH 2013 Lupburg Germany), GraphPad Prism software (version 6.05, San Diego, CA, USA)
Grunwald et al. [22]	Body scanner system incorporates both an infrared depth sensor and an RGB video camera	Thoracic, lumbar, thoraco-lumbar region.	GUI of body scanner image analysis tools	Computer-Aided Design (CAD), FEBio software
Rothstock et al. [27]	3D depth sensor	Cobb angle and Augmented Lehnert-Schroth (ALS)	Machine learning (ML)	Python 3.1 (Beaverton, OR, USA), Artec studio software (Artec 3D, Luxembourg)

Table 3. *Cont.*

Authors	Instrumentation/ Imaging Modality	Parameters Evaluated for Scoliosis Measurement	Assessment Method of Scoliosis Diagnosis	Software/ Tools Used for Scoliosis Analysis
Liu et al. [19]	2-plane view X-ray	3D coordinate of spinal curvature	A multi-scale keypoint estimation network and a self-supervision module	Pytorch platform on NVIDIA RTX 2080Ti GPU
Wang et al. [28]	Ultrasound MRI	COL	Measurements center of laminae (COL)	Custom developed software
Zheng et al. [29]	Scolioscan	Scolioscan angle	3D ultrasound imaging method: Scolioscan system	Scolioscan
Lukovic et al. [30]	*Formetric DIERS* rasterstereography scanner and digital photo camera	Cobb angle and spinal curvature	Ontology-based of the information system *ScolioMedIS*	MATLAB
Navarro et al. [31]	Digital camera (Sony Cybershot DSC-F717, 5.0 megapixels, 512 Mb of memory, 5× optical zoom and 10× digital zoom) and radiography	Digital image-based postural assessment (DIPA) angle and Cobb angle	Photogrammetry and radiographic evaluation	DIPA software and MATLAB v7.9.
Celan et al. [23]	3D laser profilemeter	Extreme points in the anteroposterior (AP) and left-right (LR) views	3D laser triangulation system	NM
Yang et al. [33]	X-ray	Bending asymmetry index (BAI)	Semi-automatic X-ray-based BAI method. 2 stages are involved, which are manual annotation and adjustment of pelvis level inclination and automatic generation of BAI values.	NM
Sikidar et al. [32]	SMART DX100	Electromyogram (EMG) and ground reaction force (GRF)	Supervised learning model	Mokka open-source software (Version 0.6.2, 64-bit, Windows, Biomechanical Toolkit)
Roy et al. [20]	Computed tomography (CT) scans	Circularity, difference between the areas located on the left and right of the spinous process (LRAsm) and difference between the ratios of width/depth on each side of the centroid of the contour (ASR).	Automatic analysis of 3D structure of human torso by quantifying asymmetry in transverse contours.	MATLAB2019a and 3D slicer software

Table 3. *Cont.*

Authors	Instrumentation/ Imaging Modality	Parameters Evaluated for Scoliosis Measurement	Assessment Method of Scoliosis Diagnosis	Software/ Tools Used for Scoliosis Analysis
Hurtado-Aviles et al. [21]	X-ray	Cobb angle	Computer-aided measurement system	TraumaMeter software (v.874, Jose Hurtado Aviles and Fernando Santonja Median, registration number 08/2021/374, Murcia, Spain)
Glowka et al. [34]	Computed tomography and digitally reconstructed radiographs (DRRs)	3D scoliosis angle	Measurement of the 3D angles between the upper end vertebra's upper endplate (three points coordinate) and lower-end vertebra's lower endplate (three-point coordinate).	DeVide Software (The Delft University of Technology, The Netherlands)

* NA—Not available.

3.5. Other Variability Used in This Study

The outcome and findings of the reviewed articles can be summarized in Table 4. There are two possible approaches that have been used for the investigation of scoliosis where thirteen studies performed their design study in quite the same pattern where the patients needed to perform quite the same procedure for the data collection and acquisition. The patients needed to execute the validated posture in front of the instrumentation or imaging modality to obtain the spinal images. But this differs from authors [18–21] where the data acquisition was collected from previous or available data from a repository collection.

It can be observed from the articles that scoliosis can be identified from multiple planes' views, which are from the frontal, sagittal, lateral, transverse, and anterior–posterior planes. The majority of the scholars studied scoliosis deformity using only one view plane, which was the coronal or frontal plane [18,21,26,28,29,31,33], while five studies used two planes, and four studies used three view planes [20,22,24,27] to assess the scoliosis deformity. The selection of a view plane during the scoliosis deformity assessment plays an important role in giving a better view of the spine.

Based on the reviewed articles, the outcome measures showed the reliability and validity of the method of the scoliosis assessment, which can be proven in the findings in Table 4. A total of five studies [18,25,27,30,32] were evaluated in their methodology through the application of performance classification, which involved the utilization of measures such as accuracy, sensitivity, and specificity. When classifying scoliosis, the majority of artificial intelligence studies [18,25,27,32] achieved above 70%, where the highest accuracy was 90.7%, and the lowest accuracy was 55%. The maximum registered accuracy level was 90.7%, whereas the minimum was 55%. It can be noted that accuracy values above 70% can be considered satisfactory, whereas there was one case that achieved low accuracy in the study [18] for algorithm 3 compared to the other two algorithms. Other than that, a variety of statistical significance methods were used to validate the method of scoliosis assessment, and this can be proven in the findings in Table 4. Seven studies were compared based on their developed method for measuring the Cobb angle where the validity of the measurement was appraised using the Pearson correlation coefficient (r-value) and p-value as evaluation measures. Most of them have satisfactory validity results that achieved an r-value of more than 0.7, which indicates a good to strong correlation level. Two studies [28,29] underwent both reliability and validity assessment, which evaluated both the intra- and inter-rater reliability using the ICC as the evaluation index, as well as the Pearson coefficient. From the reliability results where the ICC value achieved more than 0.9, it can be said that their methods had excellent reliability levels. While other authors abstained from drawing comparisons between their approach and alternative methods, they solely presented the accomplished measurement outcomes attained through their devised methodology.

Table 4. Design Study and Outcome Measures from reviewed articles.

Authors	Protocol/Design of Study	Plane/View	Outcome Measures
Dubousset et al. [24]	Patients in standing position for less than 15 min to obtain their specific 3D spinal reconstruction with the EOS system. Thoracic parameters were computed, and spinal and pelvic parameters were measured during the reconstructions.	Axial Frontal Sagittal	Mean pelvic incidence 54.3° (±14) Rotation of axial pelvic ranged between 2° and 6° Spinal parameters (Mean ± standard deviation) Cobb angle of main thoracic (61.2 ± 13°) AVR (19.9 ± 7°) Torsion index 15.8 ± 6 Proximal thoracic Cobb angle (30 ± 11°) Lumbar Cobb angle (42 ± 11°) T4-T12 kyphosis (18 ± 13°) L1-S1 lordosis (53.7 ± 14°) Thoracic parameters (Mean ± standard deviation) Thoracic volume (5056 mm^3 ± 869) SPIa (13.3% ± 1.7) SPIm (8.7% ± 1.2)
Colombo et al. [25]	Patients maintain a static stance in an upright posture at a predetermined distance from camera for 6 s. Data acquisition (sample of pictures) obtained with Formetric 4D system. Then, data underwent cleaning and normalization before proceeding to machine learning procedure.	Frontal Sagittal	Accuracy for unsupervised classifier ML for full set features achieved 61.7% and minimal set features achieved 72.2%. Accuracy for supervised classifier ML for full set features achieved 87.5% and 86.3%. While accuracy of minimal set features achieved 83.7% and 85.5%.
Yang et al. [18]	Subjects need to stand naturally for data acquisition conducted using multiple cameras. The patient's back was captured disrobing above hip. Data collected from 3240 patients with images of labeled back and entire spine standing posterior–anterior X-ray images or ultrasound images, which were used for training validation dataset. For external validation, 400 images were used for the process. Both training and external validation were performed for three algorithms, which are cases with curve $\geq 10°$, cases with curve $\geq 20°$, and curve severity grading.	Frontal	Performance of DLAs was measured with accuracy, sensitivity, and specificity, which the results are shown as below: - Algorithm 1: Accuracy = 75%, Sensitivity = 80.67%, Specificity = 58% Algorithm 2: Accuracy = 87%, Sensitivity = 84%, Specificity = 90% Algorithm 3: Accuracy = 55%

Table 4. Cont.

Authors	Protocol/Design of Study	Plane/View	Outcome Measures
Yildirim et al. [26]	Patients' back surfaces scanned with 3D hand-held scanner in three distinct positions (P1: stand with arms hanging at the sides, P2: stand with arms extended, P3: bend forward). Patients required to stabilize their body position as much as possible while maintaining normal breathing. Distance patients with scanner adjusted according to the distance indicator in Artec Studio software and 3D surfaces of the patients acquired.	Frontal	The RMS and Cobb values in the thoracic were observed to have a significant correlation coefficency (r) (P1 = 0.80, P2 = 0.76, P3 = 0.71) and lumbar region (P1 = 0.56, P2 = 0.65, P3 = 0.63);
Grunwald et al. [22]	Patients need to maintain static and vertical stance with their arms slightly abducted in front of the scanner. The scanning duration took no more than 10 s.	Coronal Transverse Sagittal	Correlation coefficients of $\rho s > 0.87$ indicates strong correlation between Cobb angle and lateral deviation, between Cobb angle and rotation of the vertebrae. Parameters have potential to offer supplementary information.
Rothstock et al. [27]	Patients need to be positioned in vertical stance with their arms slightly extended away laterally from the torso on an electronic tumtable for full torso 360° 3D scanning. Reconstruction of 3D trunk surface was performed with 3D software for data acquisition. Data analysis and classification were performed in terms of radiographic analysis and 3D surface topography.	Coronal Transverse Sagittal	Accuracy classification for curve severity = 90%. Accuracy classification for ALS = 50–72%.
Liu et al. [19]	Data acquisition of 400 full spine radiography images in anterior and lateral views from 200 patients. The dataset images were resized and partitioned into two sets, training set (340 images) and validation set (60 images). Conventional augmentation method applied to the dataset. (Add Gaussian noise and rotated up to 10 degrees randomly).	Anterior–posterior and lateral	Average precision, AP = 81.5 AP with regarding both AP and LAT views. Pearson correlation coefficient (ρ) = 0.925. Statistical significance test: p-value = 0.02134. Null hypothesis states that there is no significant difference in the AP between proposed method and the average outcome of the other established method. Requires verification in real-world scenario.
Wang et al. [28]	Ultrasound scan was performed with following parameters: a frequency of 2.5 MHz, an 18 cm penetration depth, gain of 10%. Patients' backs palpated and marked from C7 to S1 using a water-soluble marker for the scanning process. The patient laid on the scanning couch in supine position and received a total of 6 scans that were evaluated by 2 raters, with each rater with 3 scans.	Coronal	Has significant intra- and inter-rater reliability to measure the coronal curvatures. (Both with ICC, (2, K) > 0.9, $p < 0.05$) There was no significant difference ($p < 0.05$) found in COL method in ultrasound during measurement of coronal curvature at supine position. Bland–Altman method evinced an accord between these two methods, and it was found that Pearson's correlation coefficient (r) has a high value (r > 0.9, $p < 0.05$).

Table 4. Cont.

Authors	Protocol/Design of Study	Plane/View	Outcome Measures
Zheng et al. [29]	Subjects stands in front of the Scolioscan according to the locations of the four supporters at the scanner. Subjects scanned using the Scolioscan probe along the screening region.	Coronal	Scolioscan angle measurement shows a remarkably commendable intra-rater and intra-operator reliability with ICC larger than 0.94 and 0.88, respectively. The angle measurement between Scolioscan angle and Cobb angle provides moderate to strong associations with R^2 greater than 0.72 for both thoracic and lumbar regions. It was observed that Scolioscan angle tends to slightly underestimate the extent of spinal deformity compared to Cobb angle.
Lukovic et al. [30]	System developed with the aid of an ontology-based module that implements four fundamental steps, which are specification, conceptualization, formalization, and implementation.	Frontal Sagittal	The system has capacity to classify spinal curvatures and produce statistical markers about spinal curvature frequency, degree progression, and Lenke classification system.
Navarro et al. [31]	Photogrammetry method: Patients subjected to a photographic register in orthostatic posture and have the same position as the radiograph method for the upper and lower limbs. The spinous process of the C7, T2, T4, T6, T8, T10, T12, l2, l4, and S2 vertebrae was marked using double-sided tape to indicate as reference anatomical landmarks. Radiologic method: Patients assumed a relaxed orthostatic posture with the trunk pressed against the grid and kept the upper limbs at the side of the body and the feet while radiologist obtained the full-spine radiographs. Inspiratory apnea maintained during the process of the radiograph.	Coronal for photogrammetry and anteroposterior for radiography	Thoracic, lumbar, and thoracolumbar scoliotic curve topographies were used to categorize the analyses. All the areas of the spine had high correlations (ranging from 0.72 to 0.81) and significant correlation coefficients (between 0.75 and 0.88). The mean difference was quite near zero, while the root mean square error ranged from 5 to 11 degrees. The area under the curve, which ranged between 95% and 99 percent, was outstanding and noteworthy.
Celan et al. [23]	Patients in upright standing position and leaning against a foam affixed to the wall during the measurements. Arms were allowed to hang freely near body while holding their breath.	Transversal Frontal	The distances between the extreme points of the spine in the AP view were found to be marginally different between the groups ($p = 0.1$); however, the distances between the LR extreme points were observed to have a greater significant difference in the scoliosis group compared to the control group ($p < 0.001$). The quotient LR/AP was determined to be statistically different in both groups ($p < 0.001$). Thus, this indicates that the method is proficient enough to differentiate between scoliotic and healthy subjects based on statistical differences.

Table 4. Cont.

Authors	Protocol/Design of Study	Plane/View	Outcome Measures
Yang et al. [33]	Patients underwent X-ray scanning in three adopted postures, which were anterior–posterior (AP) supine, left and right bending.	Coronal	Between BAI and S-Cobb, the correlation value was $R^2 = 0.730$ (p 0.05). Out of 30 patients, 1 case was proven to have been incorrectly diagnosed while using the Lenke classification before and has now been corrected. All scoliotic curve types were correctly identified.
Sikidar et al. [32]	Dataset was obtained while the subjects were in static pose (standing), and approximately 2 to 6 trials were captured during gait (walking) per subject, contingent on the subject's level of comfort. Placement of markers adopted from Helen Hayes protocol at a sampling frequency of 500 Hz.	NA	The classification accuracy for SS, MS, and HC groups was 90.6%. The proposed model has capability to detect AIS in its early stages and can be utilized by medical professionals to strategize treatments and remedial measures.
Roy et al. [20]	Data collected from the study conducted by the radiology department and underwent analysis of CT images.	Sagittal Coronal Transverse	Patients with thoracic scoliosis have larger values for both LRAsm and ASR, which the degree of asymmetry was more pronounced in thoracic than in the lumbar region. Lumbar scoliosis patients have smaller values for both LRAsm and ASR, which the asymmetry was less pronounced in thoracic than in the lumbar region. Circularity factor does not provide any indications of scoliosis-related asymmetries.
Hurtado-Aviles et al. [21]	X-ray images collected from a digital image repository.	Coronal	Utilization of the software TraumaMeter (mean bias error (MBE) = 1.8°, standard deviation (SD) = 0.65°) depicts a lower intra-observer measurement error compared to the conventional manual Cobb angle (MBE = 2.31°, SD = 0.83°). The MBE values of the inter-group (expert and novice) distributions differ significantly when using TraumaMeter or the manual method. The use of the software leads to reduction in the difference in error between the novice and expert observers in a statistically significant way.
Glowka et al. [34]	The study consists of four steps, which are: - (1) 3D scoliosis angle calculation of computed tomography (CT). (2) 3D scoliosis angle calculation of digitally reconstructed radiographs (DRRs). (3) 3D scoliosis angle calculation comparison of CT versus DRRs. (4) Reproducibility and reliability evaluation of the proposed method of X-rays (PA and lateral).	Posterior–anterior (PA) and lateral	The 3D angle measurements obtained with DRRs and CT ($p > 0.05$) were not significantly different. However, a significant difference was found between the 3D scoliosis angle and the Cobb angle measurements performed based on the X-rays. The 3D angle measurements had high reproducibility and reliability values.

4. Discussion

The purpose of this systematic review study was to evaluate the technique or mechanism for diagnosing scoliosis by examining the characteristics and metrics that are frequently employed in imaging. Analyzing the advantages and disadvantages of parameters employed in each inquiry in depth is necessary to comprehend the assessment mechanism to find possible accurate diagnostic methods. Seventeen publications were considered in the current study for thorough review. Quality evaluation functioned as the primary methodological consideration to address the inconsistent methodological reporting by ensuring that the constraints of the examined research were considered. None of the articles that were assessed received a score below 70%, which was regarded as the acceptable average.

Participants' characteristics, parameters/landmarks, assessment methods, modalities, software, and instruments utilized in the research outcomes may all be further examined in the evaluated articles. The data characteristics were varied, and there was a propensity to group data according to gender, quantity, and the details of the data (age, inclusion criteria, and exclusion criteria); thus, it limited the analysis for certain groups in this reviewed paper. The dataset suggested has a broader range of ages and is not limited to adolescents and a young age. This is because scoliosis can happen to all generations. From the details provided of the data used in the studies, most of the data confirmed have a scoliosis diagnosis from the clinicians. Thus, it is proposed to use data that do not have confirmation of scoliosis by the clinicians for variability. As we can see, researchers have established several useful methods for diagnosing scoliosis deformity. Choosing appropriate factors, such as the instrumentation, imaging modality, and parameter or landmark evaluation, is crucial to the success of the study.

In this review, most methods focus on two-dimensional or one-dimensional views, and just a few use three-dimensional views for their data. A recent study of scoliosis deformity assessment has an interest in the three-dimensional view because it gives a better and more specific view of the spine so that clinicians can grasp an accurate diagnosis of scoliosis. A three-dimensional view gives an image of the spine in three positions which are the frontal, sagittal, and transverse, which is far better compared to others because it can clearly show the abnormal angle rotation of the scoliosis that cannot be viewed in the frontal plane. The one-view plane, which is the frontal plane, is suitable for quick, early spinal deformities, but this cannot give specific and accurate information about the curve severity and the spine deformities angle. This is quite significant in decision-making by the clinicians for the follow-up treatment.

Next, various parameters or landmark evaluations in scoliosis detection were utilized in their studies. The Cobb angle is the most common metric in determining the level of scoliosis that categorizes a person as having mild, moderate, or severe scoliosis. It is also quite simple and easier for computation for all assessment approaches whether in image processing or artificial intelligence since it is just calculating angles from two points of abnormal spine curvature; however, this can be implemented in the frontal plane only. Next, the Scolioscan angle, DIPA, and 3D scoliosis angle are the improvement metrics adapted from the Cobb angle that significantly exerts evaluation in diagnosing because they are evaluated in a three-dimensional view and have the same diagnosis concept as the Cobb angle. Metrics that evaluate the curve severity of the spine by utilizing points or coordinates on the spine, such as the BAI and extreme points or 3D coordinates, exert specific diagnosis values in the curvature of the spine. Identifying the curvature severity of the spine can aid clinicians in planning treatment accurately rather than just categorizing patients into mild, moderate, and severe categories. Some papers used human anatomy for the evaluation parameters, such as the vertebrae in thoracic, spinal, and pelvic regions, and rasterstereographic measurements, which present the abnormality of the spine clearly, but these metrics are quite complex and tedious for diagnosis for study [20,23–25]. Since it is necessary to obtain and evaluate the specific characteristics of abnormal measurements and values that manifest on the spine, which are outlined in Table 3, the parameters outlined in study [24] must be assessed in each thoracic, spinal, and pelvis region, while study [25] examined 40 VRS features. Consequently, it is imperative to ensure utmost precision in order to capture comprehensive measurement particulars and mitigate the risk of misdiagnosis. However, GRF and EMG have proven to be effective metrics, but the ability of the metric to detect scoliosis in real-world scenarios is limited since the instrument used for analysis can only be used through experiments in the laboratory.

Apparently, three studies use the common imaging modality of X-ray, and two studies use MRI or CT scans to acquire spine images. MRI or CT scans set out higher quality images than X-ray, but still, radioactivity from CT scans should be considered since X-ray has low radioactivity, which is safer and cheaper. MRI is advantageous in terms of radiation exposure due to its utilization of a magnetic field during the scanning process, which proves to be safer when compared to plane radiographs and CT scans. However, it is most commonly employed for patients exhibiting presumed atypical characteristics of idiopathic scoliosis or those in the juvenile phase, where radiation is not a viable option for conducting scanning [5,36]. Both CT scans and MRI scans contribute to high precision in image quality and enhance medical diagnosis. Unfortunately, these scans are accompanied by a hefty price tag and are limited to patients with congenital and severe curvatures, and they are commonly utilized subsequent to the diagnosis of patients using X-ray scanning. Clinicians commonly use X-ray imaging for scoliosis detection, and it is particularly suitable for first-time diagnosis or detection of scoliosis in its early stages. Several studies [37,38] have proven that X-ray can be a good modality accompanied by advanced algorithm mechanisms in scoliosis diagnosis. Another 11 studies implemented new and atypical modalities in obtaining the spine image that need to consider the cost-effectiveness and image quality obtained when using the modalities. The image quality used is very important, as it can affect the outcome of diagnosis, and thus modalities that can yield high-quality images are the best; however, other factors, such as radioactivity and cost, need to be considered for the assessment. Therefore, the choices of imaging modality depend on the needs and requirements during the diagnosis.

From the assessment methods of scoliosis diagnosis in Table 3, researchers have come up with different diagnostic methods that have certain limitations. As we can see, it is found that some studies implemented back surface topography techniques in the diagnosis to obtain the measurements, as they can reduce the exposure of radioactivity to humans. Methods in this review that implement this concept are rasterstereography, photogrammetry, 3D reconstructions of the spine and rib cage, 3D structure analysis of the human torso, and a triangulation system that integrates back surface analysis and landmark localization. However according to study [39], the author said that back surface topography techniques need to be performed with great precision due to the uneven and variable nature of human back anatomy. The parameters use in these notions for scoliosis measurement require more elaboration and details of human geometry, as we can see in the studies [20,22–25,31,34], and this must be followed with an advanced mathematical algorithm or image processing for the analysis. This requires the utilization of advanced instruments or tools that are not familiar to medical practitioners and may not stimulate them to use the instruments due to the distinct and complicated procedures [40].

The most current research focuses on scoliosis diagnosis using artificial intelligence and particularly image processing approaches. Image processing involves many steps, including acquisition, enhancement, restoration, recognition, and segmentation, and the steps may engage in the process according to the desired needs, and it is the process of converting an image into a digital format and then executing various operations to extract relevant information. Studies that apply artificial intelligence (AI) [18,19,25,27,32,33] to diagnose scoliosis can improve the accuracy and efficiency of the diagnosis outcomes. AI in medicine can analyze complicated algorithms and self-learning that can work in a manner comparable to human brain, and it can have several subfields, such as machine learning (ML), deep learning (DL), and computer vision [41]. Three studies [25,27,32] in this review employed machine learning where it consisted of pattern recognition and analysis that can improve with experience from provided datasets. This can be supported with another study [7,42] in which a machine learning algorithm, such as a regression linear and support vector machine, has successfully detected scoliosis in the early stage. Study [18] diagnosed scoliosis using deep learning as an assessment mechanism, and the DL algorithms are Faster-RCNN and Resnet, which are commonly use in the medical field [43]. However, this study only classifies the scoliosis according curve severity grading and did not give specific measurements on the abnormality of the spine curve; thus, this is not quite suitable and does not help health professionals to plan treatment since they need specific data regarding the diagnosis. According to numerous studies [43–47], deep learning may be a strong technique with a high reputation in biomedical segmentation; however, there are several limitations in terms of execution and process resources in this vertebral segmentation study. Computer vision is a process through which a computer learns and comprehends information and understanding from a sequence of images or videos [41], and refs [21,22,29,30] employ this approach. This is the highest level of difficulty since it involves building an autonomous system that can detect, diagnose, and process the provided data and then analyze them accurately, which then portrays the analyzed information to the user. Thus, this gives much help to clinicians and can facilitate their efficiency in diagnosing scoliosis. These approaches have given ease to humans and can reduce human error, especially in precise medical diagnosis, yet the challenging journey to successfully utilized these in scoliosis assessment needs to be taken into consideration. It was revealed that diagnostic assessment studies involved with artificial intelligence had average to high accuracy performance, and regarding one case of low accuracy, we speculated that the specific DL algorithm was not suitable for the dataset images, while studies involving image processing presented that most of them had good to strong correlation when compared to the manual Cobb angle, which proves the validity of their methods, and two of these studies showed excellent reliability assessment. For studies on the computer-aided systems approach, the developed systems had lower error differences between using the system and the manual method, a strong correlation coefficient, and could classify scoliosis by its severity. Overall, in the context of evaluating scoliosis deformity that can be effectively implemented in a clinical setting, it is advisable to employ X-ray as the preferred imaging modality, specifically utilizing two-dimensional frontal and sagittal plane views to capture the spine images. This preference stems from the numerous advantages associated with X-ray, as well as its widespread use and accessibility among clinicians especially in early detection. However, it is crucial to strengthen this approach with a sturdy method that combines image processing and artificial intelligence. This combination approach is vital for addressing the limitations presented by the low resolution of X-ray images. Numerous studies compare their proposed scoliosis evaluation approach either to the method currently used by clinicians or existing approaches to demonstrate their method's validity and achieve better performance of assessment. Since the new assessment methods are validated by the authors themselves and there is no validation from real-world scenarios, it is quite challenging to compare findings from the reviewed papers since different studies employed various explicit and implicit statistical techniques for the evaluation of their proposed method. A technique to diagnose scoliosis that combines artificial intelligence with image processing research may be suggested, and the lack of research on automatically determining the degree of spinal curvature can be considered for future study.

The main limitation of this article is its lack of standardization across the studies. Each study evaluated the diagnosis of scoliosis using different parameters for measuring scoliosis and different imaging modalities, which resulted in diverse results. Additionally, the literature primarily focuses on diagnostic methods that measure the abnormal curvature of the spine, with only a few addressing the entire human anatomy. This can introduce bias into the findings. Although we followed the PRISMA guidelines for systematic evaluation, our review still has some limitations that can be addressed in future studies. The search method used for this review was restricted to English language articles, and we only utilized three databases for article retrieval. As a result, some articles may have been overlooked. The criteria for identifying scoliosis deformity were limited to imaging, excluding data from other methods of evaluation. Methodologically, when conducting literature research for quality assessment, we relied on a previously published systematic review paper for guidance. However, the assessment questions in that paper were quite generic and may not be adequate for this specific field of diagnostics. Currently, there are standardized guidelines available for conducting systematic reviews that could have informed a more thorough quality appraisal. All of these limitations can be addressed and improved upon in future studies.

5. Conclusions

The present study highlights seventeen publications, which were published from 2012 to 2022, pertaining to the assessment of scoliosis deformity. This review specifically centers on the assessment aspect, alongside other variable factors, such as the imaging modality, plane view, research design or protocol, and parameters evaluated in the detection of scoliosis deformity. The data collected in this paper satisfied the fundamental assessment requirements that could impact the ability to predict outcomes.

A wide screening of studies that performed scoliosis diagnostics focusing on imaging approaches have been provided in order to identify more accurate and suitable methods to conduct assessment of spinal deformity. The practical application that might be related to the findings obtained from this study can be used in the healthcare area where healthcare professionals, especially doctors, assess spinal deformity. These findings can ease doctors to diagnose patients of spinal deformity, specifically scoliosis, accurately. Thus, they can make a good treatment plan according to every scoliosis case and lead to patient recovery from the deformity. First, we found that there are three possible approaches addressed in the assessment method of diagnosing scoliosis, which are image processing, artificial intelligence, and building a diagnosis system, and all were successful in diagnosing scoliosis. The studies suggested that the most common approach is the image processing assessment mechanism; however, other approaches are applicable to diagnose scoliosis. Next, all the analyzed studies implemented a variety of variables in the assessment methods according to their approaches. Since there is growing in the development of more advanced scoliosis assessments in this area, new potential assessment methods can be suggested to be implemented into real-practice scenarios. Consistent evaluation methods are needed because of the irregularity and inconsistency of the evaluations from the reviewed studies for comparison so that the superiority of the assessment methods can be demonstrated. To gain a more comprehensive insight into the scoliosis deformity assessment process, various elements linked to scoliosis evaluation could be further explored to enhance and augment knowledge in this area.

Author Contributions: Conceptualization, K.S.B. and A.R.S.; methodology, N.N.A. and K.S.B.; validation, S.N.B., M.F.I. and A.R.S.; investigation, H.Y., M.F.I. and S.N.B.; resources, N.N.A. and N.A.M.; writing—original draft preparation, N.N.A. and N.A.M.; writing—review and editing, K.S.B. and M.F.I.; supervision, K.S.B. and H.Y.; funding acquisition, M.F.I. All authors have read and agreed to the published version of the manuscript.

Funding: The authors extend their appreciation to the King Salman Center For Disability Research for funding this work through Research Group no. KSRG-2022-033.

Institutional Review Board Statement: Not applicable.

Informed Consent Statement: Not applicable.

Data Availability Statement: No new data were created or analyzed in this study. Data sharing is not applicable to this article.

Acknowledgments: The authors extend their appreciation to the King Salman Center For Disability Research for funding this work through Research Group no. KSRG-2022-033.

Conflicts of Interest: The authors declare no conflict of interest.

References

1. Adam, C.; Dougherty, G. Applications of Medical Image Processing in the Diagnosis and Treatment of Spinal Deformity. In *Medical Image Processing*; Springer: New York, NY, USA, 2011; pp. 227–248. [CrossRef]
2. Adolescent Idiopathic Scoliosis: Diagnosis and Management | AAFP. Available online: https://www.aafp.org/pubs/afp/issues/2014/0201/p193.html (accessed on 13 February 2023).
3. Addai, D.; Zarkos, J.; Bowey, A.J. Current concepts in the diagnosis and management of adolescent idiopathic scoliosis. *Child's Nerv. Syst.* **2020**, *36*, 1111–1119. [CrossRef] [PubMed]
4. Kelly, J.J.; Shah, N.V.; Freetly, T.J.; Dekis, J.C.; Hariri, O.K.; Walker, S.E.; Borrelli, J.; Post, N.H.; Diebo, B.G.; Urban, W.P.; et al. Treatment of adolescent idiopathic scoliosis and evaluation of the adolescent patient. *Curr. Orthop. Pr.* **2018**, *29*, 424–429. [CrossRef]
5. Karpiel, I.; Ziębiński, A.; Kluszczyński, M.; Feige, D. A survey of methods and technologies used for diagnosis of scoliosis. *Sensors* **2021**, *21*, 8410. [CrossRef]
6. Samuvel, B.; Thomas, V.; Mini, M.G.; Kumar, J.R. A mask based segmentation algorithm for automatic measurement of cobb angle from scoliosis x-ray image. In Proceedings of the 2012 International Conference on Advances in Computing and Communications, Cochin, India, 9–11 August 2012; IEEE: Piscataway, NJ, USA, 2012; pp. 110–113. [CrossRef]
7. Shrestha, P.; Singh, A.; Garg, R.; Sarraf, I.; Mahesh, T.R.; Madhuri, G.S. Early Stage Detection of Scoliosis Using Machine Learning Algorithms; Early Stage Detection of Scoliosis Using Machine Learning Algorithms. In Proceedings of the 2021 International Conference on Forensics, Analytics, Big Data, Security (FABS), Bengaluru, India, 21–22 December 2021; Volume 1. [CrossRef]
8. Horng, M.-H.; Kuok, C.-P.; Fu, M.-J.; Lin, C.-J.; Sun, Y.-N. Cobb angle measurement of spine from X-ray images using convolutional neural network. *Comput. Math. Methods Med.* **2019**, *2019*, 1–18. [CrossRef] [PubMed]
9. Ovadia, D. Classification of adolescent idiopathic scoliosis (AIS). *J. Child. Orthop.* **2013**, *7*, 25–28. [CrossRef]
10. Scaramuzzo, L. Special Issue: "Spinal Deformity: Diagnosis, Complication and Treatment in Adolescent Patients". *J. Clin. Med.* **2023**, *12*, 525. [CrossRef]
11. Vyas, D.; Ganesan, A.; Meel, P. Computation and Prediction Of Cobb's Angle Using Machine Learning Models. In Proceedings of the 2022 2nd International Conference on Intelligent Technologies (CONIT), Hubli, India, 24–26 June 2022; IEEE: Piscataway, NJ, USA, 2022. [CrossRef]
12. Sun, Y.; Xing, Y.; Zhao, Z.; Meng, X.; Xu, G.; Hai, Y. Comparison of manual versus automated measurement of Cobb angle in idiopathic scoliosis based on a deep learning keypoint detection technology. *Eur. Spine J.* **2022**, *31*, 1969–1978. [CrossRef]
13. Roy, S.; Grünwald, A.T.; Lampe, R. A non-invasive method for scoliosis assessment—A new mathematical concept using polar angle. *PLoS ONE* **2022**, *17*, e0275395. [CrossRef]
14. Gaitero, A.S.R.; Shoykhet, A.; Spyrou, I.; Stoorvogel, M.; Vermeer, L.; Schlösser, T.P.C. Imaging Methods to Quantify the Chest and Trunk Deformation in Adolescent Idiopathic Scoliosis: A Literature Review. *Healthcare* **2023**, *11*, 1489. [CrossRef]
15. Moher, D.; Liberati, A.; Tetzlaff, J.; Altman, D.G. Preferred Reporting Items for Systematic Reviews and Meta-Analyses: The PRISMA Statement. *J. Clin. Epidemiol.* **2009**, *62*, 1006–1012. [CrossRef]
16. Gunasekaran, K.; Basaruddin, K.S.; Muhayudin, N.A.; Sulaiman, A.R. Corrective Mechanism Aftermath Surgical Treatment of Spine Deformity due to Scoliosis: A Systematic Review of Finite Element Studies. *BioMed Res. Int.* **2022**, 1–14. [CrossRef] [PubMed]
17. Ku, P.X.; Abu Osman, N.A.; Wan Abas, W.A.B. Balance control in lower extremity amputees during quiet standing: A systematic review. *Gait Posture* **2014**, *39*, 672–682. [CrossRef]
18. Yang, J.; Zhang, K.; Fan, H.; Huang, Z.; Xiang, Y.; Yang, J.; He, L.; Zhang, L.; Yang, Y.; Li, R.; et al. Development and validation of deep learning algorithms for scoliosis screening using back images. *Commun. Biol.* **2019**, *2*, 1–8. [CrossRef] [PubMed]
19. Liu, T.; Wang, Y.; Yang, Y.; Sun, M.; Fan, W.; Bunger, C.; Wu, C. A multi-scale keypoint estimation network with self-supervision for spinal curvature assessment of idiopathic scoliosis from the imperfect dataset. *Artif. Intell. Med.* **2022**, *125*, 102235. [CrossRef]
20. Roy, S.; Grünwald, A.T.; Alves-Pinto, A.; Lampe, R. Automatic analysis method of 3D images in patients with scoliosis by quantifying asymmetry in transverse contours. *Biocybern. Biomed. Eng.* **2020**, *40*, 1486–1498. [CrossRef]
21. Hurtado-Avilés, J.; Santonja-Medina, F.; León-Muñoz, V.J.; de Baranda, P.S.; Collazo-Diéguez, M.; Cabañero-Castillo, M.; Ponce-Garrido, A.B.; Fuentes-Santos, V.E.; Santonja-Renedo, F.; González-Ballester, M.; et al. Validity and Absolute Reliability of the Cobb Angle in Idiopathic Scoliosis with TraumaMeter Software. *Int. J. Environ. Res. Public Health* **2022**, *19*, 4655. [CrossRef] [PubMed]
22. Grünwald, A.T.; Roy, S.; Lampe, R. Scoliosis assessment tools to reduce follow-up X-rays. *J. Orthop. Transl.* **2023**, *38*, 12–22. [CrossRef]
23. Čelan, D.; Papež, B.J.; Poredoš, P.; Možina, J. Laser triangulation measurements of scoliotic spine curvatures. *Scoliosis* **2015**, *10*, 1–6. [CrossRef]
24. Dubousset, J.; Ilharreborde, B.; Le Huec, J.-C. Use of EOS imaging for the assessment of scoliosis deformities: Application to postoperative 3D quantitative analysis of the trunk. *Eur. Spine J.* **2014**, *23*, 397–405. [CrossRef]
25. Colombo, T.; Mangone, M.; Agostini, F.; Bernetti, A.; Paoloni, M.; Santilli, V.; Palagi, L. Supervised and unsupervised learning to classify scoliosis and healthy subjects based on non-invasive rasterstereography analysis. *PLoS ONE* **2021**, *16*, e0261511. [CrossRef]

26. Yıldırım, Y.; Tombak, K.; Karaşin, S.; Yüksel, I.; Nur, A.H.; Ozsoy, U. Assessment of the reliability of hand-held surface scanner in the evaluation of adolescent idiopathic scoliosis. *Eur. Spine J.* **2021**, *30*, 1872–1880. [CrossRef]
27. Rothstock, S.; Weiss, H.-R.; Krueger, D.; Paul, L. Clinical classification of scoliosis patients using machine learning and markerless 3D surface trunk data. *Med. Biol. Eng. Comput.* **2020**, *58*, 2953–2962. [CrossRef]
28. Wang, Q.; Li, M.; Lou, E.H.M.; Wong, M.S. Reliability and validity study of clinical ultrasound imaging on lateral curvature of adolescent idiopathic scoliosis. *PLoS ONE* **2015**, *10*, e0135264. [CrossRef] [PubMed]
29. Zheng, Y.-P.; Lee, T.T.-Y.; Lai, K.K.-L.; Yip, B.H.-K.; Zhou, G.-Q.; Jiang, W.-W.; Cheung, J.C.-W.; Wong, M.-S.; Ng, B.K.-W.; Cheng, J.C.-Y.; et al. A reliability and validity study for Scolioscan: A radiation-free scoliosis assessment system using 3D ultrasound imaging. *Scoliosis* **2016**, *11*, 1–15. [CrossRef] [PubMed]
30. Luković, V.; Ćuković, S.; Milošević, D.; Devedžić, G. An ontology-based module of the information system ScolioMedIS for 3D digital diagnosis of adolescent scoliosis. *Comput. Methods Programs Biomed.* **2019**, *178*, 247–263. [CrossRef]
31. Navarro, I.J.R.L.; Candotti, C.T.; Furlanetto, T.S.; Dutra, V.H.; Amaral, M.A.D.; Loss, J.F. Validation of a Mathematical Procedure for the Cobb Angle Assessment Based on Photogrammetry. *J. Chiropr. Med.* **2019**, *18*, 270–277. [CrossRef]
32. Sikidar, A.; Vidyasagar, K.E.C.; Gupta, M.; Garg, B.; Kalyanasundaram, D. Classification of mild and severe adolescent idiopathic scoliosis (AIS) from healthy subjects via a supervised learning model based on electromyogram and ground reaction force data during gait. *Biocybern. Biomed. Eng.* **2022**, *42*, 870–887. [CrossRef]
33. Yang, D.; Lee, T.T.Y.; Lai, K.K.L.; Lam, T.P.; Castelein, R.M.; Cheng, J.C.Y.; Zheng, Y.P. Semi-automatic method for pre-surgery scoliosis classification on X-ray images using Bending Asymmetry Index. *Int. J. Comput. Assist. Radiol. Surg.* **2022**, *17*, 2239–2251. [CrossRef]
34. Główka, P.; Politarczyk, W.; Janusz, P. The method for measurement of the three-dimensional scoliosis angle from standard radiographs. *BMC Musculoskelet. Disord.* **2020**, *21*, 475-1–475-7. [CrossRef] [PubMed]
35. Wong, Y.-S.; Lai, K.K.-L.; Zheng, Y.-P.; Wong, L.L.-N.; Ng, B.K.-W.; Hung, A.L.-H.; Yip, B.H.-K.; Chu, W.C.-W.; Ng, A.W.-H.; Qiu, Y.; et al. Is Radiation-Free Ultrasound Accurate for Quantitative Assessment of Spinal Deformity in Idiopathic Scoliosis (IS): A Detailed Analysis With EOS Radiography on 952 Patients. *Ultrasound Med. Biol.* **2019**, *45*, 2866–2877. [CrossRef] [PubMed]
36. Cassar-Pullicino, V.; Eisenstein, S. Imaging in Scoliosis: What, Why and How? *Clin. Radiol.* **2002**, *57*, 543–562. [CrossRef] [PubMed]
37. Saylor, A. Artificial Neural Network for the Estimation of Clinical Parameters from X-rays of Scoliotic Spines. Master's Thesis, Widener University, Chester, PA, USA, 2020.
38. Vertebra Segmentation for Spinal Deformity Assessment from X-ray Images—ProQuest. Available online: https://www.proquest.com/docview/2570358625/F320EB77D7BE4628PQ/1?accountid=33397 (accessed on 13 February 2023).
39. Drerup, B. Rasterstereographic measurement of scoliotic deformity. *Scoliosis* **2014**, *9*, 1–14. [CrossRef]
40. Navarro, I.J.R.L.; da Rosa, B.N.; Candotti, C.T. Anatomical reference marks, evaluation parameters and reproducibility of surface topography for evaluating the adolescent idiopathic scoliosis: A systematic review with meta-analysis. *Gait Posture* **2019**, *69*, 112–120. [CrossRef] [PubMed]
41. Kaul, V.; Enslin, S.; Gross, S.A. History of artificial intelligence in medicine. *Gastrointest. Endosc.* **2020**, *92*, 807–812. [CrossRef]
42. Chen, K.; Zhai, X.; Sun, K.; Wang, H.; Yang, C.; Li, M. A narrative review of machine learning as promising revolution in clinical practice of scoliosis. *Ann. Transl. Med.* **2021**, *9*, 67. [CrossRef] [PubMed]
43. Patel, S. Deep learning models for image segmentation. In Proceedings of the 2021 8th International Conference on Computing for Sustainable Global Development (INDIACom), New Delhi, India, 17–19 March 2021; pp. 149–154.
44. Ronneberger, O.; Fischer, P.; Brox, T. U-net: Convolutional networks for biomedical image segmentation. In *Medical Image Computing and Computer-Assisted Intervention—MICCAI 2015*; Lecture Notes in Computer Science (Including Subseries Lecture Notes in Artificial Intelligence and Lecture Notes in Bioinformatics); Springer: Cham, Switzerland, 2015; Volume 9351, pp. 234–241. [CrossRef]
45. Zhang, Q.; Du, Y.; Wei, Z.; Liu, H.; Yang, X.; Zhao, D. Spine Medical Image Segmentation Based on Deep Learning. *J. Health Eng.* **2021**, *2021*, 1–6. [CrossRef]
46. Cheng, P.; Yang, Y.; Yu, H.; He, Y. Automatic vertebrae localization and segmentation in CT with a two-stage Dense-U-Net. *Sci. Rep.* **2021**, *11*, 1–13. [CrossRef]
47. Weng, W.; Zhu, X. INet: Convolutional Networks for Biomedical Image Segmentation. *IEEE Access* **2021**, *9*, 16591–16603. [CrossRef]

Disclaimer/Publisher's Note: The statements, opinions and data contained in all publications are solely those of the individual author(s) and contributor(s) and not of MDPI and/or the editor(s). MDPI and/or the editor(s) disclaim responsibility for any injury to people or property resulting from any ideas, methods, instructions or products referred to in the content.

MDPI AG
Grosspeteranlage 5
4052 Basel
Switzerland
Tel.: +41 61 683 77 34

Applied Sciences Editorial Office
E-mail: applsci@mdpi.com
www.mdpi.com/journal/applsci

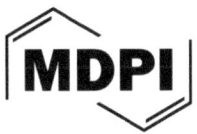

Disclaimer/Publisher's Note: The statements, opinions and data contained in all publications are solely those of the individual author(s) and contributor(s) and not of MDPI and/or the editor(s). MDPI and/or the editor(s) disclaim responsibility for any injury to people or property resulting from any ideas, methods, instructions or products referred to in the content.

www.ingramcontent.com/pod-product-compliance
Lightning Source LLC
LaVergne TN
LVHW072345090526
838202LV00019B/2484